FIELD GUIDE

Relationship-Based Care

Visions, Strategies, Tools and Exemplars for Transforming Practice

Editors

Mary Koloroutis • Jayne A. Felgen
Colleen Person • Susan Wessel

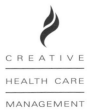

CREATIVE

HEALTH CARE

MANAGEMENT

ISBN 13: 978-1-886624-23-8
ISBN 10: 1-886624-23-2

Second Printing: October 2008
Printed in Canada

12 11 10 09 08   6 5 4 3 2

For permission and ordering information, write to:

CREATIVE

HEALTH CARE

MANAGEMENT

Creative Health Care Management, Inc.
1701 American Blvd. East, Suite 1
Minneapolis, MN 55425

chcm@chcm.com
or call: 800.728.7766 or 952.854.9015

www.chcm.com

This book is dedicated to those health care clinicians, managers and administrators who come to work every day and give of themselves through acts and attitudes of hope, compassion and care. We honor you for making such a difference in the lives of the patients and families you serve.

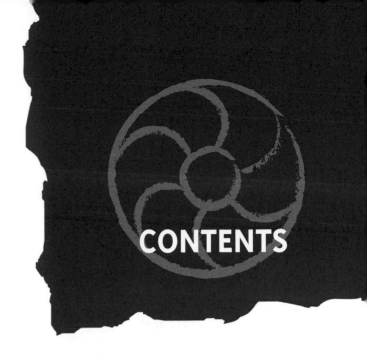

CONTENTS

PART I: VISION

PART II: INSPIRATION

PART III: INFRASTRUCTURE

Chapter 6: Embedding Relationship-Based Care into the Organizational Structure 230

Chapter 7: Embedding Relationship-Based Care at the Unit Level: Practical Considerations 255

PART IV: EDUCATION

PART V: EVIDENCE

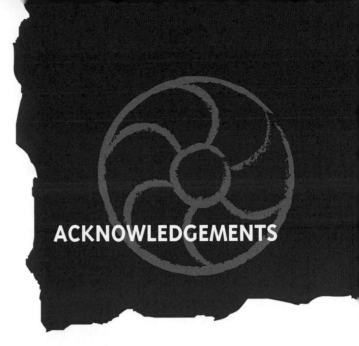

ACKNOWLEDGEMENTS

The editors of the *Relationship-Based Care Field Guide* acknowledge with appreciation your interest in this value-driven work. We at Creative Health Care Management (CHCM) have been affirmed by the response to our book *Relationship-Based Care: A Model for Transforming Practice* and delighted with how it is informing and inspiring practice changes in health care.

The dimensions and the concepts of Relationship-Based Care (RBC) have provided a framework for transforming health care. Responses suggest that RBC is being used as:

1. *an overarching concept that focuses attention on relationships (patient/family, colleagues and self),*

2. *a framework for transformation of organizational culture,*

3. *a care delivery model based on principles that shape behaviors (interdisciplinary and/or nursing), and*

4. *a way of being present in the moment in relationships with patients, families and colleagues.*

This field guide is published in response to your requests for more information and tools about how to make Relationship-Based Care live every day in organizations, groups and individuals. It is a collection of contributions from our clients and our colleagues as well as from the consultants at CHCM. It is a resource and a reference. The content is a reflection of all of our lived experiences: CHCM's expertise in facilitating the implementation of Relationship-Based Care in organizations, client exemplars and pieces authored by our colleagues.

The intention of this book is to be inspirational and informational, conceptual and practical, organizational and individual, nursing and interdisciplinary. There are paradoxes, multiple perspectives, inconsistencies, and, perhaps, unintentional errors and oversights. We acknowledge our clients and colleagues for their commitment to health care every day, and we thank them for their generous contributions to this field guide.

This field guide would not exist without the amazing teamwork of the faculty and staff of CHCM and without the extraordinary commitment of Beth Beaty, managing editor, and Chris Bjork, resources director. We extend our deep appreciation to Rebecca Smith, our writing partner, for helping us bring the *Field Guide* to life with her questions, editing expertise and unending energy. We celebrate our relationships with all of our colleagues at CHCM and beyond.

We welcome your feedback—your stories and exemplars of Relationship-Based Care—in anticipation of further exploration of the RBC experience. Join us in this hope-filled exploration of the *care* in health care.

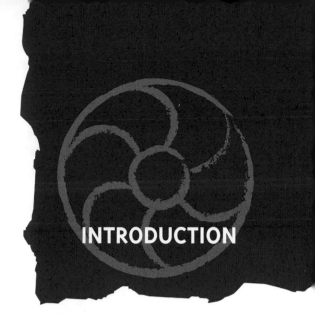

INTRODUCTION

This book exists to support every individual in your organization in his or her personal transition to practicing Relationship-Based Care (RBC). After reading this book you will have a clear sense of what RBC looks and feels like when it's thriving in a health care organization and what it takes to develop RBC in your organization. Perhaps most importantly, this book will paint you a picture of what it's like to be part of an organization that never stops evolving. Long after Relationship-Based Care is alive and thriving in your organization, it will continue to grow and change, as will everyone who embodies it.

This field guide is a companion to *Relationship-Based Care: A Model for Transforming Practice.* Developed in response to client and reader requests, it is a collection of practical tools, mind-expanding ideas and examples of RBC successes in their many forms.

Much has been written in the last few decades about "what's wrong with health care." While the writers who've taken this approach have provided the field with much-needed insights, we believe that it is now time to look more closely at what is right with health care and to build upon that. For this reason we have reflected on the best in health care today and how to transform the best of what is into the best of what can be.

Relationship-Based Care as a formalized, *implementable* culture is relatively new, but care based on relationships has been practiced as long as human caring has existed. We believe that Relationship-Based Care is based on the natural, human inclination to care for and heal others—in essence, when there are no barriers to loving care, we would express nothing *but* loving care. If our vision is to deliberately restore the sacredness to healing, we can do that best through Relationship-Based Care.

More than a philosophy that advances a specific set of practices at the point of care, RBC is, at its core, a way of "being" in an organization. Relationship-Based Care encompasses every relationship we have: with patients and families, with clinical and nonclinical colleagues, with administration and staff, with ourselves. They are all essential to patient care.

Relationship-Based Care is also a way of "being" *for* an organization. It must be integrated from the inside out. It must enter the organization through the commitment and practice of each individual in the organization. It must be advanced by every interaction, system, process and procedure at strategic, operational and tactical levels. It must be visible in every report and measurable in every satisfaction survey. It must reflect our core business: caring for patients, families and each other.

This book will help you develop the strategies and actions needed to create the knowledge-based caring relationships you want to see thriving in your organization. It is through this collective action that RBC becomes the way of being and doing business.

The sections in this book are organized according to I_2E_2, a formula for leading and sustaining change. This is the same leadership formula we use to create action plans for clients implementing and sustaining Relationship-Based Care. The design and implementation of Relationship-Based Care begins with a vision. Based on that vision, I_2E_2 asks us to consider the Inspiration (I_1), Infrastructure (I_2), Education (E_1) and Evidence (E_2) necessary to make the vision a reality and bring deep, sustainable change to health care organizations. In keeping with this formula for change, this book is divided into five parts: Vision, Inspiration, Infrastructure, Education and Evidence.

Part I: Vision

In this section, we present various reasons organizations have chosen to implement Relationship-Based Care. As the culture and needs of organizations are varied, so must be their vision for change. We discuss the mechanism within which individual ownership (personal vision) and the organizational vision intersect in such a way that deep, substantive change—cultural change—is the result.

Part II: Inspiration

In this section, we explore the importance of inspiration as a fundamental leadership action and strategy for change. Because different people are inspired in different ways, we address inspiration both diversely and comprehensively. We also discuss how to inspire others by inviting them to imagine the best that can be. True inspiration is inclusive, inviting all to participate.

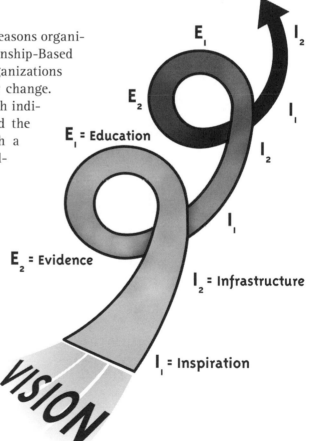

E_1

I_2

E_2

I_1

E_1 = Education

I_2

I_1

E_2 = Evidence

I_2 = Infrastructure

I_1 = Inspiration

VISION

Part III: Infrastructure

In this section we discuss how to engage direct-care practitioners, physicians, the board, executive teams and all departments in the implementation of Relationship-Based Care. We discuss how to integrate RBC into the fabric of the organization in several ways. We look at how to adapt RBC to your specific organization and link it to your vision and strategic goals. We describe the specifics of establishing and supporting the leadership teams, Results Councils and Practice Councils. We also offer practical tools to improve safety, communication and collaboration.

Part IV: Education

In this section, strategies for making learning an ongoing, everyday activity within the organizational culture are discussed. Education provides a solid foundation for RBC by preparing individuals at each level of the organization for their specific roles.

To gain the greatest return on investment of your organization's education dollars, we present educational philosophies which discuss the value of incorporating adult learning principles such as Senge's Five Disciplines, Accelerated Learning, and experiential, insight-based education. We outline educational content that successful clients have used to bring RBC alive in their organizations.

While the educational tools we offer are varied, they all direct our attention to four areas of competency. We have found that we can best support the implementation of RBC in an organization by enhancing every individual's ability to build relationships, foster creativity, think critically and provide caring leadership.

The section ends with comparisons (crosswalks) of RBC concepts, principles and processes to Magnet Standards, American Organization of Nurse Executives Care Delivery Standards, Institute of Medicine Guidelines, and the American Nurses Association Code of Ethics.

Part V: Evidence

In this section, we look at outcomes measurement. We describe what to measure, explore ways to measure it, and discuss how to use it. Too often, data is gathered, then simply gathers dust, buried in reports no one looks at twice. In RBC, evidence is used daily to keep leaders and practitioners focused, to celebrate success, and to inspire continued excellence. It is our hope that this section helps you discover a new (or renewed) passion for outcomes measurement.

We look at the impact RBC has had in organizations, and at the effectiveness of specific CHCM educational programs. We share specific tools and tips that help care givers collect evidence at the bedside. Finally, we offer the critical success factors, gleaned from experiences with and observation of hundreds of organizations as they implement Relationship-Based Care. For a more in-depth discussion of I_2E_2, see Jayne A. Felgen's book, I_2E_2: *Leading Lasting Change*.

How to Use This Book

This book was created for use in conjunction with *Relationship-Based Care: A Model for Transforming Practice*. In your quest to transform your organization's culture—whether you have already implemented RBC, are in the middle of transitioning to RBC, or are just considering whether it is the best option for your organization—the *Relationship-Based Care Field Guide* will prove to be a valuable resource.

This book is designed to be used in several different ways. It has been organized so that each part—and each chapter within each part—stands alone. You can read it cover-to-cover to get a sense of what RBC feels like in daily practice. It also works as a "drop in anywhere" book. You can refer to individual pieces to inspire yourself or others, to begin discussions at staff at meetings, or to help you articulate your vision of RBC to others.

If you've come to this guide with a solid sense of what RBC is all about, flip through it and follow your interests. If you've come to this guide to get a clear picture of what it takes to bring RBC to an organization and what RBC looks like when it's alive and thriving, we recommend a cover-to-cover reading.

The following icons are used throughout the book to highlight the dimensions of Relationship-Based Care and related concepts.

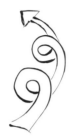

Transformational Change

Relationship-Based Care is not just another project, it is transformational change—deep and abiding change of organizations and individuals.

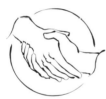

Caring and Healing Environment

In a caring and healing environment care providers tend to the needs of the whole patient—mind, body and spirit. A caring and healing environment is achieved through human connection.

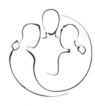

Patients and Families

Patients and their families are at the center of care and service for all members of the health care organization. Patients and families are honored as individuals and cared for with dignity and respect.

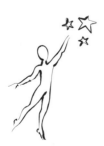

Leadership

In this book, leadership is used in the broadest sense. Anyone who knows the vision, acts with purpose and removes barriers to care demonstrates leadership. Caring and compassionate service emerges from caring and compassionate leaders.

Teamwork

Healthy teams form a support network similar to the root system of the ancient Redwood trees. Their roots systems are intertwined just below the surface, so each tree is supported by the strength of the rest. They hold each other up even in the wildest storms.

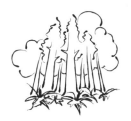

Professional Practice

Professional nursing practice is characterized by a well-defined body of clinical knowledge, proficiency in specialized skills, knowledge-based caring, and a deep understanding of the human condition. It is both the art and science of nursing.

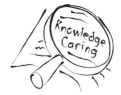

Patient Care Delivery

More than just a way of organizing work, a patient care delivery system supports therapeutic relationships, maximizes teamwork, and provides for efficient use of resources.

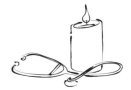

Resource Driven Practice

When practice is resource driven, managers and staff members do not think about their work as being driven by tasks and routines, but rather think about it as being driven by prioritized caring.

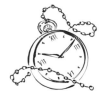

Outcome Measurement

Effective outcome measurement motivates leaders and practitioners to continuously improve the way they work and care for patients and families. To be truly motivating, data and measurement processes must be trustworthy, tangible and relevant from the point of care to the boardroom.

Welcome Aboard

The experience of transforming an organization to Relationship-Based Care will transform everyone in that organization on a personal level. Imagine, as a care giver at the point of care, having barriers to caring not only removed, but replaced with whatever it takes to actively develop accountability, continuity and clinical excellence at the point of care.

We know that you are willing to do whatever it takes to provide the best experience possible for your patients, their families and your health care team members. We are honored to offer you the opportunity to reach that goal through the formalization of Relationship-Based Care in your organization!

With never ending respect,

Mary Koloroutis   *Jayne Felgen*

Colleen Person   *Susan Wessel*

PART

I

Vision

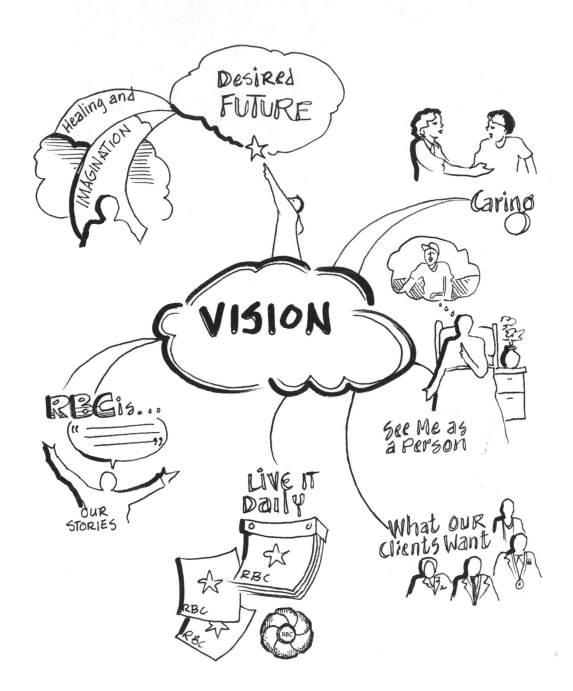

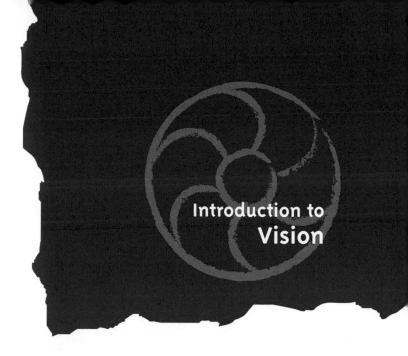

Introduction to Vision

Though Relationship-Based Care (RBC) is defined by a core set of principles and practices, it does not look exactly the same in any two organizations. Individual stakeholders within the organization define exactly how their unique pool of talent and resources will come together to create a new culture in which the care giver/patient relationship is held as sacred and every policy, process, practice and behavior functions to strengthen that relationship.

The ability to rally individuals around a viable plan for development and transformational change begins with the vision of a desired future in which everyone sees his or her own role as essential to the functioning of the whole. While it follows that everyone in an organization undergoing the deep cultural change of RBC implementation will take on new ways of thinking, being and doing, this cannot be put into place until a vision is clearly articulated.

Your organization's unique vision for RBC will emerge as you:

1. *clarify your reasons for wanting Relationship-Based Care,*

2. *develop a shared dream of what your organization will look, sound and feel like when RBC is successfully implemented,*

3. *determine the level of participation and engagement expected of all stakeholders, and*

4. *create a plan for a day-to-day practice grounded in Relationship-Based Care.*

In Part I, vision is the catalyst for transforming an organization to Relationship-Based Care. We discuss the vision as the "why" of RBC—a desire for moving beyond what is—and the "how" of RBC—what it takes to bring it to life in day-to-day practice. I_2E_2, a formula for inspiring, implementing and sustaining the vision, is introduced, and expressions of visions or dreams/desires are presented. Our hope is to make the idea of vision concrete, attainable and practical. Vision sets the direction for change by defining why it matters. It is the stepping-off place for changing a health care organization's culture into one that maintains a laser focus on compassionate and healing relationships at three critical levels: patients and families, colleagues and self.

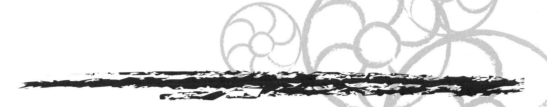

CHAPTER ONE

Begin at the Beginning

A Vision for Caring

—Ronna Fay Jevne

I have a dream—a vision of how caring could be.

Of how having been ill wouldn't mean fear and loneliness.

Where a whole institution of caring people understood that nothing is as therapeutic as recognizing the emotional pain, not just the physical pain.

I have a vision that doctors could talk compassionately. That families could talk openly. That patients could talk freely.

I have a vision that the care givers would touch patients, gently, caringly and not only physically. That all would recognize that with every touch, every smile, every word, we enter a temple. A temple so sacred, so impressionable, so beautiful that every fingerprint leaves its mark. That with every moment we enter the temple of the self.

I have a vision that care givers would share a strength—a strength that comes only from a common purpose, that comes from belonging to a community of people who believe that caring makes a difference, that custodians matter as much as physicians, that volunteers have a place beside nurses, that letters and titles matter less than kindness.

I have a vision that line-ups are no more. That people are cared for before paper. That voices convey caring before directions. That waiting rooms reflect hope rather than convenience. That death means knowing a lot of people care. That there will be no physical pain and no aloneness. That tears could give way to laughter and anger to tenderness. That joy could surface in our sadness ...

Editors' note: We have found this vision to be one of the most beautiful and compelling visions of what caring could look like day-to-day in a health care institution. Originally published in It All Begins With Hope, *published by Innisfree Press in 1991. Used by permission of the author.*

The *Why* of Relationship-Based Care:
A Vision Emerges Through Want of Something More

—Jayne A. Felgen, Colleen Person, Mary Koloroutis and Susan Wessel

> *A vision is not just a picture of what could be;*
> *it is an appeal to our better selves,*
> *a call to become something more.*
>
> *—Rosabeth Moss Kanter*

Everyone who makes the decision to implement Relationship-Based Care (RBC) is seeking to create the best possible caring and healing experience for patients, families and their care givers. Beyond that core desire, organizations chose RBC for a variety of reasons ranging from paralyzing differences among staff members to the desire to raise an already stellar standard of professionalism even higher. Just as the needs and desires of organizations are so varied, so too are their visions for change.

What follows is a sampling of the reasons organizations have chosen to change their culture through Relationship-Based Care.

One:
To Enhance a Culture
of Excellence

An organization may already have achieved recognition and awards such as Magnet designation through the American Nurses Credentialing Center (ANCC), and then decide there's no ceiling on the culture of excellence they wish to achieve. Several organizations use RBC to continue their growth through a culture of excellence (see page 561).

It is a reality in many organizations that while executive team members have a defined strategy for the overall business, they also have at least one leadership development initiative running somewhere in the organization, a customer service program in place, their nursing department working toward Magnet designation, a Joint Commission visit coming up and, as always, an unwavering focus on the bottom line. All of these things require energy and focus, but unlike any of these initiatives, RBC doesn't just address various aspects of the core business—RBC is the core business.

In an RBC organization, the continuity and quality of care giver/patient/family relationships becomes the stated objective of literally every program or initiative running in the organization. We have helped a number of organizations plagued by fragmented efforts to implement RBC as a means to provide a new, unifying focus to existing initiatives—Relationship-Based Care serves as a framework for integration.

Two: To Provide Clarity and Focus in an Organization Plagued by Fragmented Efforts

We often get calls because patient satisfaction scores are lower than desired. Leaders in organizations recognize that when patient satisfaction is down, it may be because their infrastructure is out of alignment with what they value most. One client contacted us when patient satisfaction scores were at the 11th percentile, and within 15 months of RBC implementation, the client reported scores in the 89th percentile.

Organizations know that patients and their families are appreciative when care givers establish meaningful therapeutic relationships with them—when they see them as people. Many organizations take on RBC because the subsequent improvement in patient satisfaction scores in organizations is both verifiable and impressive. The patient experience is improved.

Three: To Improve Patient Satisfaction with Care

Four: To Improve the Morale of Hospital Staff Members

People who choose to work in health care are most satisfied with their work when they know they are making a positive difference for patients and their families. Organizations experiencing low morale among staff members are often attracted by Relationship-Based Care as a means to provide role clarity and design systems to support and enhance professional roles. When this occurs, the impact on the care of patients and families is acknowledged and valued, which in turn enhances peoples' ability to have a positive impact on the care of patients and families!

Poor morale doesn't always show up in an organization as turnover. It can mean that people stay, but become visibly discontented and uncooperative. Nurses report that their greatest job satisfaction comes from providing care in relationship with patients and families. Additionally, nurses choose to stay in an organization when they experience healthy relationships with their colleagues and when there is good support and leadership from their managers. Relationship-Based Care addresses the quality of all relationships in an organization, raising the morale of hospital staff throughout the entire organization.

Five: To Improve Recruitment and Retention

When an organization is experiencing a troubling amount of turnover coupled with difficulties in attracting quality staff members, it may find hope in RBC's focus on relationships.

An organization that can honestly represent itself as one supporting care givers in their desire to make a meaningful, positive impact on the experience of patients and families, finds itself in an excellent position to recruit talented candidates. Relationship-Based Care results in staff members having a solid bond with their manager. They feel cared for and empowered to solve problems at the point of care.

Relationship-Based Care also focuses on retaining staff members by recognizing and celebrating those who build healthy relationships. Organizations that invest in staff development (rather than sign-on bonuses to get people through the door) provide something that many staff members value more than cash up front—a culture that focuses on caring for patients and their families.

Most clinicians practice at their highest professional capacity if they perceive that leaders support professional practice and that the systems, processes and procedures in place enhance their ability to practice professionally. Organizations wishing to improve professional practice value the way RBC first works to strengthen relationships between individuals and then strengthens the relationship between individuals and their work environments by eliminating barriers and interruptions to a meaningful patient/care giver interaction.

Six: To Improve Professional Practice

Sometimes leaders realize that a shared-governance model would create the kind of culture they're looking for in their organizations. They recognize that shared governance is fundamental to and supported by Relationship-Based Care. As the decentralized processes of RBC development evolve, health care team members have greater decision making power on behalf of patients and families. The entire culture changes into one that not only supports but celebrates courageous, informed decision making on the part of the people at the point of care.

Furthermore, managers experience growth and development as they refocus their energy on achieving Relationship-Based Care at the unit or department level. Managers transition from feeling responsible for making decisions and solving problems into feeling responsible for leading, coaching and developing their staff members to be decision makers at the point of care.

Seven: To Create a Culture of Empowerment

There are many organizations that have made a commitment to seek Magnet designation and have recognized RBC as a framework and methodology for the development needed to meet the 14 Forces of Magnetism (see crosswalk, page 561). Relationship-Based Care, like Magnet designation, aims to improve the patient experience through strengthening leadership, governance, professional practice and the overall role of the nurse.

Eight: To Prepare for Magnet Designation by the American Nurses Credentialing Center

Receiving Magnet designation, however, is not the end of the process. Every four years an organization with Magnet designation is reviewed. Organizations want to continue to strengthen their infrastructure and professional nursing practice. Relationship-Based Care, when implemented with I_2E_2, sets an organization up for continual review, refinement and growth.

Nine: To Foster Unity After the Merger of Two Organizations

Organizations faced with complicated mergers appreciate how the philosophies and practices of Relationship-Based Care can help organizations to remember why they are in health care in the first place: to provide quality care, clinical excellence and compassionate care for patients and their families.

In the best mergers, each organization's unique culture is honored and built upon while a common purpose is identified. In difficult mergers, people lose track of their common purpose. When RBC is used as an integrating framework as two organizations are merging, every move the organization makes is visibly tied back to the direct care of patients and families. In mergers, people typically experience so much disruption that they end up asking, "Why is all this change necessary anyway?" When RBC guides the process, the answer is "Because this change supports clinical quality and the care giver/patient relationships—and here's how...." When we discover that we are working toward the same goal, it is easier to accept changes. We feel empowered to contribute our own ideas to the new direction.

Ten: To Meet the Vision of a New CEO and/or CNO

Sometimes a new Chief Executive Officer or Chief Nursing Officer comes into an organization, desires to lead change in order to provide better experiences for patients and families, and sees RBC as the means to that end. Perhaps in a previous organization, they had experience with Primary Nursing and/or interdisciplinary, interdepartmental RBC and they want to bring it into their new organization. Many wish to leave a legacy, and RBC has proven to be both a positive and a sustainable change over time.

The Importance of a Shared Vision for Change

The phase of creating a clearly articulated vision for change is one of the most satisfying phases because it requires the organization to find its unifying thread—its compelling reason for being. A group may begin with a notion of some concrete, measurable improvements it wants to make, but members always end up digging deeper to reconnect with their very reason for being—to provide the best healing experience possible for patients and their families. And typically individuals throughout the organization get in touch with their reasons for being in health care—making an individual difference in patients' lives. Once people reconnect with their philosophical core, it is a very small leap for them to see that RBC is also a great way to achieve their business goals.

The executive team leads the process of developing an organizational vision with input from key stakeholders including the board and staff. There are many methods for developing a vision. We often use Appreciative Inquiry (see article, page 96), a process for building on what works in an organization, as a preface to individual and collective visioning. A compelling vision for the entire organization can serve as the foundation for individual departments to create their own visions with the input of all their staff members and physicians.

Relationship-Based Care can become a "rallying point" around which many other organizational initiatives and programs can focus. As already mentioned, we have found that many organizations are plagued by fragmentation of efforts. One division of an organization may be focused on redesign of the physical structure, and another on improving efficiency. When RBC becomes the central focus in the organization's culture, however, each of these existing initiatives gets tied more overtly to the way it influences the experience of patients and families. For example, when the shared vision is one in which RNs have more time at the bedside in relationships with patients, any steps taken to help RNs process paper more efficiently become steps taken to free RNs to have more time at the bedside.

When RBC becomes the guiding vision and overarching framework for the organization's myriad initiatives, all of these initiatives get linked to a stable core and common purpose. Relationship-Based Care provides a framework for meeting Magnet designation (see page 561) and Joint Commission standards, and it also keeps individuals continually involved in the evolution of their practice, thereby preventing the experience of ever feeling like they are "jumping through hoops" in anticipation of a review.

The *How* of Relationship-Based Care: Bringing the Vision to Life at the Point of Care

—Jayne A. Felgen, Colleen Person, Mary Koloroutis and Susan Wessel

The best organizational vision statements crystallize what matters most to an organization's culture. These vision statements hold the importance of relationships and compassionate, humane care for all members of the organization to claim and for the patients and families we serve to see. They provide a jumping-off point for the creation of more detailed vision statements concerning what actual practice will look like in the day-to-day. The following vision statements honor the importance of relationships:

Joy, Care and Respect

—Providence Hospital, Washington, DC

Every nurse at McKee Medical Center will experience the power of a genuine healing environment and embrace the importance of unforgettable caring moments with patients, family and each other.

—McKee Medical Center, Loveland, Colorodo

A Community of Compassionate and Skilled Caregivers Devoted to the Physical, Spiritual and Emotional Needs of Those We Serve

—Eliza Coffee Memorial Hospital, Florence, Alabama

Once the overall strategic vision statement (brief, clear, compelling) is determined, it must then become real and meaningful enough for individuals to experience in every facet of their practice. It must be made so tangible and immediate that leaders and care givers at the point of care can visualize it—and more importantly, that each can see with perfect clarity his or her own role in it. In this phase, the vision becomes personal: individual practitioners will make decisions about how to integrate RBC principles into their own practices and thus bring the vision to life.

Construct your vision with its end use in mind: It is to be used as a guiding light for all that you do for making the vision live in the daily workings of your organization.

An example of a clear vision for change in patient care in a health care organization follows:

In our organization:

- *Patient satisfaction and staff satisfaction scores are above 90%.*

- *The patient and family are satisfied because they know that their number one expressed concern regarding this episode of care is also the number one priority for their RN and the health care team.*

- *Each patient's care is managed by one RN who establishes a therapeutic relationship at (or soon after) admission, and this relationship lasts throughout the patient's stay on the care unit.*

- *The patient and family are actively engaged in the development of a care plan driven by their expressed wishes.*

- *Physicians and nurses are partners in the patient care planning process.*

- *Interdisciplinary collaboration enhances the patient experience.*

- *Patient care is attentive to the mind, body and spirit.*

- *The patient experiences caring in the way that he or she describes caring behaviors upon admission.*

Notice that these vision statements are written in the present tense rather than in the more familiar future tense. When we facilitate the development of vision statements in organizations, we ask that individuals express the details of their desired future as if they are already alive and thriving within the organization. This helps generate a clear, tangible direction, as it inspires people to get specific about how they intend to make things happen.

Here is another example of an operational vision statement, this time focusing on teamwork:

In our organization:

- *Staff members respect each other's unique contributions regardless of title or educational preparation.*

- *Co-workers are skilled in resolving issues among themselves and do not complain about other team members behind their backs.*

- *We have a culture of teamwork, with staff members offering help to each other and affirming each other's good work and contributions.*

- *Staff members speak positively about each other and the work setting and focus on finding solutions to problems that diminish the patient and family care experience.*

In order to effectively move toward something, we must have a clear picture of what we are moving toward. When we imagine in realistic detail what we wish to create, something happens to us—and to the people around us—at an emotional level. Our statements become compelling and empowering when we phrase things as if they are already happening. They take on a penetrating energy that inspires everyone involved to take action.

It is also important to note that in order for any significant changes to take place in practice, each individual must ultimately ask himself or herself, "What am I being called upon to transform?" Changes in personal practice require personal commitment.

Some examples of practical, achievable personal vision statements that have the potential for transformational change follow.

A clinical nurse manager included this statement in her personal vision:

"When I make rounds, I use appreciative inquiry to draw out the best in staff members. For example, I ask the staff to describe a satisfying patient interaction."

This same leader also included the statement:

"I approach situations with an open and nonjudgmental point of view. When I speak with staff members I listen without judgment and seek to understand before I make a decision."

A clinical nurse setting a new vision for her own professional practice wrote this statement:

"I ask each patient what his or her priority is for this shift of care and then I rally the team to meet that priority."

A CNO as a champion for integrating RBC wrote:

"I begin each meeting with the directors who report to me by asking them to describe a recent example of excellence in interdisciplinary caring for a patient and family in their service."

A COO committed to visibly leading RBC in the organization stated:

"I seek to understand the experience of the staff members in this organization so that I can support their work fully. I do this by inquiring and listening."

A board member offered:

"I open each monthly meeting with a request for a story in which a significant and positive impact on the patient or family experience resulted from our RBC efforts."

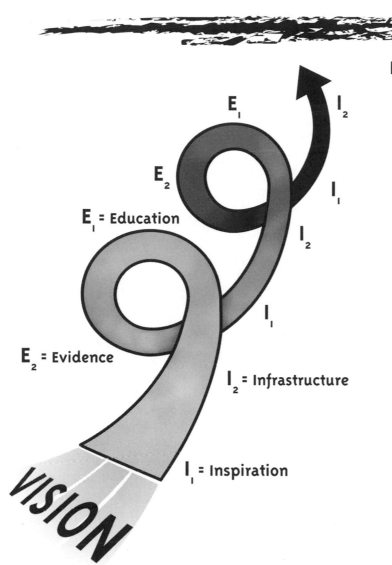

E₁ = Education

E₂ = Evidence

I₂ = Infrastructure

I₁ = Inspiration

VISION

As with any change process, professional or personal, we start where we are, figure out where we want to go, and then put together a workable plan to get there. I_2E_2 provides a formula to ensure that all planning and implementation activities for that change are comprehensive and inclusive (Felgen, 2007). When working with clients to help them implement RBC, this is the formula we use to help create each organization's "workable plan to get there."

Transformational change starts with the vision. Once an organization has discovered and committed to a shared vision for change, I_2E_2 becomes the blueprint that project leaders can refer to in order to gauge the status and progress of any aspect of the plan.

Inspiration (I_1)

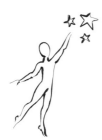

For the purposes of organizational change, the best inspiration is that which links the "new" shared vision to something that already exists within the people in the organization. Rather than thinking of the team we wish to inspire as a clean wall over which we will apply a new shade of paint, we will instead help them to see that the "new" vision is not so new—it's likely a vision they've held, and perhaps the organization has forgotten in the flurry of activity that has come to define their daily experience. If inspiration is to be lasting, it must be deep and it must align with the values and purpose of the covenant. It must bring the "new" shared vision into alignment with something that already exists in the people we wish to lead. This means communicating the vision for change, from heart-to-heart.

As a leader constructing the Inspiration (I_1) section of your I_2E_2 action plan, ask yourself:

- *How will this change enhance the integrity of our organization?*

- *How will this change improve the experience of patients and families and colleagues?*

- *What good things are already happening in the organization that we can connect to this new vision?*

- *How have we previously been successful in galvanizing others to overcome their resistance and to engage in positive change?*

- *How will we share the global vision with the organization as a whole?*

- *What inspires me most about this new vision for change?*

- *How will this change make each individual's practice more inspired and effective?*

- *How will I inspire others?*

The answers to all of these questions (and any number of questions like them) will help you target how best to inspire people in your unique organization.

Infrastructure (I₂)

There needs to be clarity of Responsibility, Authority and Accountability (see page 486) at all levels in the organization and for all roles, councils, committees and individuals.

Strategic

Every organization has a strategic plan along with mission, vision and values statements. It is crucial that the new vision becomes integrated into the existing statements and plans. The action plan to achieve RBC then becomes the method for the expression of the mission, vision and values statements and the achievement of strategic plan objectives.

Strategic thinking is big-picture thinking—it's about over-all direction, and includes broad areas of functional activity to achieve the end goals.

In strategic action planning we address questions like:

- *What can be done to support our core business and to serve our community?*

- *How could integrating the newest innovations in health care positively affect our organization?*

- *How could strengthening the visibility of organizational leaders promote a greater consensus for our vision for change?*

- *In what ways can the executive team and board link the new vision for change with visible support for RBC principles and concepts?*

Operational

The operational aspect of infrastructure deals with roles, standards, policies, organizational reporting structures, human resources, financial considerations, communication and work systems.

The operational level is where the vision comes to life in departments and units throughout the organization. Operational considerations help us clarify departmental roles, relationships, systems, schedules and assignments. Here we ask how our policies, procedures, organizational charts and systems can bring the strategic plan to life in the organization.

In operational action planning we ask ourselves:

- *What practices already in place at the department/ unit levels actively advance the vision for change?*

- *How can reporting structures be adjusted to advance the vision for change?*

- *Whose support will we want to enlist when making department, team and unit level changes?*

- *Who at the department/unit level can be tapped for leadership?*

Tactical

The tactical aspect of infrastructure deals with daily practices, routines and standards.

The tactical level is where the vision comes to life at the individual level at the point of care. In short—if it doesn't live in practice and it isn't prominent in the shift report, it doesn't exist.

While it is true that every aspect of infrastructure can be designed to advance the best possible patient/family experience, the tactical level is the level where the vision is experienced by patients, families and colleagues. The tone that is set at the strategic level and the mechanisms put in place at the operational level come to life in the hands-on practices at the point of care. There must be alignment among all these levels to overcome fears that changes will be topical and temporary.

In our planning at the tactical level, we ask ourselves:

- *How can we assist individuals to translate the strategic vision into reality in their unique relationships with patients, families and colleagues?*

- *What will it take to support each care giver and service supporter in his or her quest for the best... one day at a time, one relationship at a time?*

- *What commitments can be made to support healthy work relationships?*

- *What will I do to learn continuously to care for myself so I can provide the very best of service?*

The process of collaboratively redesigning your infrastructure to actively advance your vision for change creates opportunities for each department to express its unique translation of your vision's principles. It is vital that all innovations and expressions of the adopted principles related to the vision become embedded in the infrastructure of your organization.

Education (E₁)

Organizational change usually means that all or most of the individuals in the organization will be asked to do at least some things differently. In order to design the Education (E_1) element of the I_2E_2 formula, we assess the current knowledge and skills of our talent pool and determine what additional knowledge and skill building will be necessary to meet the vision for change.

When you offer a truly comprehensive staff development program to your workforce, people feel they are competent to not only "do their jobs," but to manage their own relationships, do their own critical and creative thinking, and make their own decisions on the job.

While programs this comprehensive can represent a fairly large investment of time, energy and money, they offer an excellent return on investment in terms of staff satisfaction and lower turnover rates.

Our Education (E_1) element comes together in response to questions like:

- *What changes are we considering that would require additional learning for staff members and managers at each level of our organization?*

- *What changes are we considering that would require additional learning for executives, medical staff or board members?*

- *What workshops would facilitate a greater consciousness and understanding of the tangible implications of the vision for change?*

- *How might we help team members better manage their own relationships during and after the change?*

- *What new critical and creative thinking challenges will staff members face during and after the change?*

Education paves the way for excellence. When individuals receive relevant, compelling training in clinical, interpersonal, critical and creative thinking and caring leadership skills, they become active participants in bringing the vision to life.

Evidence (E_2)

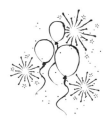

The Evidence element of I_2E_2 assesses the impact of our efforts in realizing the organization's new vision.

But while evidence shows us what impact the implementation of the vision for change is actually having on the organization, it is not to be regarded as judge and jury. It exists not to "critique" the changes, but to inspire greater commitment to the changes that have proven successful and to help redouble commitment to redesigning what has not yet proven successful.

Evidence makes visible the alignment of individual behaviors with the overall vision. In a health care organization undergoing cultural change, evidence helps us monitor the impact the new changes are making on our primary areas of concern—patient and family satisfaction/loyalty and clinical quality. Furthermore, evidence helps us to monitor the impact of related variables like staff retention scores, nurse and physician satisfaction scores, and other staffing-sensitive patient quality indicators—all of which ultimately affect patient loyalty, clinical quality and fiscal positioning.

The Evidence (E_2) section of your action plan will respond to the questions:

- *How will we determine that we have sustained our focus on the vision for change?*

- *What key process and outcomes measures are most important to capture: strategic, operational and tactical indicators?*

- *What process of data collection and dissemination will be most inclusive, efficient and compelling?*

- *How will we ensure that all evidence collected becomes available for use as inspiration in future I_2E_2 cycles?*

- *How will we measure the commitment level of the staff, managers, physicians and board?*

- *Who will manage the new data we're collecting to measure and analyze the effectiveness of this new initiative?*

- *How will we know when our vision for change is a reality?*

I_2E_2 is Designed to Cycle Continuously

As evidence is primarily compiled through measurement and evaluation, we tend to think of a body of evidence as a report card—we did what we were asked to do, our effectiveness was measured, and we got "graded" on what we did. With I_2E_2, however, evidence functions not as a conclusion, but as a springboard into a repetition of the entire formula. Evidence (E_2) provides material for Inspiration (I_1), which takes us back to Infrastructure (I_2), which takes us back to Education (E_1), and so on. That means we never get our grades and go home. It means that change is an ongoing process. It means that we inspire everyone in the organization to commit continually to the organization's vision, that we revise and improve infrastructure as needed, that we provide timely, relevant education to individuals at all levels of the organization, and that we gather evidence and use it as the inspiration to start new cycles of I_2E_2 again and again.

Reference: Felgen, J. (2007). *I_2E_2: Leading lasting change.* Minneapolis, MN Creative Health Care Management.

Relationship-Based Care Is ...

Editors' note: A key outcome for the five-day Relationship-Based Care Leader Practicum is for participants to gain clarity about the meaning of Relationship-Based Care for them individually and for their organization as a whole. We use a variety of methodologies through the five days to build clarity and confidence in leading Relationship-Based Care. One exercise is for the participants to imagine that they must convey the meaning of Relationship-Based Care in a few sentences (a 30-second elevator speech). It is our privilege to share some of their reflections as sources of inspiration.

... the foundation for every encounter in our organization. It helps us to honor the privilege we have as healers during some of the most sacred moments in the lives of those we touch. First and foremost, people will remember how we made them feel. Simply stated, it's all about relationships.

–Patricia Roach, MS, RN, OCN
Senior Vice President/Chief Nursing Officer
Faxton-St. Luke's Health Care
Utica, New York

... a model that puts the patient at the center of care. It focuses on relationships, setting the stage for therapeutic and healing relationships; the model compels us to build our universe of caring and doing around what is best for the patient. It gives us permission to examine what we are currently doing with a new lens, a new litmus test. It sets the stage for personal and professional growth for the care team and support teams. Foundational are the concepts of sacred space, healing space, centered and grounded communications. This facilitates the transformation of the environment to foster learning, reflection, nurturing of the next generation of care givers, nurturing of patients and families. Everything happens in relationships. This model acknowledges this truth and harkens us to evolve.

–Hollie Shaner-McRae, MSA, RN, FAAN
Coordinator, Professional Nursing Practice
Fletcher Allen Health Care,
Burlington, Vermont

... teamwork at its highest calling.

—Tim Ols
Chief Operational Officer
Greene Memorial Hospital
Xenia, Ohio

... a conscious action of intentional caring in all relationships within the organization that bring life to our mission and values every moment of every day.

—Theresa Weiland, BSN, RN
Director Emergency Services
St. Clare Hospital & Health Services
Baraboo, Wisconsin

... a new nursing model that frames where nursing originally came from and where we want patient care to go in our organization. It gets nurses back to the roots of why they got into nursing in the first place—because they care! In doing so, nurses and care partners intentionally choose to put the patient, family, and loved ones back in the center of their work and approach each moment by leading with their heart.

—Andrea Cochran, MA
Training & Organizational Development
University of California Irvine Medical Center
Orange County, California

... a natural progression of Primary Nursing that needs to be implemented so that the humanness of a care-giving environment will not be lost in a high-tech, fast-paced world. It will serve to renew the spirit of the care giver as much as it will comfort and satisfy the patient/family in their time of need.

—Brenda G. Larkin, MS, RN, CNOR
Clinical Nurse Specialist
Froedtert Memorial Lutheran Hospital
Milwaukee, Wisconsin

... nurses spending time to get to know their patient. Understanding and meeting the patient's needs and concerns. Integrating the patient and the family into health care decisions, planning care with the patient and family needs at the forefront. It is calming fears and frustrations; creating a circle of trust, and caring and compassion that is genuine.

–Laura A. Iacono, RN
Patient Care Director
New York Presbyterian The University Hospital of
Columbia and Cornell
New York, New York

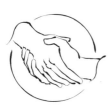

... the foundation of the patient experience–patients and families feel safe and valued.
The staff encourage and support each other.
The organization recognizes successes and celebrates.

–Anonymous

... a culture of caring where each interaction as a team is a cherished opportunity to reach out and minister to the needs of others.

–Beth Ware, BSN, RN
Director of Patient Care
Eliza Coffee Memorial Hospital
Florence, Alabama

... to own my relationship with my patients, my colleagues, and myself.

–Eunmee Shim, RN
New York Presbyterian The University
Hospital of Columbia and Cornell
New York, New York

Bringing Relationship-Based Care to Life in Daily Practice

—Colleen Person and Mary Koloroutis

A vision without a task is but a dream
A task without a vision is drudgery
A vision and a task are the hope of the world.

—Sussex Churchyard

Creating and living a vision for Relationship-Based Care that is shared from boardroom to bedside is truly transformational in an organization. Engaging everyone from the executive level through the point of care areas generates energy, creativity and involvement. Developing and living the behaviors of a shared vision provides focus and promotes success.

I. A Shared Vision For Change—What Do We Want and Why Do We Want It?

Most of us are very familiar with the concept of shared vision, as introduced by Peter Senge in the early '90s in his book *The Fifth Discipline*. Senge says, "At its simplest level a shared vision is the answer to the question, 'What do we want to create?'" The power of a shared vision is that it binds people together with a common aspiration and dream. Once this bond is solidified, individuals and teams throughout the organization own the vision and work together to bring it to life.

Shared vision and shared ownership challenge leaders to move from the paradigm of "telling and selling" their vision to actively engaging individuals and teams throughout the organization in conversations that tap into their individual values and dreams. The shared vision is "touchable." It engages individuals and teams in a creative mode—a mode that moves them from what is real today, to what they desire for their future (Senge, 1994).

Despite Senge's emphasis on the power of shared vision, it's been our experience that often organizational vision statements are created at the executive level and then communicated to the rest of the staff through newsletters and posters. The challenge becomes getting the vision off the wall and into individual daily practice. That requires individuals at all levels to ask themselves:

- *What does this vision mean in my job?*
- *What does this vision mean in daily practice?*
- *What would it mean to make this vision live in daily practice in my every action?*

Creating a clear and tangible vision for what we as an organization want to be is essential to the transformation of any organizational culture.

The vision for change is a provocative statement, written as if the vision it offers were already a reality. It answers the questions "What do we want, and why do we want it?" The shared vision does not concern itself with anything having to do with how the vision will become a reality. Concerning ourselves with how a vision will be realized draws our focus from the what and why of our intended creation. Strategic, operational and tactical action planning dealing with questions of *how* comes later.

The Eliza Coffee Memorial Hospital vision emerged from staff focus groups in which they focused on what mattered most to them and what it looked like when they were providing exemplary patient care:

> *"We are a community of compassionate and skilled care givers devoted to meeting the physical, spiritual and emotional needs of those we serve."*

This vision now serves as the focus for how RBC will be developed.

The purpose of having a shared vision is to invite widespread engagement in the process of integrating the vision into the daily practice of everyone in the organization. Transition to RBC requires a deep cultural change that begins at the level of self and transforms the individual practice of every person in

Before the vision is shared with the organization at large, it must be embodied by those who will lead the change.

the organization. If individual practice is changed in alignment with the clearly articulated shared vision, the organization itself is then transformed into exactly what it intends to be.

II. How Do We Engage Leaders and Staff Throughout the Organization in the Shared Vision?

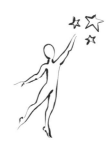

There is no power for change greater than a community discovering what it cares about.

—Meg Wheatley

Engagement comes through conversations of meaning throughout the organization. Regardless of where the impetus for Relationship-Based Care emerges in an organization, typically the executive team will authorize RBC as integral to the mission, vision and values of the organization. Before the vision is shared with the organization at large, it must be clear and embodied by those who will lead the change.

Creative Health Care Management offers a Relationship-Based Care practicum for leaders in which those who will lead the implementation of RBC in their organizations explore their own personal understanding and vision for Relationship-Based Care. A focus of the practicum is to help individuals leading the change to RBC embody the change by voicing their own personal meaning and vision for Relationship-Based Care. Below are examples of statements of personal meaning created by RBC practicum participants.

RBC is all about Caring. It occurs when the patient and family feel they have had their concerns addressed in a timely fashion by a capable and caring staff. As a staff person you know you have delivered Relationship-Based Care when your heart feels full, yet light.

—Anne Ireland, MSN, RN, AOCN
Fletcher Allen Health Care
Burlington, Vermont

RBC will spread because of all of us present today. Everyone here is a champion who will take this knowledge back and put the patient and his or her family in the center of their core business processes. Sometimes to do the right thing is not the same as to do things right.

—Jean Harry, MSA, RN, Chief Nursing Officer
Fletcher Allen Health Care
Burlington, Vermont

RBC is connected caring. Relationship-Based Care is health care; caring for the whole person, body, mind, heart and spirit through caring and healing relationships that are organized around the needs and priorities of the patient and family.

—Sheila Hauck, APRN, BC
St. Mary's Medical Center
Evansville, Indiana

Creating a clear and tangible vision for what we as an organization want to be is essential to the transformation of any organizational culture.

The vision for RBC can be introduced to the larger organization in a number of ways. Some organizations use a "kick off" in which various stakeholders are invited to hear a presentation on the philosophy and principles of Relationship-Based Care and what it has meant to the organizations that have embraced it (see page 520). The vision may also be introduced to individuals within the organization in inspirational meetings in which Appreciative Inquiry methodology (see page 96) is used to discover the best of what is currently being practiced in the organization. As these meetings always focus on the best of what is in the organization, they invariably address the internal values that cause us to perform competently and compassionately on behalf of patients and families. This focus on the best of what is and how that supports RBC provides a natural foundation to discuss what it would look like if these important values and best practices happened as the norm every day.

In every venue in which we offer the RBC vision to those who will be asked to live it, we draw individuals into a co-creation of the vision itself by inviting them to imagine the vision as it would apply to their own practice on a daily basis. This allows individuals to see the vision as evolving but reachable and to imagine themselves evolving with it.

Understanding that vision and action have to go hand in glove, we integrate shared visioning into all of our educational workshops that support RBC, including *The Caring Leader, Leading an Empowered Organization, Reigniting the Spirit of Caring, Leadership at the Point of Care* and *Work Complexity Assessment*. In each workshop, participants engage in inquiry about what matters most and what it will take to make the new vision live in practice. These experiences help people keep the vision front-of-mind so that each of them individually can be—within the scope of his or her own daily practice—the change he or she wants to see.

Vision building starts with individuals giving voice to their hopes and dreams; the collective vision emerges from conversations when leaders and staff have an opportunity to share their vision and put it into words for their unit and department. Making the vision come alive requires really looking at what it means at the practical individual level, and is addressed by putting statements of meaning together that get at the nuts and bolts of daily practice. If we have a vision of "exemplary patient care," for example, we take that vision into the practical/tactical by fleshing out the vision with as clear a picture as possible of what "exemplary patient care" looks like in each individual work role. The vision becomes real when it's lived every day in practice.

> *Vision building starts with individuals giving voice to their hopes and dreams.*

A vision is something you love enough to live every day.

—Julie Morath

Intentional questioning helps leaders to integrate the vision into every interaction they have with staff members as well as with patients and their families. Intentional questioning can help leaders draw clinicians into daily reflection about the ways in which their practice reflects the shared vision. It allows us to keep the vision alive in every interaction and to actively model the way for care givers to keep the vision alive in their interactions with patients, families and each other.

Every interaction in every venue shapes our relationships. If in our clinical interactions we ask only about problems and

III. How Do We Live the Vision in Daily Behaviors and Practice

> *Every interaction in every venue shapes our relationships.*

conflicts, we will come to believe that our work relationships exist in order to deal with problems and conflicts. If in our clinical interactions we ask about meaningful experiences of caring and healing, we will come to believe that our work relationships exist to create meaningful experiences of caring and healing for our patients and their families.

Reinforcement of the vision can be integrated seamlessly into:

- *daily questions and affirmations,*
- *daily leadership rounds,*
- *material for staff meetings,*
- *performance evaluations,*
- *reflective practice (planned and/or spontaneous),*
- *incident debriefing (positive and not), and*
- *thank-you notes.*

These opportunities encourage individuals to state what RBC means to them and what it looks like in their personal practice. Leaders then integrate the vision into every conversation. The vision provides the focus for lived behaviors to be affirmed when present as well as the focus for continued development when not fully present.

The value of leaders (positional and informal) perpetuating the vision for change continuously through their own intentional actions and speech cannot be emphasized strongly enough. Revisiting the vision in practical everyday actions carries the vision into the daily care-giving practices and assures that the vision becomes a living reality.

The challenge becomes getting the vision off the wall and into individual daily practice.

Reference: Senge, P., Kleiner, A., Roberts, C., Ross, R. & Smith, B. (1994). *The fifth discipline fieldbook*. New York: Currency.

Nursing in Utopia

—A Marie Manthey classic

Utopia is a nursing unit where the staff members are treated with respect by both the hospital that hires them and the physicians with whom they work. It is a place where the respect people have for themselves and each other means that relationships are healthy and supportive. It is a place where people understand the value of maintaining their own peace of mind.

In this Utopia, nurses are self-confident and have a sense of self-worth. They know they aren't perfect, and accept the reality that they will make mistakes. They understand that no one wants to make mistakes, but that mistakes are inevitable because they are human, and only God is infallible.

Nurses in Utopia have a sense of purpose in life and believe they have both the right and responsibility to shape their own futures.

Nurses in Utopia feel good about themselves and can therefore love their patients. They recognize and respect the interests of other nurses, patients, and physicians and respond to them appropriately. These nurses have an ability to get the job done, even within their own limitations. They are free to use the very best level of skill, knowledge, intuition, and personality strengths they possess in administering care to their patients. They understand the fundamental value and worth of their profession and are ennobled by the dignity of the human interactions they engage in during the normal course of their professional activities.

Nurses began working in this Utopia early in the nineties, when they finally learned that the essence of human growth lies in the self and that in order to grow, one must change and that each of us can only change ourselves—not anyone else.

Editors' Note: *Originally published in* Primarily Nursing, 7(5). *Used with permission.*

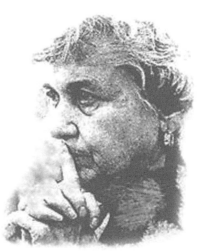

Imagination and Healing

—Jayne A. Felgen

> *Never doubt that a small group of thoughtful,*
> *committed citizens can change the world.*
> *Indeed, it is the only thing that ever has.*®
>
> *—Margaret Mead*

Editors' note: *Adapted from "Imagination and Healing ... Passion in Practice," CHCM News special edition, 1999.*

Even in today's harsh economic climate—one in which health care workers are continually being asked to do more with less—we run into great examples of individuals, units and even whole organizations in which people are harnessing their own creative imaginations to reenvision how they want to function on a daily basis. This creative reenvisioning is at the heart of all meaningful change.

Consider an example of individuals on a medical-surgical unit in a hospital transitioning to Relationship-Based Care (RBC). Weary of the continuous cutbacks in resources and disheartened by the very thought of any more incremental changes, they had little energy left to contemplate how to "turn the elephant around." So instead of focusing on how things weren't going in the right direction, they began to actively imagine what they wanted. They threw out all current assumptions and deliberately explored even the most far-fetched options. In so doing, they erased the imaginary constraints of familiar routines and controls. They began to envision an environment in which healing might more easily occur.

Picture Mary Lou, the patient, entering the double doors to a busy medical-surgical unit and instantly sensing an unexpected serenity. Quiet classical music was playing in the hallways, at workstations and in each patient's room. Calm earth tone paint, art, and textured woven crafts depicting nature adorned the walls. An oasis of lush plants surrounding a gently flow-

ing fountain invited her to the end of the corridor—a corridor uncluttered by carts, wheelchairs, gurneys or buzzing call lights. The impact was immediate and profound. Mary Lou was greeted by a staff member and escorted to her room where she was fully oriented to the unit before meeting "her" nurse, Judi, and other members of the health care team.

Judi explained that the patient, family, physician and nurse would meet together daily to assess progress toward her personal plan of care. Therapies, when possible, would occur in her room or nearby on the unit. Any pain she would experience would be aggressively managed with such artful interventions as positioning, massage and relaxation techniques in addition to timely analgesic medications. Naps and six hours or more of uninterrupted sleep should be expected nightly. A sofa bed in the room was there to encourage her husband or children to feel welcome at any time during her specific visiting hour plan (a plan mutually determined by the patient and the team). Explanations and detailed health teaching would be provided for her and the family to prepare for the transition to self-care at home. A full bed-bath would be provided in the evening after her surgery, including a soothing lavender massage to facilitate maximal rest. Evening baths and massages were proudly offered as "signature" features of care on this unit. Mary Lou learned that rest and sleep would be priorities during her stay so that early ambulation could enhance the speed of her recovery. Judi also assured her that brown sugar would definitely be on her tray as soon as she was able to eat oatmeal. Mary Lou was in heaven!

This comprehensive change of practice was designed, planned and implemented in just 90 days. These managers and staff demonstrated the ultimate in resourcefulness—driven by their passion for patients and their commitment to make a difference! These champions were also artisans. They created a professional practice design that was intended to replicate the best of what they had learned from other colleagues as well as their own knowledge of their unique patient population. But perhaps less practically, though more profoundly, they redesigned their practice to match their dreams as practitioners of what a care setting might be like.

A wise person once said, "A mind once stretched by a new idea, never regains its original dimensions." As you ponder the idea of transforming your work area into one of healing, ask yourself and your colleagues, how might our "ideal" unit be even better? As a patient on your unit, what tangible reflec-

Patients in hospitals today are in very acute to critical condition. This means that they are in a high state of dependency and vulnerability. It also means they feel anxiety and often, a loss of self.

tion of your "signature" practice would I experience? As a colleague on your unit, what would be obvious to me about your passion for patients?

Create a dialogue with your colleagues about your collective vision for a transformed patient environment. Post the "picture" created by this scenario in the staff room and then ask yourselves, what would it take for each unit in this hospital to design its own signature practice?

Margaret Mead quotation courtesy of the Institute for Intercultural Studies, Inc., New York.

Perhaps the greatest gift of Relationship-Based Care is that it increases the possibility that care givers will partner with patients in their own healing.

A Personal Interpretation of Relationship-Based Caring

—Matt Marchbanks

The following personal vision was voiced spontaneously by an environmental services veteran at a recent Environmental Services Council Meeting. We were all moved by the vision, found it very powerful and profound. Subsequently, I read it at our "Wave 2 Get Smart" session and there was great applause from the 150 people present.

I saw the following for patients and our environment before Relationship-Based Care:

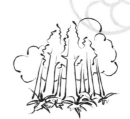

The facility and all of its departments were a large brown woven basket with a flat bottom.

As items were dropped into the basket they caught and bounced off each other and landed on the bottom. The bottom of the basket represented the Environmental Services Department.

We were always scrambling to pick up after everyone else, move items, complete requests that no one else knew who or how to handle. Many things were being partially completed or completed poorly.

My vision for after Relationship-Based Care is fully instituted:

The facility and all of its departments are a large colorful woven basket with a semi-curved bottom.

All departments are interwoven, receiving equal respect from each other for their work performed. Everyone knows what they should do and how they can help each other, and they work together to maintain a pleasant atmosphere and provide complete care for all patients.

Music begins where words end.
—Goethe

See Me as a Person

—Mary Koloroutis

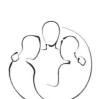

> *Have you ever felt like nobody?*
> *Just a tiny speck of air?*
> *But everyone's around you*
> *and you're just not there.*

You might expect to hear these words from a child who's been tucked away and forgotten in an orphanage in a third-world country. You might expect to hear them from a frightened, injured child hospitalized in a war-torn region of the world. But these words were written by a 9-year-old boy experiencing illness and care in a hospital right here in the United States.

Let's face it; this child has captured what it feels like to be vulnerable and in an institution—any institution—anywhere.

Most acute care is provided within institutions, and it is a reality of institutional care that rituals, routines, tasks and numbers create the context in which care is provided. While this isn't a particularly good-feeling notion to focus on, doing so helps us to fully understand one of our biggest challenges in health care:

We are called to work as healers—as individuals participating in some of the most meaningful, significant personal interactions one can ever hope to be part of—*in institutions.*

Thought

Well over a decade ago, in a *Reigniting the Spirit of Caring* (*RSC*) workshop, a patient participant distilled her desire for compassionate care into the five words *"See me as a person."* I've been doing *RSC* workshops for more than 14 years, and being seen as a person with unique needs, experiences, feelings and responses—not a bed number, a diagnosis or a procedure—is by far the most common need expressed by patient participants throughout all of the workshops.

The call to see the personhood in each patient is a sacred trust extended to us; we are called to care for people during their most significant human transitions. Every episode of care is significant, and often life altering to the patient and the family. Whether it seems routine to us or not, we must never lose track that *it's never routine for the patient.*

Patient participants in our workshops speak with emotion about their care experiences, and this is true whether their care was as recent as the last few months or decades ago. One patient participant tearfully told us about the heartbreak of giving birth to an infant son with a critical heart defect. Her child was immediately transferred away from her to a neonatal intensive care unit in another hospital. Though the birth occurred over thirty years ago, she described the experience as fully and clearly as if it had happened yesterday. She told us of her loss, her fear, and her sense of failure as a mother. She described watching the other postpartum mothers with their babies in their arms while her arms were empty. She shed more tears as she described a particular night nurse who *saw* her, who recognized her heartache and sat with her and comforted her throughout the night. At one point, this compassionate night nurse held her and softly sang her a lullaby. She described feeling invisible to other nurses and to her obstetrician who seemed insensitive to her loss and treated her as though she were any "routine postpartum patient." When we asked her what mattered most to her in receiving care, she replied, "being seen as a person."

Imagine that you are entering a hospital for care. Nothing is familiar and you are keenly aware that you are out of your element. People start telling you what to do—nicely, of course—and you notice the extent to which others are making decisions on your behalf. ("You need to get out of your clothes and put this on; would you like my help?") Now add to this that you are in physical pain—make it a moderate pain, but one you don't know the cause of yet. You are helped to the bed and told what a call button is and how it works, but you have no real sense of how much anyone expects you to use it or what

There is always time for eye contact, for smiling. There is always time to call someone by his or her preferred name.

A patient participant distilled her desire for compassionate care into the five words, "See me as a person."

Holding in your mind that nothing within the care experience is routine for the patient will help prevent you from allowing it to become routine for you.

the response will be like when you do. Some of your family members are with you, but they look as uneasy as you feel. You realize at this point that you haven't taken a deep breath for many minutes and are very glad you're about to lie down.

Patients typically are in fear and pain by the time they get to us, but when they enter an institution, that fear and pain are compounded by the experience of feeling displaced. That feeling of displacement creates a desire in every patient to feel more in control of his or her own experience. Feeling displaced makes us want to know what's happening, to feel that something around us is familiar, and most of all to experience that we are seen by those around us. Patients in hospitals today are in very acute to critical conditions; if they were not, they would not be there. This means that they are in a high state of dependency and vulnerability. It also means they feel anxiety and often, a loss of self.

It matters, of course, that we see patients as people, but everything else about how we see them matters too. Part of our inherent agreement with patients is to see them as "whole," even though they may be feeling "less than whole" due to the experience of stress and crisis. In seeing the person as a whole being with inherent dignity and worth, we see her as she truly is, not as a reflection of her illness or trauma. Our focus on the person's wholeness is a focus on her as she truly is.

There is an unspoken agreement that one human being makes with another every time a patient/care giver relationship is formed. Ultimately our work as healers is to help patients restore themselves, and the first step in that work is always to help them reclaim their self-determination.

Perhaps the greatest gift of Relationship-Based Care is that it increases the possibility that care givers will partner with patients in their own healing through establishing caring relationships. There was a time in the long history of patient care that we thought of ourselves as administers of healing—as if we were a group that took actions to benefit them. Relationship-Based Care takes the hierarchical separation of care giver and patient out of the equation through the therapeutic relationship. There is collaboration between patients and care givers that both acknowledges and bolsters the self-determination of the patient. We know that patients ultimately heal themselves.

Our job is to provide patients with every encouragement, condition and situation so that healing can happen.

In some ways, we must assume that the patient's request—"See me as a person"—is an unfinished sentence. We can reasonably extend it to mean, "See me as a person even when I'm in too much pain to say 'please' and 'thank you,'" "See me as a person even when my son is telling you how to do your job," and in many ways the most challenging of all, "See me as a person even though I don't expect to be seen as a person when I'm in this place, in this condition."

Word

In fast-moving environments our language can become habitual, and in our verbal "short-hand," we may fail to show respect for the dignity of our patients and their families. When we refer to a patient as a bed number or a diagnosis, or label patients as difficult, noncompliant, or "frequent flyers," we deface them. Even if a label itself is not derogatory, it sets us up to distance ourselves from the personhood of the patient and instead see them as objects. Our language can set up subsequent care givers to see patients in a specific way, rather than to make their own connections with each individual. We contaminate each other's relationships with our labels whether they are unkind labels or not. Labels of any kind create a prejudicial situation under which we may "dismiss" our patient, if only momentarily.

As I began this discussion with the voice of a child, the following story from another child teaches us the true lesson underlying this discussion. Mourine Evans, a nurse leader at Children's National Medical Center in Washington, D.C., shares this story when she is talking about the importance of caring for our patients and each other. She asked her preschoolers in Sunday school the following question: "How do you know you are loved?" A 4-year-old boy answered immediately, "By the sound of my name in your throat." Our charge is to convey honor, respect—love—by the sound of the other's name in our throat.

All of the language we use with our patients matters, as does our nonverbal communication. Sitting at eye level with

"How do you know you are loved?"

"By the sound of my name in your throat."

patients conveys our willingness to stop everything else in order to focus on them. It also conveys our knowledge that "standing over" people or talking with them from the doorway or on the run does not communicate respect. Choosing language and behaviors that reflect our desire to partner with patients in their own self-healing says we believe in them and hold them in regard.

Deed

Every patient/care giver interaction is a test of our core dignity and human compassion. Florence Nightingale taught us that nursing is a noble profession, but that it is up to nurses to make it so. We as care givers can keep our own dignity only insofar as we act to preserve the dignity of those in our care.

> If our focus is on "things to do," it will be clear to our patients that our focus is not on them.

Patients tell us that every act of caring and compassion matters to them. They are keenly aware of how they are being touched, and they appreciate gentleness. They are keenly aware of the precariousness of their own dignity—of the possibility that they could so easily be embarrassed, humiliated or exposed at the hands of someone who sees bathing them or changing their bedpan as a "task." If our focus is on "things to do," it will be clear to our patients that our focus is not on them. Holding in your mind that nothing within the care experience is routine for the patient will help prevent you from allowing it to become routine for you.

One of my favorite patient care stories was told by my mother. She had been in the CCU for many days. She'd experienced a massive coronary and was just beginning to notice her surroundings. She felt extremely vulnerable; every part of her body ached. On this day a nurse said to her, "Today when you have your bath I'm going to take some extra steps to make sure you feel clean and cared for." Those words alone conveyed that he saw her as a person, that he saw her discomfort and vulnerability. The nurse soaked a number of bath blankets in warm water and covered her body with the soothing blankets and gave her time to bask in their calming comfort. As my mother told this story as a guest in our workshop, she said that this nurse's compassion and generosity in taking extra measures to comfort and gently tend to her is something she will never forget. He provided the extraordinary in the ordinary, and created a condition in which she could begin to heal.

A healer is no passive observer. A healer sees people whose bodies are disintegrating, whose lives have lost their safety. ... It is the impulse to commonplace courage and everyday heroism that the healer formalizes into a life's work.

—John Poppy *The Nurse as Healer*

We work in environments in which there is rarely enough time to accomplish everything. But there is always time for eye contact—always time for smiling. There is always time to call someone by his or her preferred name. There is time to talk and interact kindly. There is time to touch gently. There is always time to treat patients as people.

When patients tell us their stories at an *RSC* workshop, we reflect on what they have told us using Kristen Swanson's Five Caring Processes (see page 323). Our patient and family participants immediately see the truth in the processes. Keeping these processes front-of-mind acts as an inoculation of sorts against routinized interactions that may result in patients feeling unseen. The Five Caring Processes—maintaining belief, knowing, being with, doing for, and enabling—provide us with a framework for making choices about what we do and why.

Caring for patients as people takes intention and conscious interaction. It requires the seemingly contradictory calling of one to be a healer within the context of an institution. Those of us who have spent any time at the point of care know that while patients may have a hard time overcoming that contradiction, committed care givers do not.

References: Swanson, K. (1993). Nursing as informed caring for the well-being of others. *Journal of Nursing Scholarship*, 25(4), 352-357.

Every patient/care giver interaction is a test of our core dignity and human compassion.

There is always time for eye contact, time for smiling, time to call someone by his or her preferred name, time to talk and interact kindly, time to touch gently. There is always time to treat patients as people.

Exemplar: Relationship-Based Care at Saint Elizabeth's Regional Medical Center

—Kim Moore and Peg Pierson

Vision

Several years ago, following hospital-wide reengineering, a need for healing and getting back to the basics of nursing was identified. A Healing Environment Steering Committee was formed to determine "What is a healing environment?" and "How can we promote a healing environment more consistently for our patients, families and each other?" Three elements of a healing environment were identified: therapeutic interventions, physical environment and therapeutic relationships.

Inspiration

Consistent with a shared leadership approach, the Steering Committee was composed of direct-care providers as well as nursing leadership. Literature reviews were conducted, findings reported and discussed. This mind-opening experience was empowering and it was from these discussions that a shared vision was created, with the conclusion being "Why would we not proceed with creating a healing environment when we know it's the right thing for our patients and for our staff?"

Education

The concepts of Primary Nursing and Healing Environment were endorsed, and education was begun. A series of two 4-hour Primary Nursing classes was held for all RNs and LPNs, focusing on the Primary Nursing model and expanding on the elements of trust, respect, communication and support. Once the introductory classes were completed, the information was shared in new-associate orientation.

Infrastructure and Evidence

Clinical skill is the foundation of therapeutic interventions, and one way we foster staff advancement and growth is through encouragement of national specialty certification. Examination fees were a barrier preventing some highly skilled practitioners from pursuing certification. A policy revision overcame that barrier; Saint Elizabeth's now pays the fee when nurses register for examination. A net gain of 28 nurses achieved national specialty certification in the past two years. Dorothy del Bueno's Performance Based Development System model is employed to assess and develop competency for all nurses. Our Clinical Ladder program also fosters professional development and is a powerful recruitment tool.

We focus on Relationship-Based Care through our Clinical Ladder program, where nurses wishing to advance submit exemplars of performance in the provider, teacher and advocate roles, all with a focus on the relationship within which care is delivered. "Tree of Life" dry erase boards in each patient room evolved from the Healing Environment initiative (see below). The boards allow patients and families to communicate important information to care givers (e.g., significant others, preferred name, what brings them joy and provides support).

Lighting, noise control and color were identified elements of a physical environment. As our hospital expansion was planned, and because of their healing environment work, nursing was involved in selecting an architect who had established a reputation for developing designs promoting spirituality and healing. Our proudest example of nurses leading the way occurred in our Neonatal Intensive Care Unit. Staff identified concepts in the literature that were found as being con-

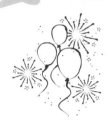

ducive to quality developmental care, better health outcomes, promoting privacy, controlling noise and reducing the risk for infection. Implementation of the family/patient-centered design has resulted in positive feedback from families, physicians and staff alike.

Trust, respect, communication, and support for our patients, families and for each other are crucial to therapeutic relationships. Creating an atmosphere of collaboration and support between all providers is consistent with our attention to therapeutic relationships. The expectation that all members of the health care team be treated with respect was articulated and enforced. We recognized that strong nurse/physician collaboration supports both a healing environment for staff and improved outcomes for patients. The positive impact of our efforts is evidenced in our most recent physician attitude survey. The survey demonstrated improved physician perceptions of overall quality of nursing care, level of professional skill and competence, nurses' use of good judgment about when to call the physician, and how well nurses, doctors and other staff worked together as a team.

Efforts to enhance therapeutic relationships and focus on nurse recruitment and retention resulted in improved retention. Turnover was costly and loss of experienced nurses could impact quality care. Rather than rushing to offer financial incentives, a Continuous Quality Improvement process was undertaken in 2001. Our Building Bridges program and a dedicated new-hire coordinator evolved to integrate new graduates clinically and socially. A positive work environment focus not only attracted new hires, but appealed to veteran nurses. Nurse turnover plummeted from 14.2% to 7.8%, and new grad from 31% to 3.5% in 4 years. Efforts contributing to a positive work environment for nurses impacted turnover rates throughout the organization, reducing turnover for all associates from 21.5% to 11.7%.

While low nurse turnover rates are one measure of nurse satisfaction, we also assess satisfaction of all associates. Organizational climate assessments are conducted regularly, and we recently added the National Database for Nursing Quality (NDNQ) Nurse Satisfaction survey. The Jackson

> The survey demonstrated improved physician perceptions of overall quality of nursing care, level of professional skill and competence, nurses' use of good judgment about when to call the physician, and how well nurses, doctors and other staff worked together as a team.

Organization (TJO) recognized Saint Elizabeth's with an award for outstanding associate satisfaction scores ranking number one in organizational client assessment in large-sized facilities based on 2004 survey data. Overall, Saint Elizabeth's associate satisfaction ranked at the 97th percentile of TJO clients. Saint Elizabeth's associates ranked at the 96th percentile of TJO respondents on the question related to employee retention.

The Jackson Organization also examined Five Top Predictors of Nurse Retention, comparing Saint Elizabeth's mean scores with those of other TJO respondents. Saint Elizabeth's scores ranked at or above the 95th percentile for three of the top five predictors. Saint Elizabeth's NDNQ Work Satisfaction Index scores were in the top quartile of hospitals surveyed.

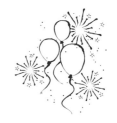

A highly valued measure of the job we're doing comes from patient satisfaction surveys, where Saint Elizabeth's clinical departments repeatedly rank high compared with other facilities surveyed by The Jackson Organization. Fourteen clinical areas within Saint Elizabeth's were honored this past year for scoring at or above the 75th percentile within that national database. Further, Saint Elizabeth's believes so strongly in patient satisfaction that we tie these scores directly into our associate compensation plan.

Sustaining the Culture

"Healing environment" quickly became a common phrase throughout our organization, and many departments wanted to contribute. Senior management, including the CNO, evaluated our system wide culture and considered how a healing environment initiative would fit. A true sustainable cultural transformation occurred when the work that began in nursing became our system wide Embrace the Spirit service excellence initiative.

PART

II

Inspiration

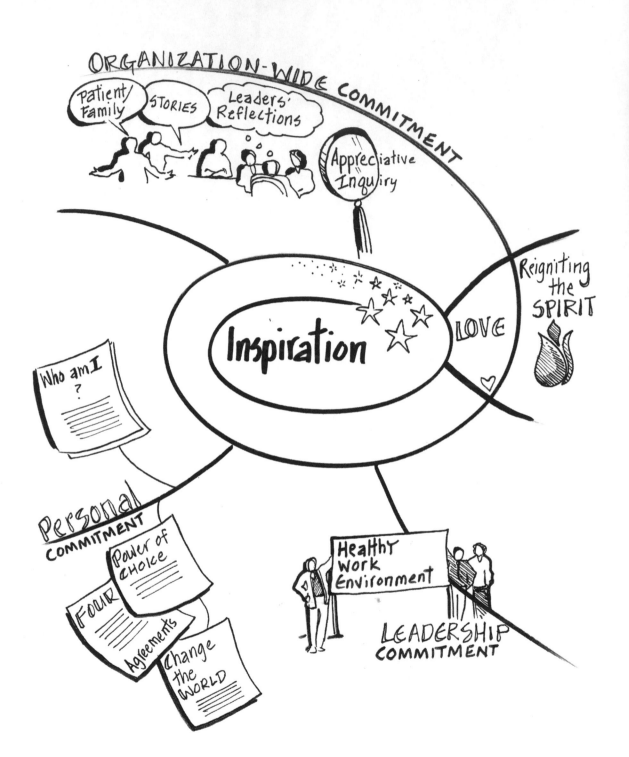

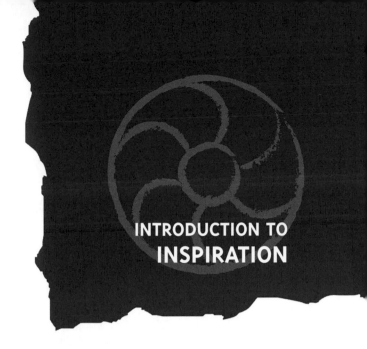

INTRODUCTION TO
INSPIRATION

Some would dismiss the notion of inspiration as too intangible to be of real value to concrete organizational change. It is much easier to see how redesigning an organization's infrastructure, educational programs, and measurement and evaluations processes would all be essential to the transformation of an organization's culture. But we know from experience that inspiration is the key to unleashing our energies for substantive, sustainable change. Inspiration gives us the energy that helps us change habits, mindsets and mental models—the energy that helps us get up every day determined to achieve our goals, to find meaning in our work, and to move purposefully toward our desired future.

In its archaic form, *inspire* means "to breathe life into." Inspirational leaders breathe life into their work, their teams, their organizations and their communities. When inspiration is strong, work that may once have seemed routine takes on new energy that gets breathed one to another. Inspirational leaders engage others in building a vision; they model the change by living the vision each day. After all, we can only teach commitment by being committed, we can only teach effective communication by communicating effectively, and we can only teach Relationship-Based Care (RBC) by modeling healthy relationships every step of the way.

In *Part II: Inspiration*, contributing authors explore inspiration as the means to provide the energy essential for transformational change. Four respected authors, teachers and thought-leaders reflect on the meaning of inspiration as it relates to human behavior and change. Examples of inspirational leadership are then offered along with methodologies for practicing it.

Part II: Inspiration also reminds us that leadership is not always all about leading other people. As positional leaders we may tend to think more about how to bring people along with us than about why we are on the road in the first place. If we want to inspire others to follow us, our best first step is to be inspired ourselves. If each of us could maintain a "laser focus" on what we love about our work, we would create work environments where people are clear about their purpose, feel free to express their passions, and find countless ways to thrive professionally every day. Our own visible love for our work is perhaps the most powerful inspiration we can offer to those around us.

Part II: Inspiration also helps to make the elusive notion of inspiration more tangible. We hope that after reading the contributions in these three chapters, leaders from the bedside to the boardroom will feel more prepared and skilled in recognizing, understanding and using inspiration to bring about positive changes in their organizations.

CHAPTER TWO

Inspiring Organization-Wide Commitment to Relationship-Based Care

Inspiration: Four Leaders' Reflections

—Mary Koloroutis

Inspiration is an extremely personal concept. We are each inspired in unique ways through the work we do, the way we see the world, the relationships we have, and the beliefs that sustain us. I had the privilege of holding a conversation with four respected leaders in which they shared their insights on inspiration. I am honored to share the thoughtful reflections of Marie Manthey, Richard Leider, Sandra Seagal and Christina Baldwin in the pages that follow.

Marie Manthey

Background: Marie Manthey is the founder of Creative Health Care Management (CHCM) and the author of numerous works, including The Practice of Primary Nursing. She is a recognized and celebrated leader of leaders. She has been a source of inspiration for many of us as we navigate the complexities and challenges of providing compassionate and humane patient care in an ever changing health care system. Marie has an amazing way of forging the future and leading with hope and creativity while keeping both feet firmly planted on the ground and staying in tune with what is basic and real and true, no matter what.

Inspiration is such an important and somewhat elusive concept. Early in my career I wouldn't have thought I would be talking about this now. Now it feels very normal and logical to be concerned about inspiration.

Inspiration is about connecting with very fundamental core values in an authentic way.

I think inspiration is about connecting with very fundamental core values in an authentic way. For me inspiration is not about "rallying around the flag" and the "rah rah rah" of anything—in fact I turn away from that kind of drama. For example, I know I feel very deeply about the positive values that the United States of America represents, but I rarely have an American flag flying out in front of my house because it doesn't feel nearly as meaningful to me personally as the values it represents. For me, authenticity is a huge part of inspiration.

I don't know when I really began to think about the inspiration of our work. I think early on in my career I thought about concepts like having a heart, having compassion, commitment to the work—to the value of the work. I am not exactly sure when it changed for me into a richer, deeper meaning of this concept of inspiration. Inspiration is a very personal concept—it's about truth telling—about being true to something that is really important.

On People Who Inspire

Inspiration is a very personal concept—it's about truth telling—about being true to something that is really important.

Mary Jo Kreitzer and Joanne Disch [Directors of the Center for Spirituality and Healing and the Densford International Center for Nursing Leadership at the University of Minnesota respectively] are very authentic—true to their values and not afraid to speak truthfully to those values with clarity and intelligence. When someone helps me understand the deeper meaning of this work, I feel inspired.

I remember reading a short story by Leo Tolstoy, *The Death of Ivan Ilych*. This was before Elisabeth Kübler-Ross and Hospice, when caring for someone who was dying was a very standoffish event. As a nurse or health care worker especially, you just didn't really want to talk to people who were dying. In *The Death of Ivan Ilych*, the person taking care of him wasn't a nurse professional or anything like that, but was just a simple peasant who let him talk about death when nobody else would. There was something about the truth behind that story that never left me. There was such a depth of value being expressed in that story. Even before I thought much about any of this, I knew, "That was true, that was right, that was the way it was supposed to be." So, when I look back in my career to some of the ways people inspired me and others, it was by hitting that inner chord—that's something that is true.

There was also an article by Sister Madeline Clemence Vaillot entitled "Existentialism: A Philosophy and Commitment to Nursing," published in the October 1966 issue of the *American Journal of Nursing.* I've just recently talked about it again at a conference, so I have it at my fingertips. That article was a mind turner for me. There are certain times like that when something has been written or said that gave me permission to reach into deeper meanings.

On What Inspires Manthey in Her Work and Life

There's not much difference between what inspires me in my work and what inspires me in my life. My life and work have been integrated in terms of fundamental values. I go to a church that is probably the only church I would go to in my faith because it expresses values that are consistent with my conscience. I cannot support a church whose values are less true to our highest calling than mine. Therefore, in my life, my involvement in religion is almost a peripheral aspect of inspiration because my personal spirituality is deeply held and what I find in my work is so big. What inspires me in the work are the stories, the real-life experiences. It is always about people for me. I would much rather read the metro section of the paper where the human relations stories are than the financial or sports pages. In our work we have incredible, intimate access to people's lives. The stories of what we do always inspire me.

Ultimately our work is to lead and inspire in a way that still allows people to be true to themselves.

What inspires me in the work are the stories, the real life experiences.

On What It Takes to Achieve Long-Term Change in a World of Rapid Change and Competing Priorities

In answer to this question, I was thinking of words like *having heart, commitment, deep belief*—but then I got to thinking, "but that's not enough." That's not really it. The values of some of today's political leaders are ones I don't consider to be the true values of our world. Even Hitler was a "true believer" of what he espoused, but he did not have true and good values. Whereas Gandhi also had compassion to go with his commitment and deep belief—and I would have followed him anywhere, I believe. It isn't just about the attributes of beliefs and commitment and heart; it's also about the trueness of the values—it's about the goodness of the values. Are they values that respect the sanctity of life or are they values that provide for a certain person or segment of society to have more than others?

Inspiring people to action over the long haul, when done ethically, inspires people to do well. If you are clear, if you have clarity of the truth, the vision, the rightness, the goodness in the direction that's being taken—as a leader that helps you get up every day and lead with energy, with a focus on the purpose and direction.

Back in 1922 a physician wrote about the "educated spirit of the nurse." He helped me see that all the way through the nursing profession, we have recognized both the importance of education and the importance of a spiritual connection between nurse and patient. The term *educated spirit* means to me that despite changes in nursing, there is an ancient truth in work we do. Even with constantly evolving technology and shifts in practice settings, and a financially driven, highly regulated environment, it is still about the spiritual connectivity between two human beings. It is still about one person helping another to achieve a greater level of health and even, sometimes, a peaceful death.

I once had an interesting experience at a Minnesota Visiting Nurse Association board meeting with city council members and county commissioners. The nurses were talking about what they do therapeutically in the home and why it takes a public health nurse to be able to do that. It became clear to me again that it is not just about providing informa-

I am inspired by people who use their gifts beyond their own self-absorption and offering something to the world.

To me that's the essence of nursing: the ability to interact with another human being in a way that increases our health or moves us to a more peaceful death.

tion or handing over the book of materials to the new teenage mother; it's about really assessing where that teenage mother is and presenting the materials in such a way that a change in attitude and behavior takes place that improves the health of the teenage mother and her child. To me that's the essence of nursing: the ability to interact with another human being in a way that increases our health or moves us to a more peaceful death. That's always been the essence of nursing. It seems to me that in order to achieve long-term adherence to universal human values, those of us who have been given the opportunity and privilege to express these values must fulfill our obligation to express them in such a way as to inspire practitioners to bring them into practice. So I'm really talking about keeping true to universal human values in a time of rapid change and competing priorities.

The question for me is "How do we keep growing ourselves and finding that voice to speak the truth in an age when truth telling is not necessarily welcome?" I recently looked at one of my favorite books, *Spirit Matters*, by Michael Lerner; it's about inspiration. He spoke about inspiration as a consciousness of sanctity. I think that's what we bring to health care as a company—*a consciousness of sanctity*. Part of inspiration is openness to the sacredness of what we do—and our being able to speak about that sanctity without reaching the tipping point. The "tipping point" to me is if we begin to talk like evangelists! Inspiration could easily be viewed as evangelical and easily be acted upon in that way if we do not thoughtfully consider what it means as we show up in the world as consultants, health care leaders and nurses. Ultimately our work is to lead and inspire in a way that allows—*encourages*—people to be true to themselves.

> Part of inspiration is openness to the sacredness of what we do.

Background: *Richard Leider is the author of* The Power of Purpose: Creating Meaning in Your Life and Work; Whistle While You Work: Heeding Your Life's Calling; *and* Claiming Your Place at the Fire: Living the Second Half of Your Life on Purpose. *He is also the founder and chairman of The Inventure Group, a consulting group dedicated to "helping people put purpose to work in their personal and professional lives."*

Richard Leider

Much of Richard's work focuses on the inspirational presence of people who live "on purpose"—those who are able to "discern their purpose and live it courageously."

On People Who Inspire

When I think of people who inspire me I think of three areas:

1. **I am inspired by people with the capacity to reinvent themselves**—*the ability to reframe what has happened in their lives into a new story or narrative. An example is Jimmy Carter—the "poster child" for reinventing. He lost his second bid for the Presidency and reinvented himself as more of a statesman than he was as President.*

2. **I am inspired by people who possess a sense of integrity or integration.** *They are the people who "walk the talk." Their insides and outsides match. They are credible and believable to me; I find them magnetic.*

3. **I am inspired by people who have a presence. When you are with them you have a feeling that they are there 100%.** *They are listeners rather than advice givers. From research we know that 55% of communication is body, 38% mood, 7% words. In the people I am describing here, body, mood and words align. It's another way into integrity.*

On What Inspires Leider in His Work and Life

In my work, I am inspired by people who live "on purpose"—those who have purpose-filled lives. My own work, my sense of purpose, is to help people discern their purpose and live it courageously. This means using their gifts and talents on things they feel a passion for in environments they want to be in. It means using their gifts beyond their own self-absorption and offering something to the world. In a nutshell, success is often measured by money and material things. My version of *Lifestyles of the Rich and Famous* would be *Lifestyles of the Rich in Purpose*. People who live "on purpose"—daily, weekly, throughout their lives.

As for what inspires me in my life, I have been taking people on walking trips to Africa for the past 24 years. Every year I put it on my Web site and people sign up to go, and they probably think signing up is all it takes. But I interview people who want to go and I choose those who inspire me—those who are living purpose-filled lives. So I find myself sitting around the fire with people who are inspirational to me. It is deeply fulfilling.

On Leaders Who Inspire

Many in the public eye inspire me. I have already mentioned Jimmy Carter.

Another is Richard Bolles. He is a longtime friend of mine and the author of *What Color is Your Parachute?* He was fired as an Episcopal priest and used that situation as an opportunity to reinvent himself. He went around the country finding out what former Episcopal priests did with their lives and authored the book. From the success of the book, he could have gone on to major fame and fortune—becoming a corporate consultant, etc. But instead he has taken a stand for the job hunter and integrated his spirituality into his work. He reinvented himself. He lives with integrity and is someone I see as the epitome of master teacher and wise elder.

Victor Frankl, the author of *Man's Search for Meaning*, is another inspirational leader. He was a psychiatrist and survivor of the Nazi concentration camps. He took the truths he learned as a survivor and moved his learning into the world. He became a worldwide figure and is another example of reinventing oneself. He taught me the power of choice—that we can take a stand for what we care about, regardless of the circumstances we find ourselves in.

At another personal level, Rollie Larson, who is 84 years old, inspires me. He is a former psychologist as well as my mentor, friend and colleague. He has been through a number of shifts in his life and always reinvented himself with absolute integrity—beyond anyone I've met. He is a listener—he is present. One hundred percent of him is "there"—at a cellular level.

On What It Takes for Leaders to Inspire Others to Action

Leaders are only as good as their practices. Leaders who repeat positive practices day-to-day are great models of "self-

> Leaders are only as good as their practices. Leaders who repeat positive practices day-to-day are great models of "self-leadership," and the ultimate leadership challenge is self-leadership.

leadership," and the ultimate leadership challenge is self-leadership. These leaders embody their messages because their practices keep them conscious and intentional. People are hungry for leaders who embody their messages.

I teach leaders practices that keep them tuned into their own gifts, passions and belief systems—practices that help them lead authentically. Too many leaders don't have deliberate practices. We know what it takes for a good athlete to perform, and the same is true for good leaders; it takes practice.

> "The future belongs to the learners not the 'knowers.'"
>
> —Eric Hoffer

On What It Takes for Leaders to Sustain Focus and Inspire Others Over Time

Alvin Toffler, the author of *Future Shock*, written in 1970, predicted that the survival skills for the future (the twenty-first century) would be these three things:

- *Learn how to learn,*
- *Learn how to relate in a diverse world, and*
- *Learn how to choose.*

That's exactly what it takes for leaders to sustain their focus and inspire others.

Leaders must be learners. In order to reinvent themselves and lead with the times, leaders must be learners. Eric Hoffer, a longshoreman-philosopher, said, "The future belongs to the learners not the 'knowers.'" I believe this. Leaders must be curious—always in a state of inquiry.

Leaders must be relaters. Leaders who can sustain their focus know how to lead from their strengths and bring out the diverse strengths in others. Wise leaders create diverse teams and cultures, including diversity of strengths.

Leaders must be choosers. Select a Sounding Board. The Sounding Board consists of two to five committed listeners—wise elders who can help the leader think things through and sort things out and make wise choices over time. Any leader who goes it alone is not wise.

Sandra Seagal

Background: *Dr. Sandra Seagal is the co-author (with David Horne) of* Human Dynamics: A New Framework for Understanding People and Realizing the Potential in Our Organizations. *Sandra is the founder of Human Dynamics International, a company that conducts research and training in the human way of being and interacting. Sandra's work is based on evidence that when there is a lack of recognition and appreciation of the differences among personality dynamics, the result is misunderstanding, conflict, and lost individual and group potential at home, at work, and in the classroom. What Sandra and her associates teach in Human Dynamics brings new opportunities for improved communications, better teaching and learning experiences, and higher levels of human integration and development.*

To inspire is to use language as a sacred trust, for words are energies that can heal or harm.

It's my belief that the capacity to inspire is "given" to each human being. However, it is not always present because the capacity to inspire transcends the personality. Inspiration is not about "me"—it's about others.

When the personality is filled with fears and longings, excessive appetites and moods, the capacity for inspiration is not present. When the personality is in essentially good shape, when it doesn't need "fixing," when it is sufficiently objective as well as compassionate—then the capacities to inspire come forward. How does inspiration manifest?

To inspire is to use language as a sacred trust, for words are energies that can heal or harm.

To inspire is to have faith in a plan larger than our own personal needs—one that uses us in service to others.

To inspire is to embrace the lessons that are offered to each of us, as it is not so much what happens to us, but how we handle it.

To inspire is to kindle the flame of love wherever we go and with whomever we come into contact.

To inspire is to be present moment by moment.

To inspire is to know, at a deep level, that we are all doing the best we can and that there is always the possibility of new life.

To inspire is to add your candle to the light in the world and never blow it out.

To inspire is to embrace the lessons that are offered to each of us, as it is not so much what happens to us, but how we handle it.

To inspire is to embrace diversity with joy, curiosity, sincerity and sensibility. It is to "honor your neighbors," no matter the form, color, age, religion or gender.

To inspire is to know that you are one part of a much larger and remarkable world. In Human Dynamics these inspirational capacities are given the term "transpersonal," meaning "transcending the personality."

On What Inspires Seagal in Her Work and Life

As the work of Human Dynamics is an inspired work, I feel inspired when I am working, especially in groups. Human Dynamics supports the bridge between what is personal and what is transpersonal. Many times when working with the transpersonal part of our work, I experience that the people may not be able to follow my language. But there is always a *living silence* in the seminar room when this part of the work is offered.

I had a spiritual teacher who once said, "When that which is transcendent is 'living' in a speaker, the transpersonal part of everyone comes to attention!" Their personalities may not have understood the words, but the message has gone into the cells of the body. A transpersonal connection has been offered and received.

I can say that the two most common comments we receive from seminar participants in every culture (now 15 cultures) are:

- *"I am feeling good about me! I am okay as I am!" and*

- *"I loved the transpersonal morning session!"*

In many cases, while the personalities could not follow the words, "the life behind the words" was registered.

Meditation inspires me; music does; books that are somewhat esoteric; biographies of people who have lived their lives in service to others. Actually, almost everyone inspires me because I can feel the potential in them! When I think more about this, there are actually two major sources of inspiration for me: people and nature.

In the natural world, it is particularly plant life that inspires me. And within plant life, it is primarily trees and flowers. I think I would have enjoyed being a landscape architect because I can stare at a petal on a very small flower for a very long time. It seems so remarkable! I guess I love the natural systems:

- *The first system in our world was nature.*

- *The second system was the natural living human systems.*

On the people side, I say again that it's almost everyone who inspires me, but there are those close to me that I have "lived with" for a very long time, and they stand out, i.e., my dear husband David; my three wonderful children; my two young grandchildren; and people like you, Mary, who offer such beautiful qualities and always in support of others.

On Leaders Who Inspire

Gandhi and Martin Luther King stand out first. It's because they offered themselves fully for the betterment of mankind. Each had a very strong presence—a very strong connection to the unseen world—to their own souls. They were living inspirations! When they spoke, their words were real and alive! The words again are *only* the point when the speaker has "lived them"—then they go out as "healing energies."

This makes me think of a verse in Scripture that I remember: "In the beginning was the Word, and the Word was with God, and the Word was God." I have often thought about this line, and while I have no idea if my way of understanding this is correct, my interpretation is "In the beginning was the Word and the Word was with God, and the Word was *Living*." I have linked this to our everyday experiences: When someone is speaking, if the words are living and positive, they become positive healing energies because the speaker has *experienced* the words—has lived the words. This becomes inspired language and positive energy for others. Gandhi and Martin Luther King "lived" their words as catalysts for positive change.

There was also Reginald Denny. During one of the riots (in Los Angeles) he was pulled from his truck for no reason, and he was beaten and clubbed and left on the road to die. Fortunately, he was picked up by an ambulance and the doctors saved his life. He very likely could have died on the road.

There was an interview with him many months later when he was "healed" and he was interviewed on TV, and what was amazing was that he did not feel any anger toward those who almost killed him. He did not even need to forgive them. He did not have to forgive them because he had not blamed them. He had compassion and understanding for them and their lives and their sorrows. I could tell by how he spoke that he was completely authentic. There are people who have never forgiven anyone or anything—and certainly have not forgiven themselves. This man inspired the world and certainly opened the hearts of many! So that story is about the "Ordinary Man," and there are others like him.

When people carry each other's stories, they inspire each other to better performance, and they know how to help each other in moments of stress and crisis.

On What It Takes for Leaders to Inspire Others Over Time

In terms of leadership, the personality has to be conscious, mature, strong as it is sensitive, balanced, flexible and given to a purpose that is qualitative and that serves everyone! Body strength and health are critical because leadership is hard work and requires sustainment across time—sensitivity includes the capacity to sense, feel or intuit the "lay of the land" (often this is not obvious).

Leaders who can inspire others need to be connected to a purpose that transcends themselves—meaning a purpose that supports one's self, while the identified outcome serves the community as well.

A question arises for all of us, leaders and nonleaders alike. The question is: *"What is it to be a human being?"* If we can agree on answers to this question, we can begin to educate people in all fields (as well as children) with tools and practices that support "being human." This is not only for leaders. This is for everyone.

Can it be that we are all angels having a human experience? Is this behind what it means to be human? Is being human, in part, a journey toward transcendent direction and movement into the future?

I just came across a passage from Joe Jaworski's book *Synchronicity: The Inner Path of Leadership.* In it he says:

"My capacity as a leader comes from my choice to allow life to unfold through me." He goes on to say, "Successful leadership depends on fundamental shifts of being, including a deep commitment to the dream and a passion for serving versus being driven by the pursuit of status and power." Jaworski quotes Michado, a Spanish poet, who says, "Wanderer, there is no path. You lay the path in walking."

Ultimately, this is our life. What choices will each of us make that serve the human condition?

Christina Baldwin

Background: *Christina Baldwin is the author of many books, including* Calling the Circle: The First and Future Culture; Life's Companion: Journal Writing as a Spiritual Quest; *and* Storycatcher: Making Sense of Our Lives Through the Power and Practice of Story. *Christina is known for her groundbreaking work in the fields of group process, personal writing and spirituality. She is co-founder (with Ann Linnea) of PeerSpirit Inc. Christina has been teaching the use of the circle practice (described in* Calling the Circle) *to facilitate dialogue and create a sacred space for human interaction and to accomplish important tasks or goals together.*

For me, inspiration is a rising up of creative response and reaction to my own thoughts and to what is going on around me. Say I'm participating in a meeting and we are trying to make some wise and important decisions. I'm not sure what to say or do that would be helpful. I take a breath and all of a sudden I "know" what I want to contribute, and when I offer it, my idea sparks other people's ideas; synergy begins to spin between us. Pretty soon we've made decisions that "feel right" to all of us. We are satisfied with ourselves, perhaps even elated. Inspiration is contagious and generative. Once inspiration stirs in us individually it jumps from thought to thought; or in a group, it jumps from person to person. The meeting changes: We are out of the box, we tell each other we are inspired ... and, if we're wise, we experience gratitude for what has come alive between us.

Inspiration is one of life's mysteries: The impulse to call, to ask for help, is met with response–the impulse to guide. Is this internal? External? Is inspiration a psychological or spiritual experience? Or is it the bridge between psychology and spirituality, between what we generate from our own thought processes and what is given to us by grace? I don't know what inspiration is. I don't take credit for having it; I give thanks.

Inspiration is one of the oldest recorded human experiences. We see the body stance of "man," arms extended, arms raised, kneeling in supplication, gestures we recognize as universal expressions of the call for help painted on cave walls going back 30,000 years. We think we know what this means because we still do it ourselves. The shaman calls for animal or spirit guides to guide her in healing; the psalmist calls out to the Old Testament God, "What is man that thou art mindful of him?" In her journals, written during World War II under horrific conditions, Etty Hillesum writes of her spiritual growth and says, "A desire to kneel down sometimes pulses through my body, or rather it is as if my body has been meant and made for the act of kneeling." We are made for the act of calling—made for the act of receiving—made for inspiration.

People are fascinated by this mystery. We admire it in each other, tell stories designed to kindle it, and are profoundly grateful when it occurs in our daily lives. But there's also an edginess to inspiration; it often asks us to take risks, to step into new territory within ourselves or with each other. Maybe that's why we don't listen to it all the time. Maybe we cherish stories of inspiration so much because they have the power to increase our capacity to receive inspired guidance and to act courageously in response.

On What Inspires Baldwin in Her Work and Life

I believe most people want to finish the day with a sense that they were somehow able to tap into guidance and to make moral and values-based choices in whatever the day required of them. So what inspires me in my work is to create conditions that support inspiration. These conditions need to contain respect for "call and response." They need structure that fosters social safety and that encourages us to speak authentically, and to be listened to, witnessed and given a spatial sense of time to attune to the response rising up within us, or coming from another member of the group.

These conversational conditions occur when we change how we meet, what we say and the way we listen. In profes-

> The gifts of our personal lives don't need to be grand, only offered.

sional settings, this is accomplished by including story and reflection in the pattern of the meeting. When people expand the conversation to include personal stories, or stories that inspire them to collaborate more deeply, the conditions for inspiration are present. We all want to know that it's not easy for any of us to keep faith with the course of our lives, to bring heart to work, to replenish ourselves, to provide support for each other, to mentor, to parent, to wonder what is happening in the larger systems of which we are a part. Stories of our challenges and successes at facing them are profound teaching tales that inspire each other. Once inspirational understanding from these stories is alive in a group, that group can accomplish greater tasks, move through issues more efficiently and holistically, and switch into crisis response with a sense of trust in each other's good intentions.

Recently, my PeerSpirit partner and I were facilitating a staff retreat for the nurse leader team at a trauma hospital. After a day of business planning, we spent the second morning sitting outside in the sunshine in a circle of lawn chairs while each nurse leader responded to the question "How did you decide to become a trauma care nurse?" Over the course of two hours, the group listened respectfully to deeply personal stories that were the foundation of their career. One woman had had a sister die of an aneurism and experienced the tenderness of a good nurse at that moment; another had been a patient and thought about the kind of nursing she had wished for herself; one had lived through trauma and wanted to provide nursing from the wisdom gleaned from experience. There was much laughing and crying and the pleasure of having one's own story and struggle responded to in heartfelt ways. This team will function differently for a long time—they see the source of each other's strengths and vulnerabilities. When they have to slip into high-management mode, they will trust each other, and question, and make better decisions together.

It saddens me how little we do this in our work lives—even in health care settings, where teams need to be grounded in each other's stories so that they can make good decisions together in the moment. When people carry each other's stories, they inspire each other to better performance, and they know how to help each other in moments of stress and crisis.

When people expand the conversation to include personal stories, or stories that inspire them to collaborate more deeply, the conditions for inspiration are present.

I'm really talking about keeping true to universal human values in a time of rapid change and competing priorities.

Facilitated council is one way to elicit inspiration, but it can happen informally in any moment in life when we're willing to engage. One day on my way into the grocery store I saw a rather haggard young mother standing by her cart, and though her children were tugging on her, she didn't move. I made eye contact with her, smiled a little and felt compelled to ask, "Are you all right?" and her story burst out of her.

"The checkout girl gave me more money than she should have," the mother said. "There was a ten-dollar bill stuck to a one and I walked out with it. Now I'm scared. I should give it back but I'm afraid to go in there."

Here was a woman in moral dilemma; she certainly looked like she could use the money, but she knew it wasn't right to take it. She needed someone to talk to, and when she told me her story it put me into the dilemma with her. Now we had a chance to inspire each other—or not. Three little kids were watching.

"Let's go in together," I volunteered.

> To give each other hope, we need to tell each other the stories of a million moments when ordinary people make extraordinary choices.

What we make of the world depends on ordinary people facing moments like this and making decisions that inspire their self-esteem, create a sense of communal accountability, and provide moral models for their children. And to give each other hope, we need to tell each other the stories of a million moments when ordinary people make extraordinary choices. The courage of that woman to return ten dollars is equal to the courage of a corporate executive correcting company fraud, or a government rectifying its social policies. And then we pass along the good news.

It is quite possible that fifty years from now, a father will be saying to his son, "You know, your grandmother raised us on little money in a world where it seemed everyone else was rich. She bought our clothes at the thrift store and paid for our groceries with food stamps. One day, I saw her return a ten-dollar bill because she knew it was the right thing to do, and I learned …" Why do I think this moment will survive in inspirational story? Because I have these stories in my own family and so do you. Story has a will to survive and a power to serve as a universal teacher.

On Courage and Inspiration

There is a kind of fearlessness that takes over when we are inspired to be our best self and do what we know is right. We step out of ourselves and enter a process that is led by guidance—and in this process I believe help surrounds us. It's that relationship thing again—the call and response aspect of inspiration. There is a moment when courage is required—like jumping into cold water—the fear is in the hesitation, the debate; then if we leap there is only commitment. We come up sputtering, but as we start to swim, the water warms around us and we are warmed by our activity. I don't like cold water, and even though I know I'll feel better once I just jump, I hop along the water's edge full of debate within myself. Finally, I'm in—and once again the process works. I think the choices toward integrity and inspiration are often like this: We see the situation, we go through our process of decision making, and then we either walk away or jump in. When I jump in, I am always met; I rise to the occasion with inspiration about how to help.

We live right now in a social environment that focuses on fear, and I think it's the message itself that is creating the most dangerous situation because fear separates us from inspiration. Fear can change the dialogue so all I hear are my anxieties, my judgments and my assumptions. Fear removes me from that state of listening and engagement in which inspiration can use me for good—and I have to find my way back to the courage to jump in and get to work in the situation as it is. That's what I want: for life to use me for its own good. And that's the conversation I want to be in with people: Do you know what you want to donate your life to? How are you doing with that? What kind of support do you need right now? What's the legacy you're hoping to leave behind you? How can we help each other find the courage to sustain ourselves in this journey?

On What Sustains Baldwin

I work intensely with people, holding our stories, our dilemmas, our longings ... so when I need to replenish myself I head right to nature. Nature gives me the ability to see the human story as part of the planetary story. Nature allows me to put human concerns into a larger context—for example, geologic time. Maybe this planet isn't all about us; maybe this is

> We live right now in a social environment that focuses on fear... fear separates us from inspiration.

> Fear removes me from that state of listening and engagement in which inspiration can use me for good—and I have to find my way back to the courage to jump in and get to work in the situation as it is.

the planet of the stones, the planet of water. When I go down to the beach at the edge of my neighborhood and walk with my dogs at the end of a day, I can see the towers of Seattle on the far shoreline—little rectangular blips that appear to be less than an inch tall. And on clear days I can also see Mount Rainier towering over the city—a huge shimmering presence that dwarfs all signs of human endeavor. The mountain is covered in glacier and looks serene on the horizon, but it's a volcano, one of seven in the Cascade Range. I am glad there are forces beyond human control and far more powerful than human concerns.

I am often moved to tears in nature, and I go to her for signs and signals that I'm on the right track. When I'm on a conference call and we're at a pivotal point in a conversation and an eagle flies through my line of sight, I notice. I note what we were saying when the eagle graced the conversation—sometimes I share this event, sometimes I just hold it privately. Once recently I was encouraging a colleague to take hold of the power of her message and a small earthquake rumbled under the building where the group was meeting. Everyone's eyes got really wide and she shouted out into the room, "Okay, I get it! No more bumps!!!" Nature talks back in ways I interpret as encouragement, inspiration, solace and support.

> Nature talks back in ways I interpret as encouragement, inspiration, solace and support.

On Leaders Who Inspire

When I was a girl living at the edge of Minneapolis, I needed to discover how people grew up to lead very different lives than the ones modeled around me. *How do people find a different path?* So starting in about 1960, I began a lifelong habit of reading memoirs. In those days, I read biographies of women—every book I could get my hands on. I read about Queen Victoria, Madame Curie, Katharine Hepburn and Ingrid Bergman. At that time, Eleanor Roosevelt was writing columns in *Ladies' Home Journal* and Margaret Mead was writing in *Good Housekeeping* magazine.

I began to piece together the possibilities for being female and taking leadership and authority over my own life. These iconic women became my first "inspirators." It was a big leap for me, and it's often been a strenuous journey because I grew to expect I'd make my life one that contributed publicly in some way.

More recently, I most often find myself inspired by people whose names are known primarily in their own communities. They are people who come to the circle and share their courageous life journeys. People who speak of their willingness to keep on keeping on, and whose lives model constant innovation. They are people who think and do. They live their beliefs. They are fulfilling their destinies.

We tend to think of destiny only when someone turns out to be famous or takes on a role of huge public significance, but I believe we all have a destiny to fulfill. The heart of our inspiration for each other occurs when we talk about what it's like to recognize and claim personal destiny. We all struggle with this. In the movie *Kundun*, the biography of the early life of the Dalai Lama, there is a moment when the young man turns to his brother and asks plaintively, "Do you ever wonder if they got the wrong boy?" "No," says the brother … but the exchange illustrates how universally strenuous it is to live one's destiny.

Joanna Macy calls the time we are in "the Great Turn." John Brantner calls it "the Hinge of History." Clarissa Pinkola Estes declares, "Everyone living was born for these times." Many people seek to articulate the sense that we are living through a great point of choice in the species. The world changes for good when moment by moment we make choices that call out the best in us and inspire us to contribute whatever we have come to contribute. The gifts of our personal lives don't need to be grand, only offered.

My friend Terry was an Outward Bound instructor and middle school physical education teacher in prime physical condition when, at age 32, she was struck by a car while bicycling on a sunny Saturday afternoon. While she was still in the air, she recalls vividly, she heard a voice telling her, "This is your spiritual awakening." She hit the ground after falling from the hood of the car that had rammed her and suffered a severe bruise of her spinal cord at T12. She is paraplegic and uses a wheelchair most of the time for mobility. We met when she joined a group of 20 participants on a kayaking trip along

> The world changes for good when moment by moment we make choices that call out the best in us and inspire us to contribute whatever we have come to contribute.

the Missouri River in South Dakota. She brought her own specially adapted kayak, maneuvered herself through 3 days of camping, and inspired the group with her presence. A year later, we met again in the circle of the nurse leadership team, where she encouraged her colleagues to share their stories, and shared her own. "It's that 32-year-old inside me," she says, "who guides me in my work here at the hospital—who remembers what it's like to lie in a hospital bed unable to imagine adjusting to what's left of your physical capacity. I roll in and maybe they see possibilities beyond where they are now." What Terry brings into the room with her is a true story: a woman living with physical disability, and a nurse leader with skills to help patients and colleagues. She's not Christopher Reeve; she's not famous; she's herself, and that is inspiration enough.

> *The desire to pass along what we are learning in helpful ways is the core impulse of leadership.*

When we distill our lives, I think the desire to pass along what we are learning in helpful ways is the core impulse of leadership. That's how Margaret Wheatley defines it when she says, "A leader is anyone willing to help at this time." When I need some inspiration I turn to the people around me and ask a question that leads to story.

- *What is your spiritual awakening?*
- *How do we lead with integrity?*
- *Tell me about a time when vulnerability was your most important teacher.*
- *Tell me a story about a time when things looked dark and someone made the right decision to turn the situation around.*

What comes out of listening to such stories can inspire me for months. The number of people who are dedicated to helping at this time is beyond counting.... I think we're going to make it through the Great Turn!

Soul + Science = Healing

—Peter E. Person

In college, years before I became a physician, I worked as an orderly in the hospital near my home. I spent my weekends passing out food trays, changing linens and helping patients into and out of bed. It was also my job to bathe our male patients, including a 50-year-old patient with metastatic bone cancer named John.

I bathed John once a week for nearly a year. During that time, John would always ask about my family and my schoolwork, but conversation would eventually turn to fishing and hunting, two subjects he dearly loved. By the year's end, I could smell the damp maple leaves John tramped through on the way to his deer stand each fall. I knew the precise location of every secret fishing hole on his favorite lakes. And I knew that no matter where life took me, I would never forget the wisdom I gained from my time with John.

In that hospital room, alone with a dying man, I learned how to listen. Without knowing it, John taught me that my ears were the greatest tool I would have at my disposal when I became a physician. In medical school, I would learn the science I needed to treat and cure my patients. From John, I learned how to help them heal.

When I talk to others about our mission as a health care system, I've gotten into the habit of writing "soul + science = healing" on a sheet of paper. It illustrates my belief that true healing requires more than just clinical medicine. It requires that we tend to our patients' emotional and spiritual needs

Editors' note: *While meeting with his leadership team, Dr. Peter E. Person, the CEO of Miller-Dwan Hospital in Duluth, MN, was asked how he became such a good listener. He shared this story in response.*

In medical school, I would learn the science I needed to treat and cure my patients. From John, I learned how to help them heal.

> You don't need an MD behind your name to make a patient feel special. You need an open heart, a ready ear, and a conviction that you're here to make a real difference in someone's life.

as well. And here's the real beauty of this—it allows us all, regardless of our job title, to play a role in the healing care of our patients. You don't need an MD behind your name to make a patient feel special. You need an open heart, a ready ear and a conviction that you're here to make a real difference in someone's life.

I believe most of us choose health care careers because we want to feel connected to a cause greater than ourselves. We want to know that our work makes a difference, that someone's day will be just a little bit easier because we were in it. Our ways of doing this are as unique and individual as each of us, but the important thing to remember is that we share a common mission: We're here to bring the soul and science of healing to the people we serve.

People trust us to protect their physical well-being. They trust us to hear and honor their stories. They trust us with their very lives. We can honor this trust by treating our patients and our work with a real sense of awe, responsibility and respect. Our patients deserve nothing less from us—and we deserve nothing less from ourselves. Keep up the great work.

> We're here to bring the soul and science of healing to the people we serve.

Caring: Core Value, Currency, and Commodity ... Is It Time to Get Tough About "Soft"?

—Jayne A. Felgen

Is it time to get "tough" about something many regard as "soft"?

What if the key to the financial health of our health care organizations, the remedy for staff recruitment and retention challenges and the means to achieve patient and family satisfaction is a simple but essential factor: caring?

What if the straight path to a favorable bottom line is a laser focus on the core of our business: patient care?

What if caring were the currency with which we build a reputation of wealth and prestige, admired by the public and professional community for the value we bring?

What would it take to elevate caring to a position of prominence within the organization's mission, vision, values, culture, leadership and clinical practice?

What if caring were valued as a competency as relevant as clinical-technical and critical thinking skills?

What if caring could unleash the potential to favorably improve the economic position of each of our health care facilities?

There is an abundance of care in health care! And, sadly, it is often invisible. While caring lives in the hearts of care givers, in the midst of the increasing focus on task completion, technical innovations and best business practices, leaders' attention and staff behaviors have not always been focused on caring practices and their moral and economic value (Felgen, 2000).

Editors' note: *Originally published in* Nursing Administration Quarterly, *27(3), September 2003. Used with permission.*

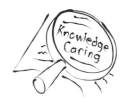

Our leadership imperative is to make clear the organizational mission, to create environments in which staff are inspired and expected to develop and implement caring professional practice principles. One step in that direction is to discover and hold up those practitioners who already model the essence of caring. Leaders must continually direct the organization's focus to what matters most in our organizations, the caring and healing relationships at the point of care.

The intent of this article is to share two caring exemplar stories, begin a dialogue about caring from the perspectives of recipients of care, and offer a practical platform from which renewed leadership efforts to exceed the expectations of patients, families, and colleagues can be launched.

Nursing: The Finest of the Fine Arts

Nightingale described nursing as "one of the Fine Arts; I had almost said the finest of the Fine Arts."

Proud and wise nurses nod knowingly when they encounter Nightingale's description of nursing as "one of the Fine Arts; I had almost said the finest of the Fine Arts" (Nightingale, 1860): These nurses have come to realize the powerful impact nurses in all manner of settings have made on human lives. The impact on patients and families has been particularly positive and meaningful when the practitioner has purposefully employed the principles of caring in their practice.

Art rises above the ordinariness of life experiences and creates remarkable expressions of creativity, boldness, clarity, and subtle or overt beauty that make lasting impressions to be savored again and again. Great works of art are priceless.

Just as priceless are the experiences of patients, families, and co-workers when care giver relationships are infused with passion and purposeful caring.

The Mary Johnson Story

Four years ago this chronologically gifted author was engaged in a family health drama not unlike many of us face, sandwiched between concerns for our children and our parents.

In the middle of a 2-day work visit with a client in North Carolina, I received a call from my husband in Pennsylvania to alert me of my mother's hospitalization in Ohio. Despite having no clinical background, he calmly explained that Mom was now on the telemetry unit with her acute CHF, cardiac arrhythmia and COPD having been stabilized during several hours in the ED. After a brief pause he continued to explain that recent tests affirmed a recurrence of my father's bladder cancer.

From the hotel room at 7:15 p.m. I called the switchboard operator in my hometown hospital. She, in turn, connected me with the Unit Clerk on the telemetry unit. I introduced myself and explained that I was the eldest of MLW's children, that I was a nurse, a former CCU/ICU nurse. And, despite a history of holding it together in crises, I was losing it and feeling unusually anxious about Mom's condition. Could I speak to Mom's nurse?

She replied that their nurses worked 12-hour shifts and that her nurse was in report and could not be interrupted. I asked if she'd consider writing the nurse a note and slipping it under the door, so the RN could make that decision. Chuckling, she exclaimed that that was not an option, but I could call back in fifteen minutes on the 1-800 line.

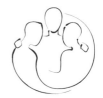

After pacing the floors and sobbing, I regained my composure and, fully "loaded for bear," called again. The *UC greeted me and thanked me for calling back so promptly because Mom's nurse, Mary Johnson, was waiting for my call.*

Mary introduced herself as an RN and Mom's nurse. She continued, *"I understand that you are the eldest of Mrs. W's five children and you're a nurse. Please tell me how recent your critical care experience has been, so I'll know at what level to begin our conversation."*

Amazed, I replied that although it had been several years since I actively delivered care, I had taught arrhythmias and cardiac pathophysiology. I was most out of touch with the gadgets.

Without hesitation she began a thorough review of clinical findings, test results, treatments, and their effectiveness. Then she asked, *"Jayne, what more do I need to know to give your Mom the very best of care?"* I shared that we learned yesterday that Dad's bladder cancer test results were positive again. *"Do you think that may be playing a part in your mother's stress?"* Absolutely!

"Jayne, is there one thing I could do for your Mom that she would most appreciate?"

Undoubtedly, a backrub would most please her. As thin as she is and with arthritis especially painful in her spine and hips, and lying for several hours in the ED on a litter, she'd greatly appreciate a massage.

Then, Mary asked, *"Jayne, what can I do for you?"* I gasped and when I had recovered from my surprise, I answered that she had just done it. She added, "I can only imagine that if I were in your shoes, I'd be wondering if I should go or stay. There are no certainties, but I believe your Mom is out of the woods clinically. Only you know if your Mom needs you or your family to visit right away. *Please give me your number so I can call you if her condition changes. If you can't sleep, call me anytime between now and 7:30 a.m. I will not consider your call an interruption."*

Mary then transferred the call into Mom's room. After a very brief hello to Mom, whose shortness of breath was profound, I spoke to my youngest brother and began to translate what I had learned. I was immediately distracted by background activities at the hospital and asked what was happening now. He replied, *"It is Mom's nurse ... she's giving Mom a backrub."*

Mary Johnson had accurately assessed that I was also in need of care. Her questions had been provocative and purposeful in uncovering what most mattered. And, she immediately transported that learning into her practice.

Dialogue

This story is extraordinarily rich, particularly when we conjure up a busy telemetry unit at the beginning of a shift. We can explore it and discover more than the obvious lessons by using the Four Quarters Reflection exercise from Dynamic Dialogue practice. Designed to elicit multiple perspectives from any experience, Dynamic Dialogue is an innovative and interactive learning methodology that integrates principles and techniques from storytelling, dialogue, action learning, Jungian psychology and drama. One aspect of Dynamic Dialogue poses a series of questions to uncover deeper insight. The responses listed are my initial reactions and are offered to begin a dialogue which may continue within your organization.

1. What cycles, trends, or patterns did you observe in this story? What was occurring between the lines, seemingly invisibly?

    - *Shift report was viewed as a legitimate fact-finding process important to crafting a unique patient plan of care.*

    - *The unit clerk perceived herself as part of the team, listening and following up promptly.*

    - *The RN welcomed the family into the patient care planning process and recognized that as part of the patient's support team, we held information salient to her role as advocate and coordinator.*

    - *A mutually respectful relationship was established in moments.*

    - *Responsibility for managing Mrs. W's care was accepted and communicated.*

2. What about this story and its players deserves appreciation? What lesson is it designed to teach us?

    - *Mary Johnson's clear focus and use of resources in MLW's golden hours, those first hours after admission.*

    - *Provocative and thoughtful questions that conveyed purpose and caring principles.*

    - *Critical thinking was excellent! Mary Johnson chose to attend to first things first; namely, a backrub before other interventions.*

    - *Mary Johnson knew that open sharing of information was in the family's and patient's best interests.*

3. What feelings did you experience and where in your body were these feelings experienced?

    - *Early frustration, anxiety, pain, and fear.*

    - *Relief, gratitude, safety, and comfort.*

    - *Respect, cared for.*

    - *Hope.*

    • *Experienced feelings in chest including palpitations when anxious; in eyes when overwhelmed with emotion including tears; and laughter that accompanied relief.*

4. What great truth emerged? What actions are you compelled to take in response to this experience?

    • *Caring is a legitimate art form. Mary Johnson and others like her are artists, treasures.*

    • *The care team consists of other professionals as well as nurses.*

    • *Caring at this rich level can and does occur despite the system, not because the system routinely supports or expects this level of caring and its effective and practical application.*

    • *Commitment to highlighting the priceless value of a therapeutic, caring and accountable relationship established by RNs with patients and their families as the ultimate expression of their professional role.*

    • *Commitment to facilitate research that seeks to measure the impact of accountable, caring patient-professional relationships, models of care that encourage and expect caring professional practice, care delivery systems and leadership behaviors that support caring principles, and organizational cultures that value caring as their business mission and strategy.*

Caring Theories

This story of the fine art of nursing can also be savored through the eyes of caring theorists. Jean Watson's model of Human Care focuses on the interpersonal relationship between patient, family, and nurse. She calls for both personal and cultural transformation, and describes the tenets and significance of the paradigm shift in her "Era III" transpersonal caring-healing framework (Swanson, 1999). Elements of this framework are evident in Mary Johnson's practice. From that initial single caring moment, a caring-healing consciousness was experienced across the miles in a manner so compelling that the memory continues to inspire.

There is evidence as well of practices consistent with Kristen Swanson's mid-range theory outlining five processes present in any caring relationship (Swanson, 1999). Mary Johnson went the extra mile and created a sense of hope. She centered on the family, sought the family's story and made every attempt to understand this event in our lives. She was emotionally present and listened with attention. She preserved dignity, acted competently, and provided comfort. Finally, she facilitated the passage through this life transition by explaining, informing, generating options, validating and supporting.

The questions posed to the family by Mary are consistent with findings in Madeline Leininger's work regarding cultural care diversity and universality (Leininger, 1994). This work affirms the universal experience of caring as behaviors that convey respect for/about, concern for/about, helping, assisting, facilitating, attending to details, actively listening, being present, feeling a connection, protection, touch, comfort measures, and adjusting the environment (from 2001 ICN notes, as published in CHCM News, 5(5), Sept. 2001).

Several of the concrete behaviors outlined in Sharon Dingman's The Caring Model were also in evidence (Dingman, et al., 1999). Dingman prescribes the use of five intentional interventions as a guide for daily practice. They include: (1) asking patient/family their preferred name, (2) introducing self and explaining their role in care, (3) *sitting* for 5 minutes with patient and family to plan care, (4) using appropriate touch as defined by the patient, and (5) connecting the organization's mission statement with the patient's plan of care.

Nurse Johnson's practice integrated several of these behaviors, the most noteworthy of which included a 15-minute phone conversation with the family of a patient not yet seen and which occurred immediately following coming on duty and completing shift report!

Perhaps the most compelling comparison that can be made is between the behaviors demonstrated by this nurse and those outlined in "Through the Patient's Eyes". (Gerteis, et al., 1993) In this Picker Study patients and families described care as

Mary Johnson went the extra mile and created a sense of hope. She centered on the family, sought the family's story and made every attempt to understand this event in our lives. She was emotionally present and listened with attention.

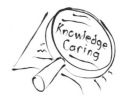

Patients and families described care as healing when care attended to mind, body, and spirit, when they experienced a relationship with their healer, and when they were actively engaged in care decisions.

healing when care attended to mind, body, and spirit, when they experienced a relationship with their healer, and when they were actively engaged in care decisions.

Mary Johnson established a relationship with the patient's family in that first golden hour when insightful assessments matter most for patient-specific care planning. She recognized that the daughter was also in need of care and involved her in these initial plans. The choice to give the backrub to Mrs. W. as the first physical intervention on her shift was arguably as effective for the mind and spirit as it was for the body!

The Mary Johnson story tells the tale of caring from the perspective of a patient's family, a view not always regarded as important in our focus on task completion for patients. The next story uncovers caring in the workplace and details one powerful leadership intervention used to create an environment of healing-caring in another community hospital.

The Bernie Story

Bernie was one of 35 participants in a retreat experience authorized by leaders in a Pacific Northwest community hospital to rekindle the spirits of staff and managers to care for themselves, their colleagues, patients and families.

During introductions Bernie announced to co-workers assembled in the welcoming circle, *"My name's Bernie. I work in the maintenance department. I'm here because my boss told me to be here. Our hospital's creating a healing environment, so I guess my role is to heal the toilets."*

Thus began a 3-day odyssey in which this group's unique sense of humor and passion for patient care emerged in remarkable ways. Over the subsequent hours and days members of the group bonded during creative exercises to renew themselves including reflection, journaling, small group activities, music, dance, play, art, hand massage, imagery and action learning sets.

Similar to the experiences of other groups, stories told by patients and families who were invited guests on the second day were the highlight of this time away. The guests shared their personal experience of health care describing what had

been most caring, and what might have been more caring. The dialogue deepened during small-group interviews.

The participants progressed from initial uncertainty about what to expect from this retreat, through introspection, to learning they shared values with colleagues and to generating possibilities and plans for making an impact back in the workplace. Retreat participants always report individual transformation and a renewed commitment to focus on what matters most for patients, families and their co-workers. Bernie's journey was no exception.

In the closing appreciation circle Bernie announced, "I owe each of you a profound apology for my flip introduction three days ago. One nurse in this room and another back at the hospital made all the difference in the world to me and my family as we struggled this year with my father's failing health and death. You saved us. So, the truth is, *I show up for work every day devoted to making sure you nurses have what you need, in working order, before you even know you need it!*"

Bernie's message had a palpable effect, and there was not one dry eye in the room.

Bernie was the same person on day three as day one, wasn't he? But what had changed? What made it possible for his deeply held values and his sense of purpose to be publicly expressed? What will it take in our organizations to make it safe to talk about what's important in our lives and our important work?

Caring Across the Generations

This same retreat format was experienced in another hospital, this one in the Midwest. Here the retreat was also one of several strategies employed to support an organizational commitment to implement a Relationship-Based Care delivery model. The invitations to this first retreat were strategically targeted to staff from the pilot units involved. One of these units had a particularly high staff turnover rate. The Unit Practice Council on this unit decided to openly address their interpersonal issues related to staff dissatisfaction. They invited novice and expert nurse pairs to attend the retreat together.

The patients, family and physician who comprised the panel on day two voiced their needs and they echoed those previously mentioned: respect for the *human* and *being* rather than doing as functions of caring are most appreciated.

Again, the farewell comments on day three were telling. One novice nurse exuberantly shared that she had learned caring theories in her nursing program. She could describe them, but they had never been successfully translated into actual practice behaviors. Then, as she began work, she again heard the word *caring*, but she witnessed expert nurses focusing primarily on tasks, particularly those related to patient safety. She had still not seen caring theories modeled. Now, during this experience, she was able to learn directly from patients and families what matters most to them. And, equally importantly, she learned that the expert nurses, after several decades in the profession, cared as much as she did. In turn, the expert nurses were thrilled and somewhat surprised to realize that, although there are distinct differences in the generations, there is a deep commitment to caring for patients that they share.

Evidence

We're learning that when you use scientific evidence to drive the design of health care environments and processes, you impact a wide variety of factors, from medical errors and nosocomial infections to stress and staff turnover. Research into the impact of design is yielding results in economic and clinical indicators, market share, and satisfaction numbers—results that carry weight with decision makers in health care institutions.

—Robert Ulrich, "A Better Place to Heal"

Evidence suggests that caring-healing behaviors and cultures are the currency that buys patient, family and co-worker satisfaction. One Midwest hospital which launched an organizational effort to restore pride in its practice and care back into health care experienced a five-fold gain in its patient satisfaction survey scores in the first year.

Dingman's findings support the value of identifying and evaluating unique nursing behaviors that advance patient

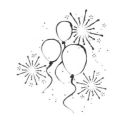

satisfaction. A study involving a for-profit hospital found that during the 3 months after intervention, and for the first time, the hospital was in the top 10% of all hospital ratings in the corporation for inpatient satisfaction. The hospital achieved best practice recognition for Overall Nursing Care, Concerns Shown by Staff and Nurses Explained Procedures. The Caring Model was the central theme for the performance improvement initiatives within the organizations that led to a successful Joint Commission accreditation survey and ultimate commendation (Dingman et al., 1999).

One unit manager reported that his staff vacancy rate dropped from 30% to 0%, with a waiting list of applicants following a care redesign that emphasized caring for colleagues and patients and their families.

Practical Plans

Visionary leaders have learned that the key to their personal success and that of the organizations they serve has been a steadfast focus on the core mission of providing the best of care, specifically by designing systems that support professionals who touch patients and families at the point of care.

The leadership practice of successful and caring executives includes inspiring staff and managers to embrace the pride and privilege of the professional nursing role, creating an infrastructure that supports empowerment of staff at the point of care, developing competencies in caring, managing relationships, and critical thinking comparable in importance to clinical-technical skills, and articulating expectations of accountability for providing exquisite care as defined by patients and families.

Caring leaders skillfully engage the entire organization in this endeavor by acknowledging that everyone has a talent to offer in this care mosaic. Their personal perception of their leadership role demonstrates an understanding that their relevance in the organization is only as influential as their ability to periodically and meaningfully touch the point of care experience. Lessons learned there drive conversations and activities that occur at all levels of the organization, board, and community.

Caring leaders skillfully engage the entire organization in this endeavor by acknowledging that everyone has a talent to offer in this care mosaic.

The caring message must be clear, consistent, and continuous.

Routinely, executive leadership team and unit staff meetings open with stories of caring describing how differences had been made. Unit Practice Council clinical case conferences highlight exemplary staff leadership experiences in the art and science of nursing that led to positive patient outcomes. Staff, students, managers, faculty and allied health professionals eagerly participate in support of their colleagues and the common mission to serve.

Performance measures include equal weight for behavioral competencies as for clinical-technical and critical thinking. Caring behaviors are modeled at all levels of the organization. Caring outcomes are integrated into professional and employee rewards program criteria.

Caring executives actively partner with local schools of nursing in all of these endeavors. As partners, nurse leaders in service and education ground the next generation of nurses and nurse managers in the meaning and implications of caring theories and practice.

Committed leaders understand that renewal of spirit is a personal journey. These leaders invest wisely and support their greatest asset: their staff. They discover the funds to support time away for staff and managers to reflect purposefully on the incredible work that is nursing.

Conclusion

Caring deserves greater value in the health care marketplace. Human resource packages aside, caring has its greatest value when it lives in the organization, in daily interactions, in job descriptions and performance appraisals, and it is a precious commodity, visible or invisible.

Care givers feel most appreciated when the significance of their efforts is acknowledged as meaningful. It takes courage to care! Bonuses and salary increases are always welcomed, but when caring exists in every fiber of the fabric of their work environment, nurses feel cared for, relevant and empowered to do what they do best ... care for others.

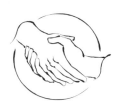

Caring leaders at the bedside or in executive suites give us hope and energy to accomplish what matters most, caring for another human being when they are at their most vulnerable.

Staff will always remember a nurturing colleague or leader who supported their growth personally and professionally. Patients and families will always remember who was there for them when they most needed help managing a health crisis. Nurses will always care.

Caring is the currency. You can bank on that!

References: Dingman, S., Williams, M., Fosbinder, D., & Warnick, M. (1999). Implementing a Caring Model to improve patient satisfaction. *Journal of Nursing Administration*, (29)12, 20-37.

Gerteis, M., Edgman-Levitan, S., & Daley, T. L. (1993). *Through the patient's eyes: Understanding and promoting patient-centered care.* San Francisco: Jossey-Bass.

Felgen, J. (2000). The patient as CEO: Passion in practice. *Journal of Nursing Administration*, 30(10), 453-456.

Felgen, J., & Kinnaird, L. (2001). Dynamic dialogue: Applications to generational diversity. *Seminars for nurse managers*, 9(3), 164-168.

Leininger, M. (1994). *Transcultural nursing: Concepts, theories and practices.* Columbus, OH: McGraw-Hill.

Nightingale, F. (1860). *Notes on nursing: What it is, and what it is not.* Mineola, NY: Dover Publications.

Swanson, K. (1999). Nursing as informed caring for the well-being of others. *Journal of Nursing Scholarship*, 25(4), 352-357.

Ulrich, R. (2002). in Balchik, G. A better place to heal. *Health Forum Journal*, 45(4), 10-15.

Watson, J. (1999). *Postmodern nursing and beyond.* Edinburgh: Church Livingstone.

Appreciative Inquiry Applied:
Using the Reflective Practice Cycle to Inspire

—Colleen Person

Once the decision is made to bring Relationship-Based Care (RBC) to an organization, we begin the process of discovering how best to customize its principles and practices to the individual organization. This requires uncovering the best of what currently exists in the organization, harnessing the generative energy of those already moving in the right direction, beginning a dialogue about the changes coming in the organization, and then designing—with the input of the same individuals within the organization who will bring RBC to life—a workable plan to do so.

As I consult with organizations seeking to implement RBC, I adapt and integrate Appreciative Inquiry methodology, action learning, storytelling and reflective nursing practice into a Reflective Practice Cycle in order to inspire and generate information for use in the later, more specific design of RBC within the organization. The Reflective Practice Cycle, grounded in Appreciative Inquiry (AI) methodology (Cooperrider and Whitney, 2000), focuses on current strengths rather than focusing on problem areas. The Reflective Practice Cycle is carried out in four "rounds," as indicated in the model on the left.

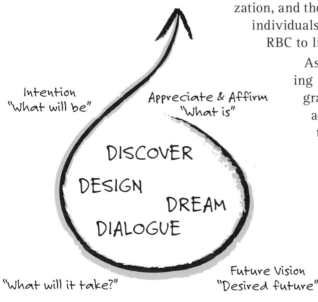

Intention
"What will be"

Appreciate & Affirm
"What is"

DISCOVER

DESIGN

DREAM

DIALOGUE

"What will it take?"

Future Vision
"Desired future"

The Four D's of the
Reflective Practice Cycle

The first three rounds—**Discover**, **Dream** and **Dialogue**—help us to create a clear picture of what is valued most by those in the organization, to generate a clear and inspiring vision for change, and to engage in meaningful, generative dialogue about the future. In these three rounds we answer the questions:

- *What is the best of what's currently happening in the organization?*

- *What is our desired future?*

- *What will it take to achieve our dream?*

The fourth round—**Design**—answers the question "What will be?" It pulls together what is discovered, envisioned and discussed into an organization-specific plan that will help determine how RBC will be adapted and customized within the organization. The findings from this round guide the adaptation of the RBC principles which drive all future organization-wide and unit-based action planning.

The individuals, the stakeholders, the essential constituents who will participate in the Reflective Practice Cycle are determined by the leaders bringing RBC into the organization. We guide those selecting participants to think inclusively—all who will be affected should be represented. We have had organizations send as few as 20 and as many as 200 participants—but always representing a diverse mix of stakeholders from disciplines and departments across the organization. We typically convene small groups of approximately 20 to 25 people in two-hour sessions over two days and engage them in the 4-D Reflective Practice Cycle of Discover, Dream, Dialogue and Design. The Reflective Practice Cycle gets a wide range of individuals engaged in owning the transformation to RBC right from its very inception.

Participants come away feeling inspired, eager for RBC to become a reality in their organization, and enthusiastic about spreading the word about RBC to their peers. The Reflective Practice Cycle helps stakeholders to feel truly ready to move forward with RBC, as it invites them to recount the successes they've already lived in day-to-day practice. They come away with a clear sense that they can bring RBC to their work areas, in part because they recognize that they have already been

Participants come away feeling inspired, eager for RBC to become a reality in their organization, and enthusiastic about spreading the word about RBC to their peers.

doing it in the best practices they describe and that the principles of RBC are in complete alignment with the very reason they are in health care in the first place—to care for patients and their families with compassion and connection.

Round One: Discover

In the first part of this round, we use appreciative questions to discover common values and the best of "what is" within the organization. We have individuals introduce themselves, not only by the traditional name, role and length of service, but also by stating what they appreciate about the organization. Common values emerge, as do the unique aspects of the "personality" of the organization. Even more importantly, a positive and engaging, inspirational tone is set. People are able to say out loud what they appreciate about the culture of their organization. The improvement in the energy of the group is always dramatic.

Invariably the key themes from the patient care stories include therapeutic presence, caring behaviors and an individual relationship with the patient and family.

In the second part of this round we raise topics for further inquiry with questions crafted in advance using Appreciative Inquiry in the following areas:

1. Patient/Family Care—the core of our business,
2. Teamwork—how we accomplish our work, and
3. Professional Competencies—the knowledge/skill basis of our work.

Examples of questions used for each topic are:

Patient Care: *Please share a story of patient care that was especially meaningful to you. How did you contribute to the successful outcome?*

Teamwork: *Describe a time when you were part of or observed an extraordinary display of cooperation or teamwork. What were the behaviors that made it possible?*

Professional Competencies: *Share an example of professional competencies that had a significant impact on a patient outcome in your unit or department.*

With each of these topic areas, small groups of four to six people are given time enough for each person to share a story of excellence, personal value and meaning related to the topic. There is typically a pause for reflection as it may be a new experience for participants to share what they're proud of in their work environment. Very soon, however, the stories begin pouring out along with laughter over humorous or exhilarating experiences and often tears over the memory of meaningful relationships. People reconnect at an emotional level with the sense of privilege they feel in caring for patients.

After individual storytelling, the small groups share a story of particular significance to them with the whole group, and the essence of these stories is captured by the facilitator on a flipchart in mind map form. The entire group then identifies the key themes and behaviors that exemplify meaningful patient care, teamwork and professional competency. These themes and behaviors become the findings and principles which will drive the planning for what Relationship-Based Care will look like in their organization. Participants own these findings as "achievable" because they come from their own experience.

Invariably the key themes from the patient care stories include therapeutic presence, caring behaviors and an individual relationship with the patient and family. Participants report that these stories are inspiring and moving to them.

Teamwork stories emerge from the multiple perspectives of individuals coming together as a team in the interest of patients and families. The behaviors described are always those consistent with a culture of caring for one another within a context of mutual trust and respect. The behaviors frequently represent personal responsibility, ownership, "taking initiative; doing what needs to be done." A classic teamwork story is one of an emergency situation where everyone just showed up and "did the dance of competency," doing all that could be done for the patient. These are stories of extraordinary knowledge and courage.

The stories of professional competency bring the impact of clinical knowledge and skills on patients and families into conscious awareness. The storytelling helps participants to reflect and verbalize what they did and why and to realize the impact of their actions on patient outcomes. This causes a shift in group focus from the task-based nature of work to knowledge-

They take the findings with them in their hearts and heads. Each subsequent discussion they engage in becomes a subtle contribution to the eventual design of RBC.

based work which includes both clinical and caring competencies. Themes that emerge from this line of inquiry include a heightened sense of professionalism, a value for evidence-based practice and a strong desire for continuous learning.

Round Two: Dream

The next step in the Reflective Practice Cycle is to Dream—to envision the future, the next generation of excellent care for the organization. Participants are paired in a structured, facilitated visioning exercise. There are three rotations of partners with decreasing amounts of time allotted for each rotation. Each person in the pair is asked to describe his or her vision for the future of excellent patient care in the organization—to offer his or her own "I Have a Dream" speech. Partners are to listen with attention with the expectation that they will feed back what they've heard to their partners in their own words. In the second rotation, with a new partner and less time, each is asked to share the dream and what it will take to make it a reality, again with feedback. In the third rotation, with a new partner and even less time, each is to share his or her dream and the steps he or she will take to make it a reality.

Participants often find this exercise as challenging as it is exhilarating. They are surprised by the challenge of listening with attention—not saying anything, not offering advice—and hearing what's said thoroughly enough to repeat it. After this exercise participants report that their dreams become clearer and clearer through the process of saying them out loud and hearing them validated and paraphrased by the other person. They become increasingly adept at articulating the essence of their dream in a few words—which then empowers them to continue to speak with confidence about their dreams to others in the organization.

When the content is reviewed, participants are amazed at the commonality of themes. Positive energy and excitement build as participants come to understand that they are not alone in their hopes and dreams, that their individual actions do make a difference, and that there is widespread agreement within their organization that when we work together, "we can do it!"

The ideas from the Dream phase are captured on the flip-charts, and along with the Discover themes they serve as the focus for the next two rounds: Dialogue and Design.

The impact of the first two rounds can best by summarized in a quotation from Meg Wheatley:

> *"There is no power for change greater than a community discovering what it cares about."*
>
> (Wheatley, 2002, p. 46)

The next round in the Reflective Practice Cycle is Dialogue. Dialogue occurs throughout the process of bringing RBC to an organization—during the initial conversations with leaders, during every step of the Reflective Practice Cycle, during the design phases with leaders and staff and in inspirational and educational workshops throughout the implementation process.

The intent of engaging in dialogue—and of doing so before we undertake the actual implementable design of RBC within the organization—is to put immediate and amplified attention on the best past performances of individuals and teams throughout the organization. This allows the best of "what is" in each organization to be integrated into each organization's customized RBC principles.

The purpose of this round of the Reflective Practice Cycle is for participants to answer the question "What will it take to achieve our desired future by doing more of what works?" This round can be structured in different ways, depending upon the composition of the group. The conversations can occur in the same small groups that have been together for the first two rounds, or if several members of work groups are in attendance, they can convene a small group to share themes that emerged in the Dream round that are specific to their area and then engage in a dialogue about what it will take to achieve their dreams in their service areas.

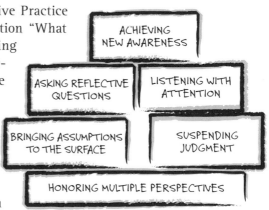

ACHIEVING NEW AWARENESS

ASKING REFLECTIVE QUESTIONS

LISTENING WITH ATTENTION

BRINGING ASSUMPTIONS TO THE SURFACE

SUSPENDING JUDGMENT

HONORING MULTIPLE PERSPECTIVES

Dialogue refers to a purposeful conversation built on:

- *honoring multiple perspectives,*

- *suspending judgment,*

- *bringing assumptions to the surface,*

- *asking reflective questions,*

- *listening with attention to achieve new awareness, and*

- *building common understanding.*

In this round, themes typically emerge around individual contribution, affirmation and appreciation, leaders and staff working together with a shared vision, staff resources, equipment, supplies, education and commitment over time.

The biggest challenge is in coming together around a common statement or two describing a desired future—one that conveys their true ideal for their organization. In keeping with AI methodology these statements are most effective when they are written as:

- *Narrative statements proposing the ideal;*

- *Provocative statements that stretch the organization beyond its norm, stated "as if" the statements were current reality;*

- *Affirmative statements, using vivid positive imagery; and*

- *Statements of belief that constitute the ideals of the organization.*

(Whitney, Trosten-Bloom, & Cooperrider, 2003)

These statements build bridges between the best of "what is" and the best of what will be. They can be simple and effective like the statement of intention embraced by Providence Hospital in Washington, DC:

"Living our mission of joy, care and respect in every relationship every day."

Another client, St. Francis Hospital in Topeka, Kansas, wrote the following statements of intention:

- *Leaders and staff working together with the shared vision, commitment, communication, and persistence over time;*

- *Broader understanding and appreciation of one another and other departments;*

- *Affirmation of success;*

- *Provide resources, education, and information;*

- *Personal acceptance of own impact with continuing affirmation of behavior.*

These statements of intention became powerful drivers at St. Francis Hospital over the course of the development of their care delivery model. They chose to revisit the first statement regularly to keep on course when things got challenging.

All of the statements of intention created in Round Three become part of the findings that are used in the organization's future planning for Relationship-Based Care. The statements also serve to refocus, to ground, to redirect when the progress isn't smooth.

Round Four: Design

After the first three rounds, we have collected (and recorded as mind maps) findings that serve to define the unique characteristics of the organization. In the Design round, participants gather all of their findings for integration into the design planning at all levels in the organization for the implementation of Relationship-Based Care. This way, when the organization's RBC principles are eventually drafted and adopted, it is apparent to all involved that it was their vision, values and voice that shaped what RBC will ultimately look like in their organization.

It appears to be a natural outcome of the Reflective Practice Cycle at the personal, individual level that participants go back to work and begin designing—informally and unofficially—what RBC will look like in their immediate surroundings. They take the findings with them in their hearts and heads, and each subsequent discussion they engage in becomes a subtle contribution to the eventual design of Relationship-Based Care. In this way, the work of Design begins with the simple and powerful statements of intention that individuals make at the close of the organizational assessment—and later at the close of inspirational/educational workshops such as *Leading an Empowered Organization* (*LEO*), *Reigniting the Spirit of Caring* (*RSC*), or *Leadership at the Point of Care* (*LPC*). This Design work continues well into implementation as individuals decide at the beginning of a shift what they intend to do when they enter a patient's room or what they will do given a patient's needs and their own resources of time and talent.

At an organizational level, Design occurs not only in the informal, ongoing, generative manner described above, but also through design of a comprehensive architecture for change. Design intensifies when leaders and staff begin engaging in the process of creating their unit-specific Relationship-Based Care action plans. Design continues when behaviors that demonstrate the best of what we are and can be are exhibited, affirmed and appreciated. It grows when staff members share stories of meaning with one another in continuous reflective practice, both formal and informal.

Or they can be as comprehensive as this template that Regions Hospital in St. Paul, Minnesota is using to develop its Relationship-Based Care model. Used with permission.

> There is no power for change greater than a community discovering what it cares about.

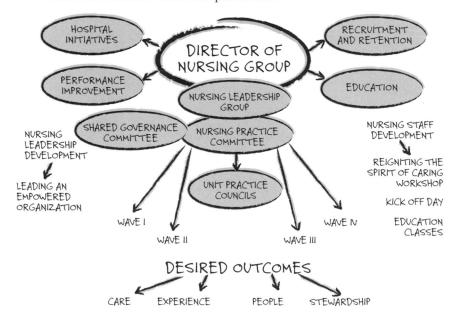

The power of the Design round is that it:

- *Grounds us in the best of "what is" in the organization,*

- *Focuses us on a collective desired future,*

- *Offers a clear sense of what it's going to take to bring RBC to life,*

- *Engages leaders and staff from the beginning in a positive, energizing way, and*

- *Provides inspiration, the first step of I_2E_2.*

When all rounds are completed participants are energized and inspired, and we as facilitators have learned what we need to know to ensure that all future planning will reflect the deeply held values of those in the organization. These specific, concrete actions follow the Reflective Practice Cycle and are embedded in the infrastructure:

- *The findings generated in the Reflective Practice Cycle drive the customization and adaptation of RBC principles for each element of the care delivery model.*

- *These principles are approved by the Results Council (if organization-wide) or Nursing leadership (if nursing only).*

- *Unit/Department Practice Councils develop action plans to achieve the principles.*

- *Action plans are evaluated, refined and implemented (and evaluated and revised as needed throughout implementation.)*

The Reflective Practice Cycle ensures that positive energy, engagement, ideas, learning and innovation guide every step of the process.

Cycles Are Continuous

Although this article is primarily about how the Reflective Practice Cycle enables us to collect findings early in the transition to RBC, the Reflective Practice Cycle can be used effectively at any stage in the transition process. Though we do draft organization-wide and unit-specific action plans and work carefully to carry them out, all effective transitional processes benefit from periodic review and revision. Those stakeholders who do not participate in the organization's first Reflective Practice Cycles often have a chance later to add their voice, and we have seen information generated in these later sessions put to use very directly in rethinking and revising existing plans.

At virtually any stage in an organization's transition to RBC, it can use the Reflective Practice Cycle to collect more findings using Appreciative Inquiry. In fact some organizations have repeated Appreciative Inquiry focus groups during the continuous performance improvement phase as a qualitative measure of progress.

The Reflective Practice Cycle is a powerful process for transformational change—to initiate change, to drive change in an affirmative approach, to "course correct," to stimulate the next cycle of development. Our clients have validated the basic tenet of Appreciative Inquiry: "What you want more of already exists ... do more of what works!"

References: Cooperrider, D., and Whitney, D. (2000). *Collaborating for change: Appreciative inquiry.* San Francisco: Berrett-Koehler.

Whitney, D., Trosten-Bloom, A., & Cooperrider, D. (2003). *The power of appreciative inquiry: A practice guide to positive change.* San Francisco: Berrett-Koehler.

Wheatley, M. (2002). *Turning to one another: Simple conversations to restore hope to the future.* San Francisco: Berrett-Koehler.

Inspiration: How It Works and How to "Work It"

—Donna Wright

How It Works

Inspiration is the first step in the long-term transformation of groups. Understanding how inspiration works is essential for everyone in health care. Inspiration provides the spark that keeps us moving toward our shared vision.

Simply defined, to inspire means to draw forth or bring out. But inspiration, like many other concepts, is more complex than what we often imagine. Once it is broken down into its essential components, however, it can be understood and used effectively to transform groups and organizations.

Phase One: The Basics

There are three main elements in this model. In this first phase of the model, we see the three basic elements necessary for inspiration to occur:

- *an individual to be inspired,*
- *a setting—a group or environment—in which an individual can be inspired, and*
- *something for an individual to be inspired toward.*

Element #1: The Individual

Inspiration always starts with the Self. For each of us, there was some "spark" that led us into the field of health care. For some of us the spark was bold and clear—unmistakably

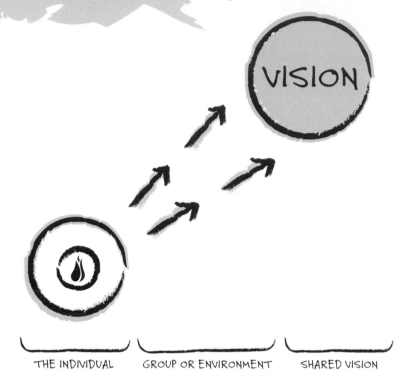

Wright's Model of Inspiration (Figure 1)

THE INDIVIDUAL   GROUP OR ENVIRONMENT   SHARED VISION

directing us to seek out a career in the caring profession. For others it was a quiet flame that we may not completely understand even as we read this, but we feel a pull to do what we do every day. And for still others, the flame has come and gone. Where we once felt inspired by our work, we may now feel burned out and tired. In any case, anyone has the potential to be inspired, and in every case, inspiration works essentially the same way.

Element #2: The Group or Environment

As we work, we move into groups and we work in an established (though ever evolving) environment. As we strive to reach a goal, we may encounter support and encouragement along the way, and we may also encounter negativity and barriers that hinder us from reaching our goal.

Element #3: The Shared Vision for a Desired Future

This is the reason we press forward on a daily basis. The vision for a desired future may be shared by a small group of people or a whole organization. It may be clearly articulated or

Inspiration provides the spark that keeps us moving toward our shared vision.

some vague notion of who or how we want to be. This element provides the reason for forward movement.

In this phase, illustrated by Figure 2 below, further elements emerge. As individuals begin interacting with each other in their environment, those individuals can find themselves backed, buoyed, fortified and further inspired by a combination of external motivations, personal and professional encouragements, and their own realization of their ever increasing competencies. These inspirations sometimes come through the actions of someone directly seeking to inspire individuals, but they can also be the natural benefits of moving through a healthy, supportive environment.

Notice the light inside the circle representing the flame of desire of being called to a profession or work. This represents the light of each person's internal desire to do meaningful work. If this is in alignment with the shared vision—we have a match.

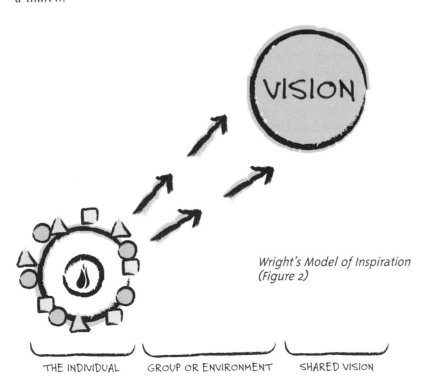

*Wright's Model of Inspiration
(Figure 2)*

THE INDIVIDUAL   GROUP OR ENVIRONMENT   SHARED VISION

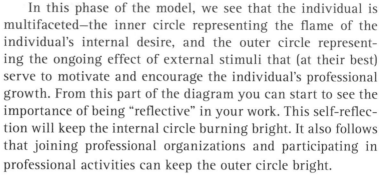

In this phase of the model, we see that the individual is multifaceted—the inner circle representing the flame of the individual's internal desire, and the outer circle representing the ongoing effect of external stimuli that (at their best) serve to motivate and encourage the individual's professional growth. From this part of the diagram you can start to see the importance of being "reflective" in your work. This self-reflection will keep the internal circle burning bright. It also follows that joining professional organizations and participating in professional activities can keep the outer circle bright.

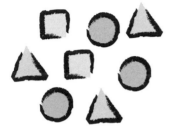

Competencies

An additional aspect of this phase is the role that an individual's own competencies play in his or her movement through the professional environment. These competencies—measurable indicators of the growth and development of individuals in their practice—are necessary to maintain and sustain inspiration because they help individuals to attain the required knowledge and skills to achieve their vision and instill greater confidence that they are prepared for the journey to their goal. Individuals will need a variety of competencies to do this. In any field, these would be competencies that focus on ways to implement the desired vision, deal with any negative energy that gets in the way of the vision on a daily basis, and sustain personal energy to continue moving actively toward the vision.

As each of these competencies is essential to an individual's success, each is therefore essential to helping individuals sustain inspiration on the way to their goals. The acquisition and development of competency is a lifelong learning process.

Inspiration can also be fostered through the ongoing journey of examining and reexamining our personal choice to be part of the health care profession. If inspiration is to be part of this journey, then reflection must be its focus. This means asking "why" and "what" questions about the profession and our involvement in it, instead of asking "how to" questions. We need to seek out reflective opportunities. There is great inspiration to be had through regular participation in reflective activities.

This next figure illustrates what the inspired individual encounters on his or her journey to the desired vision. Some days, the journey to the vision is not a clean, easy sprint. Along the way, we will often encounter conflict, usually in the form of communication issues and negativity. Unfortunately, we will always have these barriers as a part of our daily work. What we find in our work environments can either help us maneuver through these common barriers or it can add to the difficulty of moving to the goal.

Some environments are very healthy. They focus on strategies from Marie Manthey's Commitment to My Co-worker (Manthey, 2000) like maintaining mutual trust and affirming each other's contributions. They are environments in which the actions of those in leadership align with the overall organizational philosophies. They are environments in which communication and conflicts can be addressed openly and honestly—environments where relationships take center stage.

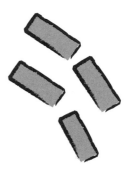

Barriers

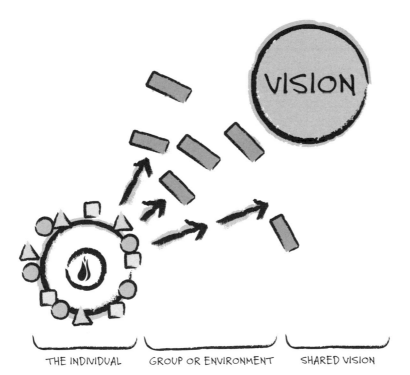

Wright's Model of Inspiration (Figure 3)

THE INDIVIDUAL   GROUP OR ENVIRONMENT   SHARED VISION

But some environments are not so healthy. Sometimes communication is strained and conflict is not addressed. Tension builds and mistrust creeps in. People misinterpret intent, and conspiracy thinking starts to take over. This can create unhealthy teams up and down the organizational chart.

Before we can help sustain the inspiration of individuals in these barrier-laden environments, we must first understand the scope of what they're dealing with as well as how well prepared individuals are to deal successfully with those around them. Determine whether individuals on your team know how to influence others who express negativity and indulge in conflict. Determine whether the environment's negativity and conflict are so overwhelming or out of control that the average person cannot succeed. Determine who, if anyone, has so continually tried to deal with negativity and conflict that he or she has become too tired to try anymore. Be as realistic as possible about what is really going on before determining what supports to offer. Adequately preparing people to break through these common barriers is essential to keeping inspiration alive.

Phase Four: Celebration

When our efforts each day meet our vision, we can provide further inspiration by acknowledging this achievement with celebration. This is a very important element for keeping us inspired every day. Celebrations can be planned or spontaneous, formal or informal, large or small.

Take the time to celebrate all along the journey. Successfully maneuvering through the barriers we encounter is cause for celebration. And while it is obvious that reaching our vision is cause for celebration, reaching for our vision with notable creativity and renewed enthusiasm can be cause for celebration too. Celebrating our daily triumphs can include:

- *Reflecting on our caring for our patients,*

- *Celebrating our commitment to each other and our ongoing improvement of our team efforts, and/or*

- *Taking the time to care for ourselves and celebrate our courage to do so.*

(Readers already well versed in Relationship-Based Care will notice that we have just restated the three pillars of RBC, expressed through the art of celebration.)

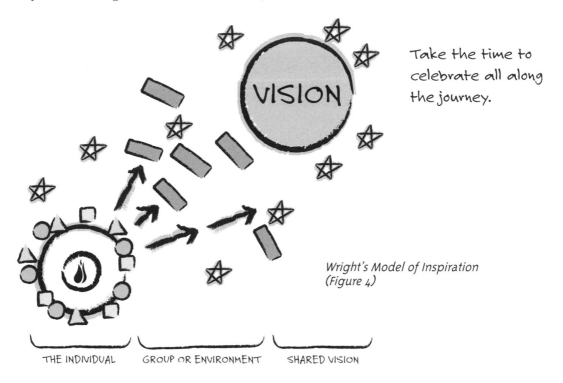

Take the time to celebrate all along the journey.

Wright's Model of Inspiration (Figure 4)

THE INDIVIDUAL   GROUP OR ENVIRONMENT   SHARED VISION

How to "Work It"

The secret for most leaders to be successful in inspiring people is to first understand all of the components of the inspiration model. Without this fundamental understanding of inspiration, organizations are likely to take actions that actually undermine the inspiration of its individuals. Before we discuss the best way to "work" inspiration in an organization, let's look at an example of a scenario in which a group experiencing challenges with inspiration is offered a solution that falls well short of its mark:

- *Your staff looks burned out, and on top of that, customer satisfaction outcomes are low.*

- *You want to increase customer satisfaction, so you plan to do a series of classes on customer service.*

Sounds reasonable enough. However, this approach assumes that the individuals on the team either do not know how to do good customer service or do not have the desire to practice it. This "solution" directly challenges the first part of the Inspiration Model—"the individual"—and most detrimentally, it makes a negative presumption about what "the individual" lacks.

What if, in this situation, the individuals are very inspired themselves and desire to give good customer service, but the reason they are failing is because of some environmental barriers? They try to advocate for the patient, but they get shut down. They try to be creative, but time will not allow them to do so. They try to find different approaches, but others in their environment continually tell them, "We can't do that"—"Policy won't allow that"—"They wouldn't let us."

If this is true, the effect you intend to achieve with the customer service training class may send staff members the message that you believe they do not care, or even that they are inept. It may also communicate to them that even though they have been trying to tell the organization that systems are failing or the environment is not conducive to their (and the organization's) desired outcomes, leaders are not interested in their feedback and have gone ahead with training programs to focus on the individual's knowledge of customer service only. In this situation, we may actually create a larger problem than what we had before.

Leaders need to first diagnose the actual barriers to inspiration. (It may be the people who are in distress, but that doesn't mean it's the people who are the problem.)

Leaders need to first diagnose the *actual* barriers to inspiration. (It may be the people who are in distress, but that doesn't mean it's the *people* who are the problem.) Once this is done, we can creatively look at ways to address whichever part of the model is compromised while reinforcing what we are already doing well.

"Working Inspiration" by Demonstrating Respect for the Individual's Contribution

It is Element #1—the Individual—that should be addressed only when the following conditions are present:

- *An individual has forgotten the reason he or she was called to the profession—lost the internal fire.*

- *An individual experiences lack of engagement in the profession through burnout—lost his or her connection to the profession itself.*

It is only in situations like these that it is in any way helpful to address a solution to the individual directly.

In these situations, individuals can benefit tremendously from opportunities to renew their commitment to their profession. Reflection is the focus. This is an ongoing journey of having "Why" in discussions about the profession and our involvement in it, not asking "how to" questions. These individuals need reflective opportunities, and though not all individuals lose their "fire," it is beneficial to offer reflective activities on a regular basis. (Please note: these are not focused on education for skill building but rather are events focused on self-reflection.)

Individuals can also benefit from joining local or national professional associations or organizations. Participating in these organizations' activities—attending conferences, volunteering for projects or committees—can be very inspiring for individuals.

Once we understand the Model of Inspiration well enough to know that we are not dealing with uninspired individuals, we can approach the problem in the previous example (remember the group who is experiencing burnout and lagging customer service scores?) with questions rather than answers. The first question to ask of the group is not "What are our biggest customer service problems?" but rather:

- *"When do you feel we achieved good customer service?"*

- *"What needs to be in place to achieve this high level of service?"*

- *"How can we create this level of customer service again every day?"*

This is a good example of using Appreciative Inquiry technique. (see page 96).

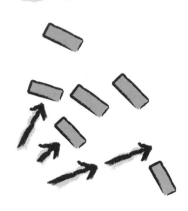

"Working Inspiration" by Tending to Conditions in the Environment

It is Element # 2—the Group or Environment—that needs to be addressed when the following conditions are present:

- *People do not have the skills to deal with the negativity and conflict in the environment.*

- *People do not know how to influence others who express negativity and conflict.*

- *The environment's negativity and conflict is so overwhelming or out of control that the average person cannot succeed.*

- *People have continually tried to deal with the negativity and conflict and have become too tired to try anymore.*

In these situations, it is helpful to address a solution with an entire group. Foster healthy work environments by equipping each individual with the tools to deal with whatever negativity and conflicts arise daily. This means developing skills related to persistence, empowerment, "letting go," governance, shared decision making, dealing with killer phrases and other healthy communication skills. This is not competency development related to the job's technical skills and tasks, but developing skills to recreate our environment and manage it every day.

Use Appreciative Inquiry to examine as a team what has worked in the past and how we can recreate those situations again in the future. This leads to discovery of strategies to deal with interpersonal issues each team faces and it guarantees each group will develop custom strategies to deal with its unique issues.

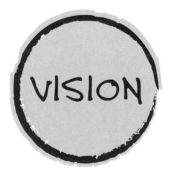

"Working Inspiration" by Refocusing on the Vision or Goal

It is Element # 3—the Vision or Goal—that needs to be refocused on when the following conditions are present:

- *Everyone is inspired and working together well, but they all seem to be moving in separate directions. Management/Leadership responses to employee behaviors and actions are inconsistent or incongruent with previously articulated expectations.*

It is under these conditions that it is most helpful to harness the inspiration already in place and refocus individuals on their shared purpose. Leaders help others "stay the course" by their own role modeling as well as the questions they ask and the behaviors they affirm.

To keep us from getting off course from our vision, leaders need to be very aware of how their own follow-through (or lack thereof) influences the work culture. If leadership does not commit to, articulate and follow through on the organization's vision, no one else will either (see page 453). When we are inconsistent, we create instability in our vision. To assure that leaders stay focused on the vision, many have begun to do quality improvement monitoring in relation to their own leadership responses and to create reports that summarize the organization's overall leadership responses. This is a healthy leadership response to keep us on target.

If leadership does not commit to, articulate, and follow through on the organization's vision, no one else will either.

"Working It" Together

A comprehensive understanding of the Model of Inspiration helps prevent wasted efforts and unintended insults that could result from implementing programs to reinspire an already inspired staff when it's the leaders who have lost their focus.

Solving our issues takes staff and leaders working together. This group effort creates empowerment and ownership for everyone involved. It also gives people a chance to examine every day what they do well—not just what their challenges are.

Once we understand how inspiration works, we can deliberately "work it" to keep us moving together in the same positive direction every day. When armed with knowledge and understanding of this model, we can achieve our goals, no matter how complex they may be. Inspiration gives us the fire to make it happen.

Reference: Manthey, M. (2007). *"Commitment to My Co-workers,"* (Wallet card/poster, Creative Health Care Management.)

Engaging the CEO and Executive Team Through Patient and Family Stories

—Mary Koloroutis

The capacity to watch over and guard the well-being of others is an important gift, and one that is learned with great difficulty.
For it is one thing to see the situation others are in, but it is quite another to care enough about them to want to help, and yet another to know what to do.

—The Sacred Tree

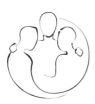

In the late '90s, I was director of Professional Practice at Abbott Northwestern Hospital in Minneapolis, MN. We practiced many of the principles of Relationship-Based Care (RBC) and worked with an executive team who was highly committed to the provision of high-quality, compassionate patient care. After experiencing the power of patient and family stories in a three-day retreat designed for nursing staff, the CNO and I decided to recreate that experience with the executive team so that the members would gain further insight and more direct and personal understanding about what mattered most to patients and families receiving care. The CNO paved the way, and the executive team agreed to use an entire two-hour Executive Council meeting to listen to the personal stories of six patients and family members who had experienced care in our organization.

As the six patients and their family members told stories about their care, we were all moved by the depth and power of their experiences and the trust they extended to us in sharing so openly. They gave specific examples of the things that mattered most to them, such as a gentle touch when one woman was feeling especially vulnerable and afraid, a nurse's advocacy when they were worried about a procedure and the implications, a listening ear in the middle of the night when one man was feeling very alone and already missing his wife, who was dying. They described the little things that mattered most, like knowing who was caring for them, a tissue box within reach, trusting that the care giver would help them stay steady as they weakly transferred from the bed to the chair after extensive surgery. They described experiences of feeling seen, of being touched, of being protected, of being respected and treated with regard and dignity. They also shared moments in which they did not experience care—the rushed nurse who did not look at them when she spoke, spoke in terms they did not understand, and conveyed that she was "too busy" to help right now. The transport attendant who talked loudly to others in the elevator (while forgetting the person on the cart) and seemed to find every bump in the hallway to run over as he took the patient to the procedure room. The receptionist who would not look up as a family member stood by the desk needing assistance. Fortunately, their experiences of "noncaring" were much less frequent than their experiences of compassionate care and, while upsetting, were not earth shattering because the patients and their families reported encountering so many more staff and care givers who were gracious, compassionate and present.

After brief stories were told to the whole team, we divided into six smaller groups so that each patient and family member could interact more personally and directly with each member of the executive team. The patients and families were encouraged to explain their stories in further detail in these small groups, and the executive team members were encouraged to inquire about whatever they wanted to understand more completely. These small groups then reported what they had learned back to the whole group, and we talked about what was learned and the meaning to all involved.

The response to the experience was stunning. The CEO said that it was the best executive meeting of his career and that he hoped there would be future opportunities to engage with patients and families in such an intimate and meaningful way. The executive team members reported learning the following:

> The CEO said that it was the best executive meeting of his career and that he hoped there would be future opportunities to engage with patients and families in such an intimate and meaningful way.

Compassionate, knowledge-based care is what makes the care experience excellent, and it makes a profound difference in the ability of people to recover and heal.

1. The quality of the relationship between the nurse and the patient and family has a significant and often pivotal influence in the way they experience care.

2. Patients and families expect *top-notch clinical quality as a minimal standard*—a baseline! Compassionate, knowledge-based care is what makes the care experience excellent, and it makes a profound difference in the ability of people to recover and heal.

3. When the care experience is compassionate and humane, patients and their families report high levels of satisfaction and loyalty to the organization, the care givers and their physician.

4. Patients' and families' stories were about caring, touching, comforting, supporting and advocating. The stories related times in which care givers helped when someone was feeling uncertain, vulnerable, afraid or in crisis. The stories described times in which people felt "safe and seen" within strange and even life altering circumstances.

5. The care experience is complex from both a clinical and a human perspective. We must expect and support high-level interpersonal competency development for care givers and others who touch the lives of patients and families. Interpersonal skills are as critical for high-quality care as technical/clinical skills.

The experience of bringing the executive team and patients and families together to engage in a meaningful dialogue about the meaning of caring exceeded my expectations. Some crucial lessons are:

1. It is important and extremely valuable for the executive team to interact with patients and families at a personal level. By setting up the experience and structuring the process interaction, the team had the tools and support to make a personal connection and learn from the stories.

Interpersonal skills are as critical for high-quality care as technical/clinical skills.

2. The experience of patients and their families, as told by them, connects us with what matters most, to the human experience which is core to our mission and central to our business as a health care organization. Such stories must not remain unheard, and it is particularly powerful to hear them directly from the people receiving care and

even more powerful to engage in a dialogue about what it means for them, for future patients, for care givers, for our organization and for our community as a whole.

3. Patients and families are moved and impressed when an organization's leaders want to listen to them, want to understand their experiences, and want to support compassionate care for all patients.

4. Patients and families say sharing their stories is therapeutic and healing for them. They experience healing and resolution for themselves and great hope in being asked to share their knowledge so that we (health care professionals) learn and continually strive to create the best possible and most compassionate health care experience for all people who come to us for help.

5. When patients and families have experiences like this one, they tell others in the community, which strengthens the reputation of the organization as one that cares about the quality of the health care experience for the patients and families served.

6. Meetings like this require a small commitment of time and yield big rewards for all involved.

Reference: Four Worlds International Institute. (1984). *The sacred tree*. Twin Lakes, WI: Lotus Light Press.

CHAPTER THREE
Inspiring Leadership Commitment

Adapted from "Creating and enhancing healthy work environments," CHCM News (2002), 6(2), 1, 3.

Creating and Enhancing Healthy Work Environments

—Colleen Person and Bonnie Marsh

As we reflect on conversations we've been involved in about what comprises a healthy work environment, a few themes emerge: People are calling for a new type of leadership, renewed individual accountability and healthy interpersonal relationships.

Leadership

> "A leader is anyone willing to help at this time."
>
> —Margaret Wheatley

The call for a new type of leadership is not necessarily a call for new leaders. Nearly anyone can learn to lead effectively if he or she is willing to trade our current leadership model—one built on competition, expertise and dominance—for one in which leaders look realistically at the world around them and hold a vision for an improved future. The new view of leadership starts with who we are and how we show up in the world and the workplace. In the new model, leaders know, share and live their vision and values. Effective leaders are outcome-oriented and recognize that calling others to partnership is essential to achieving those outcomes. They demonstrate an understanding that meaningful work is the greatest motivator and that meaningful conversations are prerequisite to bringing out the best in everyone. They set the expectations for a positive culture and articulate what behavior is expected and what behavior is unacceptable.

Individual Accountability

Individual accountability from each and every one of us is essential in the workplace, regardless of our specific roles and responsibilities. Each of us has vital contributions to make in creating a life-affirming work environment. Those contributions must consistently be positive and proactive. When we acknowledge that each and every one of us has the capacity to make a significant difference by accepting responsibility for our own attitudes and behaviors, as Meg Wheatley writes, "all hope breaks loose." Each of us has phenomenal capacity for making caring and creative contributions to achieve the desired outcomes of the group. It all starts with asking yourself "What can I do?" Your unique contributions and your renewed commitment to what you can do make you the quintessential building block to the future you desire.

It all starts with asking yourself "What can I do?"

Healthy Interpersonal Relationships

The third call in creating and enhancing healthy work environments is for healthy interpersonal relationships. Colleagueship develops through sharing values, caring for one another and treating each other with mutual respect. In a healthy work environment, less than positive contributions are dealt with in a timely, coaching fashion by colleagues giving respectful feedback in the interest of the whole. What we do and say and how we do and say it is as vital to our work cultures as the very air we breathe—it can drain, sustain or enrich us. Each of us is responsible for creating our own culture whether that be a culture of the 3Cs (committing, caring and collaborating) or a 3B culture (bickering, backbiting and blaming). When everyone's positive contributions are expected, valued and affirmed, teamwork and creative problem solving are enhanced and the culture thrives and grows.

With these three key ingredients—leadership, individual accountability and healthy interpersonal relationships—work groups have the capacity for creating and enhancing an environment that provides positive, productive, meaningful work experiences. We encourage each of you to engage in meaningful conversation with one another to create the work environment you desire.

Colleagueship develops through sharing values, caring for one another, and treating each other with mutual respect.

Leading an Organization-Wide, Interdisciplinary Approach to Relationship-Based Care

—Matt Marchbanks

As an organization starts the journey to develop consistently great patient care, RBC creates the framework to stay organized and focused.

I have been very fortunate to spend my career in many different arenas, which allows my perspective to be much more diverse than just health care. I have been in health care for more than 11 years and have come to the realization that Relationship-Based Care (RBC), when implemented from an interdisciplinary approach (involving all members of the health care team), is the way to maximize the healing potential of every patient. Large health care systems may already be "patient focused" but Relationship-Based Care unleashes the full caring potential of all members of the team and can address and fix long-standing process issues.

I was very fortunate to work at Walt Disney World in the late 1980s. The expectation that *leadership is a choice* is a very powerful message at Disney. Empowerment is a great word but cannot reach its full potential if the culture is not conducive for empowerment to emerge and consistent in supporting it. When teams are led instead of managed, human caring can attain amazing things. This leadership must become the fuel that drives health care, as our business is helping people whose health is in a compromised state.

A "no excuse" leadership style is simply the act of creating an environment where individuals can achieve "unrealistic" expectations for great patient care. Relationship-Based Care, rolled out from an interdisciplinary perspective, creates a seamless organization of caring professionals. Patients do not care about the organizational structure of the facility; patients care about being cared for by competent, compassionate people who literally hold their lives in their hands.

Relationship-Based Care cannot be completely experienced by every patient until all members of the organization are supporting and nurturing the relationship with the patient. In our organization, we use "provocative statements" to create visions at all levels—visions that can become reality. The energy of every employee is needed to attain one common goal and to drive clarity of the RBC mission. A great example of a provocative statement that we have used to help our vision become a reality is:

Inspiration and genuine compassion come from caring human beings, not titles or positions.

> "Relationship-Based Care will become the strategic framework for Faxton-St. Luke's Health Care to achieve the corporate goals and address process issues that prevent personalized patient care for every patient."

As an organization starts the journey to develop consistently great patient care, RBC creates the framework to stay organized and focused. Values, good or bad, define a culture in any organization. Focusing on the value systems allows the organization to change the existing culture. However, values alone cannot redefine or change a patient care delivery system—the principles from RBC have the same correlation as values to a culture. As health care professionals understand and apply the principles of RBC, the full potential of a unit or individual is realized. The RBC principles must be internalized and owned by every member of the team. Only then does the patient experience coordinated care that is beyond description. This coordinated care is based in compassion and empowered employees focusing on making a difference for the patients and their families, in areas that are most important to them.

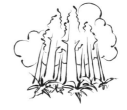

The structure of the Unit Practice Council (UPC) and the Results Council allows the organization to stay organized and focused, while engaging all departments. Because of tighter budgets, support areas in today's health care organizations are forced to manage with a "one size fits all" mentality. Creating a Support Practice Council (SPC) allows the support areas to interact with all of the UPCs in a coordinated fashion. This structure also supports early Waves as they systematically expand their areas of influence and contribute to systems and process improvement throughout the organization. Ultimately, all support areas will create their own specific councils within their work areas, but the SPC should remain intact to offer a coordinated big picture focus to create a best practice support system. This type of thinking creates a synergistic partnership between support departments to maximize all needs for our patients. The SPC will create new levels of thinking so that today's challenges are addressed with tomorrow's thought process. In other words, how do you solve a current issue if the thinking stays consistent with the environment that created the opportunity for improvement in the first place? This type of thinking will also drive us to new organizational efficiencies.

As all areas begin to review, adapt and implement the principles, the organization can move from a flashlight-type (diffused) approach to a laserlike precision for every patient's needs. If all professionals don't nurture the relationship, how can the needs of the patient be fully realized? This question underlies why so many people say you need to get out of the hospital so you can get better. Every health care professional can make a difference in the stay of a patient, not just the nurses and physicians. Inspiration and genuine compassion come from caring human beings, not titles or positions. We must create a culture where the smallest acts of kindness and caring can be reproduced and celebrated daily. One's technical ability does not correlate with his or her ability to be compassionate or empathetic. It is imperative that leaders do not confuse the two distinct skill sets.

Professionals outside of nursing and medicine must play a vital role in nurturing the relationship with the patient. The key for our organization was to use the Creative Health Care Management formula for change, I_2E_2, to create the framework and structure (see page 25). Human beings by nature tend to focus their mental energy outside of their own sphere of influence. This mindset can actually take on a life of its own and then the smallest tasks can appear to be overwhelming. Using I_2E_2 as a framework for change in our organization has created momentum and a focused clarity for what is most important

> Every health care professional can make a difference in the stay of a patient, not just the nurses and physicians. Inspiration and genuine compassion come from caring human beings, not titles or positions.

for the patient and has facilitated all of us working together instead of feeling alone in patient care.

Using Appreciative Inquiry (AI) is imperative as the journey of RBC begins, especially in the early stages of the Results Council and Unit Practice Councils. Creating an environment of Appreciative Inquiry (see 96) helps individuals bury their baggage as it can sometimes be easier to just be negative or fly "below the radar." Great leaders use Appreciative Inquiry even if they do not know the specific AI work or refer to what they do as AI. They simply ask the right questions (focusing on what works rather than what doesn't so that more of what works can happen) because the question determines the answer and the mindset. If used properly and often, it can help the implementation of RBC go much more smoothly, while defusing potential negative encounters. It is much easier to focus on what is wrong. Health care in this respect is no different from every other industry, this is what most professionals have to do daily—figure out what is wrong. This is why AI has to be consciously interwoven into the daily life of every leader in the organization.

Relationship-Based Care creates a "no excuse" environment where the unexpected and unrealistic occur for great patient care. As every department and care giver focuses on every patient, our culture will become a patient-centered model of excellence. The vision is one where all patients are received instead of being "handed off." As every area focuses on receiving patients, it will become evident to our patients that we are ready for them and welcome them. It is much like a relay race where each runner touches the baton together before the passer lets go. This type of teamwork prevents the "baton" or patient from being dropped. In a relay race, once the baton is dropped the race is over. How do patients measure their experience if they are constantly handed off, instead of being received in every area of the organization?

RBC creates a "no excuse" environment where the unexpected and unrealistic occur for great patient care.

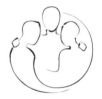

Exemplar: Inspirational Leadership

—Karen S. Hill

*The simple act of touching someone is a powerful way
to begin healing loneliness and isolation.*

—Dean Ornish

Editor's Note: *Previously published as "Re-igniting the Spirit" in* Journal of Nursing Administration, *April 2006, 36(4); 167-169. Reprinted with permission.*

Background: *This article is reprinted with permission from JONA April 2006. Written by Karen S. Hill, MSN, RN, CNAA, BC, FACHE, Vice President/Nurse Executive, Administration, Central Baptist Hospital, Lexington, KY, it appeared in the Inspiration Point Department of JONA which highlights a nursing leader who demonstrates the ability to inspire and lead change through a project. As noted in the article Dr Banister's project, "Nursing and Hospital Morale Initiate" (HMI), was developed in conjunction with Creative Health Care Management.*

The focus of this month's Inspiration Point department is Gaurdia Banister, PhD, RN. Dr Banister is the Vice President of Nursing at Providence Hospital in Washington, DC. She received her bachelor of science in nursing from the University of Wyoming, and her master's and doctorate in psychiatric/mental health nursing from the University of Texas at Austin. Dr Banister has received numerous awards and honors, including being selected as a Robert Wood Johnson Executive Nurse Fellow.

About the Project

Providence Hospital is a 408-bed acute care inpatient facility, which is part of Ascension Health, a faith-based health system in Missouri. In May 2000, Dr Banister assumed her current position while Providence was undergoing a significant change in its patient population. The closure of the primary provider of indigent care in the Washington area had forced a huge influx of patients with complex social, psychological, and medical needs to Providence for both inpatient and outpatient care. Nursing staff reported feeling frustrated with the new challenges presented by these patients, including increased acuity and swelling patient populations. Through focus groups with staff members, Dr Banister heard overt and indirect messages of uncontrolled stress attributed to the facility environment and physical exhaustion. Quantifiable evidence of the problem was obvious by increasing nursing turnover above national norms and nursing vacancy rates of more than 20%. Patient satisfaction also suffered and was particularly evident in the overfull emergency department, where satisfaction plummeted to the 67th percentile of their national database.

For 9 years before her transition to administration in 2000, Dr Banister served as a Director of Nursing for Behavioral Health Service at Providence. After the sudden death of the previous nurse executive, Dr Banister was promoted to her current role as nurse executive. Thus, an opportunity for mentoring from her predecessor was not an option in dealing with role transition and the job challenges. Acceptance in the Robert Wood Johnson (RWJ) Executive Nurse Fellows program in 2001 occurred at an optimal time in her career transition, according to Dr Banister. The networking and resources available through the Fellowship allowed Dr Banister to develop and institute an internal facility initiative that was focused on caring and renewal of spirit among the nursing staff in response to the feedback and data she was receiving.

Inherent in her mental health nursing background was a keen sense of connection with her targeted population, in this case, her staff. At the onset of her new administrative role, Dr Banister formally met with multiple staff nurse groups, reviewed employee survey data, and listened to front-line managers and supervisors, who also reported a sense of helplessness in traditional attempts to assist staff in the development of coping skills and improvement of turnover.

Dr Banister's project, "Nursing and Hospital Morale Initiate" (HMI), was developed in conjunction with Creative Health Care Management, a healthcare consulting company based in Minneapolis. Before her project initiation, initial quantitative data were collected, including measurement of factors such as nursing staff satisfaction with the patient, nurse and physician relationships, and the intent of staff to stay in the organization. Dr Banister also consulted with mentors such as Dr Maryann Fralic, DrPH, RN, FAAN, from FWJ, other leaders within the Ascension system, and consultants from Creative Healthcare in both the analysis of the data and the development of her plan. The HMI program started with a pilot group of staff nurses who attended a 3-day seminar focused on re-igniting the spirit of caring. Included as part of the HMI program was a wellness initiative, including seated massages offered on a rotating schedule to the staff nurses in various departments, stress management techniques, and a fitness and weight management component. One additional aspect to the program after the initial phase was the addition of a "Healing Garden," which provided the staff, nursing and nonnursing, an opportunity for spiritual reflection, meditation, and relaxation in support of the renewal of the spirit and stress management. Funding for the initial program was provided through the RWJ Executive Nurse Fellows program and contributions from a local trust.

The faculty of Creative Health Care Management focused on 3 objectives for the 3-day seminar meetings in support of the HMI project. Those objectives were to:

- *Offer specific techniques to help staff members develop a personal plan to take better care of themselves.*

- *Encourage nurses to work more effectively as a part of a team, both within the nursing work force and in their specific departments.*

- *Focus participants on the primary purpose of their roles, which is to provide better care for patients at Providence Hospital.*

The theoretical framework operationalized by Dr Banister for this initiative is the "science of caring" as defined by Dr Jean Watson.[1] Dr Banister reports that Dr Watson's concept of affiliation supported a key strategy in her plan to address stress management on the part of her staff. Dr Watson writes "The affiliation system allows feedback from others that helps to shape one's thoughts and support feelings, and to identify and reduce anxiety."[1(p184)] Refocusing the Providence nursing staff on approaches to affiliation supported the 3 goals of the educational programs: management of self, relationships with peers, and connection with patients. The concept can be summed in this quote from Dr Watson's work, "A basic assumption of the affiliation need is that people need people- for help and companionship. Affiliation behavior is a universal need and the basis for humanism." [1(p185)] A key goal of Dr Banister's project was to assist her staff to in recognizing their own need for affiliation as a coping skill to deal with the changes in the hospital environment.

A post project analysis, conducted in 2003, showed a decrease in the nursing vacancy rate to 7% and emergency department patient satisfaction scores at an all time high of 98%! Several variables measure pre and post project demonstrated statistically significant improvements, including satisfaction with the registered nurse-patient relationship and a higher "intent to stay" measurement.

The HMI has been so well received throughout the institution that the facility now supports the operational cost of the programs. The offerings have been expanded to nonnursing staff, such as the unit clerical personnel and nursing assistants, who also play important roles on the unit-based teams. Additional programs have been added to support the program, such as department and facility sports teams, book clubs, and upgrading of staff lounges to provide a more aesthetic environment for relaxation and breaks. The staff organized an exhibition softball game in support of the evacuees of Katrina, which demonstrates support of affiliation with the community. One additional component of the program is the "All About Us" effort, which provided hospital funds to allow departments to showcase unit-specific projects supporting the caring philosophy to other facility staff and physicians.

Lessons Learned

Dr Banister reported many leadership lessons learned from her role in the HMI project, including the following:

- *Stay connected to the staff. Dr Banister remarked that the inspiration for the development of the initiative came from staff discussions and creation of "wish lists."*

- *Seek nursing mentors from both within and outside your organization. This was particularly relevant to Dr Banister because a formal role transition was not possible. Dr Banister reported that networking with nursing leaders, both from within and outside the Ascension system, also allowed her to manage her own stress in addressing these difficult challenges and in providing consultative support.*

- *Seek sources of external funding. Dr Banister was able to combine 2 sources of funding to support the initial programmatic expenses. This support allowed for the measurement of outcomes and outside consulting. Formal outcome measurement and presentation by Dr Banister to key audience led to organizational support for future endeavors as a strategic priority.*

- *Be bold in your career moves Dr Banister was encouraged to apply for her current position by others within her institution. This move was definitely a stretch for her career, but one that has been a positive change for both the facility and for her, as a nursing leader.*

- *Consider hiring an executive coach. This was a strategy Dr Banister implemented to provide herself with guidance for her own leadership development. The coach selected by Dr Banister lived in the Washington area. This close physical proximity supported real-time interaction and assessment as needs arose.*

How Do You Regenerate Yourself as a Nurse Leader?

Remember to take care of yourself. Dr Banister reiterated, "You have to take care of yourself first, to be able to care for others." Dr Banister tried to include time for exercise, travel, and family activities in her schedule. She has also taken her learning to the community by being the champion for the District of Columbia Board of Nursing, Committee on Impaired Nurses. Dr Banister used her experiences from the HMI program in developing programs to assist impaired nurses dealing with stress and loss of control. She was also able to use knowledge gained from her mental health background in both her executive practice role at Providence and her leadership initiative at the Board of Nursing.

References

1. Watson J. (1985). Nursing: The philosophy and science of caring. Niwot, CO: University Press of Colorado.

Nurse Managers Manage Staff

—A Marie Manthey classic

A group of Head Nurses was recently asked, "What was the most important skill you had to acquire when your unit moved into Primary Nursing?" The responses were diffuse and wide-ranging.

The first response came from a Head Nurse who used the analogy of her experience as a parent, and was something with which all of her colleagues agreed: "I had to learn to let go of controlling what happens to patients on my unit."

One area of discussion within the group centered on the concept of "providing support to Staff Nurses without taking away independence." Head Nurses were reminded of their need to know staff strengths and weaknesses (in addition to patients' needs) even better than when they were practicing Team Nursing. They agreed upon the importance of evaluating care on a day-to-day basis, which they emphasized, "required learning how to make patient rounds, knowing what to look for, how to learn from the patient (using both verbal and nonverbal communication techniques), ascertaining the effectiveness of the Primary Nurse, and using documentation tools to evaluate staff." Each of these tasks requires the Head Nurse to assess when his or her intervention would ultimately be a help or a hindrance—in part, whether to intervene or to let go.

This theme was explored even more deeply when the discussion moved specifically to the area of "being able to step in—and knowing when not to." Most present indicated that this timing problem was very difficult to handle, and was related to a feeling of their own loss of control over patient interventions and outcomes. They agreed that the compensation for this loss of control was staff growth, which they viewed as the most positive aspect of their transition to Primary Nursing.

Editors' note: *The role of clinical manager has gone through several evolutions since this classic piece was written by Marie in 1981. Yet the nugget of truth remains, that the role of the manager is to create the environment and develop and support the staff in delivering and managing patient care. Simple, but oh, so complex as well. Originally published in* Primarily Nursing, *1(5). Used with permission.*

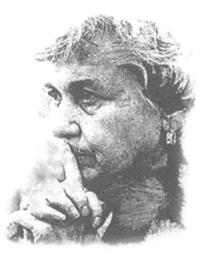

From these comments it is clear that the Head Nurses I spoke with that day knew their job—to develop their staff members and to avoid controlling patient care. It breaks down this way: The Head Nurse manages the staff and the staff manages patient care.

In order for Head Nurses to successfully make a transition to the successful day-to-day practice of Primary Nursing, the superstructure must support the role change. Too often, however, administrators expect units to change without recognizing that change has to start at the top, not at the bottom of an organizational structure. Head Nurses play the most pivotal role of all in this change process, and for this pivotal role, they need support and understanding from their managers, as well as from their staff.

What to Do About "Those People" Who Won't Come Along

—*Mary Koloroutis*

In any cultural transformation there will be those who do not want to change. It used to be that we thought of "those people"—no matter how large or small a group they represented—as serious impediments to our ability to change. Because we assigned this group's resistance so much importance, we also gave them a lot of power and attention. In many ways, we linked our own ability to transform as an organization to their willingness to change as individuals.

But we've learned a few things since then.

In any transformation to Relationship-Based Care (RBC) that engages individuals in creating their own personal vision for integrating RBC into their own practice, most people will ultimately come along. It becomes obvious to them that they are being asked to redesign their own practice—to better align it with their own deeply held (and sometimes forgotten) beliefs about compassionate caring. We have found that putting the bulk of our attention on those who do want to come along is far more productive than putting it on those who don't.

Author Peter Block speaks with blazing insight to the issue of "those people" who will not come along in his book *The Answer to How is Yes*:

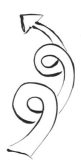

The question, "How do you get those people to change?" distracts us from choosing who we want to become and exercising accountability for creating our environment. We cannot change others, we can just learn about ourselves.

Even when we are responsible for employees or children, we surrender our freedom and our capacity to construct the world we inhabit when we focus on their change.

People resist coercion much more strenuously than they resist change. Each of us has a free will at our core, so like it or not, others will choose to change more readily from the example set by our own transformation than by any demand we make of them. To move away from the spirit of coercion, we replace the question "How do you get them to change" with—

"What is the transformation in me that is required?"

"What courage is required of me right now?"

We cannot change others, we can just learn about ourselves.

When we shift the focus to our own actions, we also have to be careful not to ask it as a HOW question. This is not a question about methodology, it is a question of will and intention. When we honestly ask ourselves about our role in the creation of a situation that frustrates us, and set aside asking about their role, then the world changes around us.

(Block, 2003, pp. 19-21)

The answer to "How do we get others to come on board?" is this: Keep your focus on where you want to go and why. Change your behavior and invite others to come along. Take your focus off "those people." This is a reversal of conventional wisdom and it is a reversal that is long overdue. We can find countless ways to identify, embrace and amplify all the good we see in an organization. We bring out the best in an organization by naming it and asking those who have had success in creating it in the first place to create more of it.

Organizational transformation happens at the level of the individual. But it's important to realize that, as Block says, we can only change ourselves—we can only really lead by example and then support, encourage, and educate others who are inclined to change similarly. This means that when we address the resistant actions of those who will not come along, we do so not because they are wrong, but because in the new context we've created, we as individual leaders are not able to ignore or condone behaviors that are inconsistent with humane, individualized compassionate care.

Again, conventional wisdom is turned on its head. We have been told for decades not to personalize our professional actions. And while we aren't proposing that anyone perceive another's behavior as a personal attack, we are suggesting that individuals act with the most personal of convictions to sustain and nurture the new vision and culture. It is acceptable for a leader visibly living the vision every day to say, "It is expected that the practice on this unit will reflect our organization's vision for Relationship-Based Care. *This means that we treat each individual with respect and we interact with patients and their families with care and compassion....*" Leading a deep cultural transformation takes courage, and courage is always personal.

If the vast majority of individuals in an organization embrace the vision and start moving visibly in the direction of it, the environment will change—even if a minority of individuals would rather things stay the same. When that happens, people will choose to move in the new direction or choose to leave and find a better fit elsewhere.

Reference: Block, P. (2003). *The answer to how is yes: Acting on what matters.* San Francisco: Berrett-Koehler.

Keep your focus on where you want to go and why, and take your focus off "those people." This is a reversal of conventional wisdom and it is a reversal that is long overdue.

CHAPTER FOUR

Inspiring Personal Commitment

Who Am I in This Work:
Using Self-Reflection for Personal Change and Growth

—Gary L. Saltus

Things always change around us.

If you are reading this book, you are probably anticipating (or already experiencing) a fundamental transition of your work culture. This fundamental transition will mean interpersonal changes; changes in each department and unit; changes in policies, processes and procedures; changes in how teams function; and most importantly, changes in care givers' relationships with patients and their families.

Change this big is always challenging. Even when the goal is both desirable and achievable, the road can be difficult. It seems that no matter how diplomatically a major change is presented to us, the first thing we hear is "Stop doing things the old way (a.k.a. the wrong way) and get ready to learn something completely new." In reality, Relationship-Based Care (RBC) is always built on the best practice that is already happening in an organization. That said, however, the changes that come with RBC implementation are as deep as they are broad and as fundamental as they are practical.

Change happens whether we are ready for it or not. It's up to us whether we embrace the change and experience transition with ease or we push against the change and experience struggle.

Knowing who we are in our work is the first, most essential step in creating a smooth transition for ourselves. If things change around us and we don't know who we are in the midst of that transition, we may feel displaced, victimized and alienated.

When we are challenged to let go of the old way of life, self-reflection allows us to gain a sense of who we are at our core so that we can gain a sense of who we are amidst the changes. A new situation in which we feel well-placed, adequate and secure comes only to those individuals who sit in self-reflection long enough to figure out who they are and what they want.

Relationship-Based Care is always built on the best practice that is already happening in an organization.

What Is Self-Reflection?

Self-reflection is an activity that falls under the category of "self-care." While self-care includes care of the mind, body and spirit, self-reflection pertains most specifically to the mind. (We all know, however, that once we "get our heads straight," we are more likely to thrive physically and spiritually as well.) In short, self-reflection is all about knowing who we are in any given situation:

Who am I? What is my work here? What can I contribute?

What do I need to 'let go of' in order to contribute to this work?

What will it take for me to stand where I am and feel as good as I can? Or would it be better for me to no longer "stand where I am" at all?

The answers to these questions are important not only to our mental, physical and spiritual well-being, but by extension to the well-being of those around us, whether we are in direct service to them or not.

Knowing who we are in our work is the first, most essential step in creating a smooth transition for ourselves.

Most of us play many roles—partner, parent, family member, co-worker, friend, community member, etc. In each of these roles we have a contribution to make and we have opportunities to receive benefit from the contributions of others. If we're tired and stressed we limit our abilities to contribute (though we still go through the motions as best we can) and we limit our abilities to receive (though we may find that we are increasingly demanding of others). If we're walking through our lives drained to half capacity and we don't take time to "recharge our battery" to 80 or 90%, then all we can give is 50%.

But try telling somebody who's running around at 50%, trying to accomplish 100% of what's required to schedule time for self-reflection. It's a hard sell in that moment.

In our work and in our lives there are countless fires to put out, and too many of us feel like we never get to do what we really want to do. We work our bodies until they drop; we let our minds spin unchecked in nondeliberate thought. But the truth is that tired, stressed-out people can usually still function. When we're overtired, we just break everything down to manageable tasks and work until we either finish them or run out of time. Our mental and emotional fatigue throws us into that task-based functioning and leaves us without a sense of "self" in our work. In that condition, it never occurs to us to ask (let alone to answer) the question "Who am I in this work?"

Unfortunately it's usually the care giver who is too tired to think beyond the tasks at hand—the care giver who would benefit from self-reflective practice the most—who is most resistant to it. Fortunately, however, it is also the care giver who is most resistant to self-reflective practice initially who usually gets the most out of it.

Self-reflection tends to lead us back to our emotional fundamentals:

> When we're overtired, we just break everything down to manageable tasks and work until we either finish them or run out of time. Our mental and emotional fatigue throws us into that task-based functioning and leaves us without a sense of "self" in our work.

- *Why did I choose this work?*
- *What do I want to get out of this work experience?*
- *What is my contribution in this work?*
- *How (if at all) am I being "fed" in this work?*
- *Is my unique contribution to the world best used in this work?*
- *Who am I in this work?*

140

It is with these questions and others like them that we begin and then deepen the process of self-reflection.

What Does Self-Reflection Look Like?

Self-reflection can be a guided activity or it can be done alone. In either case, the elements of self-reflection are typically 1) a catalyst, some new information that inspires or provokes thought, and 2) some time for quiet reflection or meaningful conversation through which we see who we are in the context of the new information.

A practice of regular reflection can start with going for a walk with music or a headset with an audio book. I would suggest books like *The Power of Purpose* by Richard Leider or *Learning as a Way of Being* by Peter Vaill or Parker Palmer's *Let Your Life Speak*. Each of these books provokes thought and challenges individuals to see themselves in new ways. Even if you don't have easy access to a discussion group, you can think about how the new ideas you're hearing about apply to you.

The overriding message that comes through self-reflection is "all is well." Even recalling past events that were not so happy can help us to remember that things really do turn out okay in the end (even when things are not so obviously "okay" when they're happening). The more we do self-reflection, the more we have this method of self-soothing at our disposal. Mental and emotional fortification comes from this self-reflection. It is, essentially, the adult journey of life.

Doing self-reflection in a group can be especially satisfying. Emotions get stirred up in a group and important discussions result. Even if it is others in the group who do the talking, everyone who stays mentally engaged benefits. In facilitated self-reflection, once an individual is done speaking, the facilitator goes to the group and asks what got "stirred up". Sometimes we need something from outside ourselves to stimulate our own thoughts. We need something to compare ourselves to, and it often helps to hear somebody else's perspective. Doing self-reflection in groups helps us to heighten our own awareness of what we don't already know, and, by taking that in and working on it with a group (or even in our own minds), we see the world and our place in it differently.

Doing self-reflection in a group can be especially satisfying. Emotions get stirred up in a group and important discussions result. Even if it is others in the group who do the talking, everyone who stays mentally engaged benefits.

Resistance to Change

Some of us enjoy self-reflection very much and are thrilled at the prospect of doing more of it or doing it in a more meaningful way. Others are not inclined to self-reflection. It may be that they don't know how to do it or that they see it as an inefficient use of their very limited time. Some of us experience true anxiety at the prospect of self-reflection. Here are three reasons why this might happen:

i. Sometimes we are stopped by the feeling that we have unfinished business.

The cure is to finish the business or to let it go, but none of that can happen until the light of our consciousness shines on it. If we don't see the mess, we won't clean it up.

There's some unfinished business that we just have to focus on finishing. Maybe it's a crucial conversation we know we have to have. Maybe we owe someone an apology. We need to be aware of how we've been creating closure for ourselves—and whether we haven't made closure a priority. If you have unfinished business, finish it. But don't make finishing your business into a long project that can then become another excuse not to move on. Finish what can be finished efficiently and then get to the work of self-reflection.

> There's some unfinished business that we just have to focus on finishing.

We might also be better off "putting off until later" something that is important. (We could, for example, deliberately put something off because we know intuitively that it isn't time yet to do a specific task or to pursue a specific goal.) By deliberately deciding to put something off until later, we finish the business "for now" so it won't be on our mind Now. The consciousness required to make a deliberate decision—even the deliberate decision to "put something off until later"—puts us in the present, allowing us to focus on what's happening now. Freeing ourselves from thoughts about projects we'd actually be better off saving for later can actually give us an energy boost, while a nondeliberate bout of procrastination will create in us the paralyzing feeling that we have left something important unfinished.

There are also things that we don't have any control over and we just have to let go of. (They're more accurately called "unfinishable" business in that they're not ours to finish.) If we focus on these things that are beyond our control, we create big energy leaks for ourselves because we're not in the present when we're worried about things we can't control. Fortunately, letting things go can finish even the most unfinishable business and free up our energies for more deliberate pursuits.

Remember also that when something is unfinished, it may well be unimportant.

2. Some of us fear that since in deep human connection we bring ourselves "warts and all," deep human connection is "all warts."

First of all, there's a lot of judgment in the idea that the "warts" are bad. When we're talking about what it means to be human, it's best to assume that it's all good and even that which appears to be detrimental is at the very worst "helpful information" and is at best, a great gift. In fact, it is often the work of self-reflection which helps us to move past our judgments (so often self-judgments) about what is going on in our lives. Self-reflection gives us a broader perspective—it gives us the ability to see things with new eyes—which invariably results in a softening of our own often too-harsh assessments of ourselves and our lives.

3. "I'm afraid to do the work of self-reflection because I'm afraid I'll find out I don't belong in my life."

While it is fairly uncommon that self-reflection will lead us to conclude that we are horribly misplaced in our own lives, it is likely to bring the imbalances and misalignments in our lives into the light of our own consciousness. And while these realizations can be uncomfortable, the discomfort caused by the new realization is nothing compared to the discomfort of the long-standing situation it reveals. The only difference is that after self-reflection we know the cause of that nagging feeling, that low-level depression, or that hair-trigger irritability that's been plaguing us (and those around us) for so long.

It's important to remember that our lives, as we're living them, are rarely if ever a perfect reflection of who we really are. But if our self-reflection helps us to see that we have a lot of changing to do before we can really live so that our outside experience matches who we really are, we still don't have to

Remember also that when something is unfinished, it may well be unimportant.

conclude that our lives as we're currently living them are a sham. We can live the life we're living now as a transition until we find out what life would be authentic to us. It's important to accept that the transition is just as legitimate as the end result. If you wake up to find that you don't belong where you are anymore (and don't know where you do belong), you can still just stay where you are and do your transition work until you find your new life. Don't blame yourself or think you're a failure for being where you are. It's another gift, as everything you've lived up until now has made this moment possible. It's made you who you are and it's brought you to your transition time—which just happens to be now.

Accepting Vulnerability

Most of us fear that vulnerability is a deep pit that will swallow us whole—that is, until we consciously experience the liberating security of it.

Self-reflective practice challenges us to be vulnerable. In our speech, we often couple the word *vulnerable* with the word *weak*, but in reality—especially in health care—vulnerability is one of the strongest characteristics we can have. It is to be cherished, rather than feared.

Being vulnerable means being honest with ourselves, saying what we're really feeling, and being able to talk about our pain in front of others. We're in a field where there is a lot of sorrow to take on if we choose to. But being vulnerable doesn't mean allowing ourselves to join others in their sorrow; it means allowing ourselves to be fully present with those in sorrow and to not be afraid to experience and show emotions. As professional care givers, we are taught not to let it get to us. And while as a heart surgeon, my job was literally to hold the hearts of my patients in my hands, I don't know that I was ever fully human until I became secure enough in my own vulnerability to let others hold my heart in their hands.

> But being vulnerable doesn't mean allowing ourselves to join others in their sorrow; it means allowing ourselves to be fully present with those in sorrow and to not be afraid to experience and show emotions.

Vulnerability is liberating and sometimes also painful and frightening. When we experience it, we let go of a thousand-pound weight; we feel lighter, and we have more energy. We feel connected to the people with whom we've shared and are able to connect with others. Doing reflective practice with others creates a bond between the person who allows you to see his or her heart and the person who holds your heart while you are sharing your innermost sorrows and joys.

Our goal is to do the work of vulnerability and to create a shared vision—a new vision around care of co-workers and care of self—together. We come together for self-reflection so we can share stories and make ourselves vulnerable, and create intimately supportive relationships.

How Best to Change

There's a concept called the Paradoxical Theory of Change, which comes from the Gestalt Institute of Cleveland (GIC). Common to any Gestalt work is that a facilitator (whether in one-to-one or group processes) creates a safe place to do the work by asking fundamental questions that keep participants focused and continually moving forward.

The Gestalt process helps us to see the workings of our lives in a new way by having us ask ourselves the questions:

- *Who am I?*
- *What do I want?*
- *What am I doing to get it?—And what am I doing to keep myself from getting it?*

These last two questions invite us to look deeply at our own behavior, but an important aspect of the facilitator's job then becomes to help participants to appreciate their discoveries about their own behavior, even when they discover that their behaviors are self-defeating. It is fundamental to the Paradoxical Theory of Change that we don't ever focus on our behaviors in order to change them. We foster awareness of our behavior, but only to see whether it's serving us or controlling us.

The Paradoxical Theory of Change is not about correcting anything, and that's why it can be a real mind-shift for health care professionals in particular to engage in it. There is no aspect of it that parallels the traditional medical model of "diagnose and prescribe." Instead, it invites us to assume that there is nothing to be fixed—that all is always well—and that it is our work to figure out who we are and then make our authentic choices based on that information alone.

We foster awareness of our behavior, but only to see whether it's serving us or controlling us.

The Paradoxical Theory of Change says that to simply set an intention and then force ourselves to behave according to that intention sets us up for a painful struggle. Instead, it encourages us to reflect upon who we are and then allow the discoveries we make in that self-reflection to lead us to change automatically.

All of us have had the experience of setting an intention and then working to change our behavior to match our intention. It sounds like a reasonable way to make changes. But all of us also have experiences in which this method hasn't worked. Many of us have set an intention to eat a more nutritious diet and then experienced that our actions have fallen short of our intentions. Many of us have set the intention to save money for some particular purpose and then experienced that our actions have again fallen short. It seems that if we're far from believing we can accomplish something, we feel we have to pull together enough resolve and courage to hit the road with real determination (this time)! But if we are far from believing we can accomplish something (or if the intentions we're setting are not in harmony with who we are), no amount of forcing ourselves into action will do us any good.

Fortunately, there's a much easier way.

Instead of resolving with determination to change our behaviors, we can find out more about who we are and what we want and then allow the changes to evolve naturally. We change because we learn more about ourselves. When we do the work of self-reflection, we become more attuned with our true selves, and since we are only comfortable when our behaviors are attuned to who we really are, our behaviors automatically change.

After we begin to change, however, it is essential to support that change with a sustained focus on who we are (rather than what we want to do.) If we lapse into old behaviors it will be because we are tired, stressed or sick. And it's at those times that it is most important to remember who we are. It's these very lapses (which we so often rush to call failures) that can be such important gifts. Through a practice of self-reflection, we can learn the practice of allowing our awareness of our lapses to bring us back to the present so that we can make

We change because we learn more about ourselves.

conscious decisions about what we want to do based firmly in *who we are.*

It's also important to remember that many of the behaviors we decide are no longer a good fit with who we are have been serving us well up until now. They've allowed us to become who we are now. Self-reflection helps us to be more balanced in our changes. It helps us to be thoughtful in our decisions rather than reflexively reactive. For now, if a behavior is still serving *who we are,* we can keep it; if not, then we will change.

When we're stuck in the doldrums, we can do two things: renew our passion for all the things we're currently doing, or find a new passion. This can still be a scary prospect, though, because we know the pain of the doldrums, but we don't know the pain of the unknown. Still, nobody can work with us and we can't work with ourselves if we're stuck in the pain of the known, because that sticks us in the past and future (as we speculate about how we got into the mess we're in or how we might possibly get out of it), which means we can't be in the present.

> When we're stuck in the doldrums, we can do two things: renew our passion for all the things we're currently doing, or find a new passion.

Without a sense of self—without a notion of *who I am in this work*—most of us are still able to plod along, but we are not in a position to really connect with anyone. True connection happens "self-to-self," so unless you have a sense of you, true connection doesn't happen. A doer of tasks can be attentive, but it takes a "self" to be present. And the practice of Relationship-Based Care requires presence.

Getting Support

Doing reflective practice with a facilitator can be very helpful, as those skilled at facilitating this type of work can pick up helpful cues from the conversation and guide individuals into deeper levels of vulnerability. My work as a facilitator of self-reflection is about being with people so that they have a new awareness that gives them a new direction in their lives. It can be very subtle—a facilitator sometimes does little more than *create the safe space for change.*

As a facilitator, I might invite participants who talk about feeling stressed to just sit for a moment and *feel* the stress—to feel the thought that "I can't do it." We might work with both

But think about it: would you inhale without exhaling? Would you tense a muscle and then never relax it? We're built for balance. Without it, we turn into a mess of knots. Even as leaders we must remember to stop always giving and learn to receive.

polarities—feeling our way through every possibility between spectacular success to dismal failure—and see where the resistance lies.

When we feel the struggle consciously, it can help us to know ease when we feel it. Take a moment to flex a muscle and then relax it. We think of the flexing as the *action* and the "release" as *nonaction*—merely as the mostly unconscious cessation of flexing. But this is physiologically inaccurate. Relaxing a muscle *completely* requires deliberate action. We may relax to some degree without perceivable effort, but if in any given moment someone were to invite us to participate in a relaxation exercise, we would see immediately that we're physiologically on "orange alert" most of the time. Right now, for example, let the chair you are sitting in support your weight more fully than it has been. Give yourself a moment to breathe deeply and really let yourself settle in. See the difference? This is a good analogy for struggle versus ease. It's not enough to recognize your struggle and decide to stop struggling. Experiencing ease takes conscious, deliberate action.

It's important for all of us to both receive and give support. We in health care get so geared toward giving that we block ourselves from receiving. But think about it: Would you inhale without exhaling? Would you tense a muscle and then never relax it? We're built for balance. Without it, we turn into a mess of knots. Even as leaders we must remember to stop always giving and learn to receive. We are of limited use to anyone if our way of being is so one-sided.

The Payoff

Self-reflection helps us to be present.

When we find out who we are, we have the presence to be gentle with ourselves even when we determine that big changes are in order. If we discover behaviors that no longer serve us, we can still acknowledge that they have served us well up until this point. If we find that a behavior is controlling us, we'll want to make the choice not to let it do that, but it is only when we know who we are that we can make that choice.

Consciously choosing what to do begins, of course, with consciousness. Self-determination is rooted in the willingness to choose in any moment. It's born out of a commitment to ask ourselves continually, "Is this behavior of mine attuned with who I am? Is it in harmony with who I now know myself to be?"

As care givers in an RBC culture, we commit to being present with ourselves, our co-workers, and our patients and families. If we are more present with ourselves, we aren't going to worry about who we are with others. In a culture that focuses on relationships, this presence—this level of self-knowing that only comes with self-reflection—is irreplaceable.

If I can know my truth—and know that it is my truth and not necessarily anyone else's—I can be much more accepting of somebody else's truth. In an interpersonal connection based on who we really are, we can move within teams with new confidence in both ourselves and others.

When we know who we are, we don't worry so much about how others perceive us. When we understand our own contribution, we don't worry so much about whether others think we are contributing enough. When we know what we want out of life, we're far more likely to notice when it's offered to us.

Self-determination is rooted in the willingness to choose in any moment.

The Power of Choice: Fostering Professionalism Through Personal Responsibility

—Michael Henry Cohen

We are never captive or powerless on the job unless we choose to be.

We are never captive or powerless on the job unless we choose to be. The perceptions of captivity and powerlessness are self-imposed and always disabling. Eleanor Roosevelt once observed, "No one can make you feel inferior without your consent." Mahatma Gandhi said of his oppressors, "They cannot take away our self-respect if we do not give it to them." It is always our own willingness to feel victimized that hurts us far more than any external forces over which we have no control.

The life of Viktor Frankl, a Jewish psychiatrist who was imprisoned in a Nazi concentration camp, illustrates that choice can be more powerful than even the worst human circumstances. Frankl's entire family, with the exception of his sister, perished in the camps. He lost every material possession, suffered from hunger, cold and brutality. Stripped to his naked existence, he faced the potential of extermination each hour.

All that remained for Frankl was the "last of human freedoms": the ability to "choose one's attitude in a given set of circumstances." Throughout this horrific experience, Frankl chose to maintain a sense of meaning and responsibility in his existence.

Without question, the camps facilitated a strong feeling among the prisoners that fate was their only master and that one must not try to influence it in any way. The temptation was

166 •

overwhelming to allow the environment to completely dictate one's attitudes and behavior. But within this context, Frankl dared to ask:

> *"But what about human liberty? Is there no spiritual freedom in regard to behavior and reaction to any given surroundings? Is that theory true which would have us believe that man is no more than a product of many conditional and environmental factors—be they of a biological, psychological or sociological nature? Is man but an accidental product of these... Does man have no choice of action in the face of such circumstances?"*

(Frankl, 1969)

I cite this example to illustrate that even under the absolute worst of circumstances, a person is not "victim" or "captive" unless he or she chooses to be.

As a hospital human resource professional, I counsel employees on all levels to help them gain a greater measure of control over their work lives. At every opportunity, I share with employees how to steer clear of self-defeating behavior and instill in them a sense of responsibility for the impact their attitudes or behaviors have on others. I view them as adults who have adult decisions to make and who must be accountable for their own actions. And I never buy into employees' perceptions that they are captive or victim to a problematic situation, regardless of how deeply troubled they are by their perception of helplessness.

Regardless of the work problem or the person experiencing it, we have three options from which to choose:

- **Accept and Adjust.** *There are some things with which we are dissatisfied, which happen to be out of our control to change. When this happens, we are wise to focus on the positive aspects of the working conditions. If we are so busy worrying and complaining about what others are doing, we have no psychic energy left to do good with what is right in front of us. Maintain realistic expectations, and don't turn everyday work frustrations into catastrophes.*

> It is not our job to identify a problem and our manager's job to fix it.

- **Become a Responsible Problem Solver.** *Become a positive agent of change. Attend department meetings. Actively and constructively participate in decision-making processes. When we have a difference of opinion with a co-worker or manager, we can talk to him or her in a direct, honest and respectful manner. We can make the choice to be cool, calm and collected, particularly when others are losing control. Remember, it is not our job to identify a problem and our manager's job to fix it.*

- **Separate Yourself from Toxic Work Relationships.** *If we can't solve a problem and accept that it is too much of a compromise on our professionalism, integrity or self-esteem, we must consider separating ourselves from our toxic work relationship. "Separating" is not necessarily quitting, however. We may want to consider transferring to another shift or work unit within the organization. But when we do exit, we need to make certain that we finish strong and "leave the campsite cleaner than we found it."*

In any moment in which we feel pushed around by our circumstances, it would do us good to remember these three choices. We are also wise to remember the example of Viktor Frankl. His genius was in his ability to recreate his experience of his circumstances through the power of his own perception.

Reference: Frankl, V. (2000). *Man's search for meaning.* Boston: Beacon.

All You Need Is Love ... Agape Love

—Scott Louis Diering

Who is a care giver? A care giver is any person who may interact with a patient or the patient's family while the patient has any needs or concerns. Anyone.

Traditionally, we think of care givers as nurses and doctors. However, in the office, clinic or hospital setting every person with whom a patient may have contact is a care giver. It does not matter what we do—security, pharmacy, housekeeping, reception clerk—if we have contact with patients, we are care givers.

An ER Story: Failing to Care

A burst of cold air followed the pair of women into the main entry of their regional medical center. As the younger one pushed the wheelchair, she said, "OK, Gramma, I'll just wheel you up to the registration desk and you can get started while I go park the car." Ms. Claire Hendricks pantomimed with her fist against her throat a few times, and Julia realized her grandmother had left her Servox (which she usually wears around her neck) in the car. The Servox is the artificial electromechanical voice box Ms. Hendricks has used to speak since her laryngectomy 6 years ago.

"I knew we forgot something. Don't worry. I'll bring it when I come back. Just show them your cards and they can get things going till I find a place to park."

Who is a care giver? A care giver is any person who may interact with a patient or the patient's family while the patient has any needs or concerns. Anyone.

Ms. Hendricks hated this feeling of helplessness, and she hated being without her voice box.

She had always been very independent and productive. Hadn't she worked side by side with Rosie the Riveter, building B-24 bombers, 60-some years ago?

Oh, well, at least they know me here, she thought. *I'll be okay without my granddaughter.*

Ms. Hendricks waited patiently at the registration window. After a few minutes, a woman sat down and began to peck at a keyboard, the blue light of the computer monitor reflecting in her glasses. Although her nametag trumpeted, "Ask me! My name is Rebecca! I care!"

"Insurance cards, driver's license or other form of picture ID," croaked Rebecca, staring at her computer monitor, pecking away. Ms. Hendricks produced the requisite documents and waited patiently.

Ms. Hendricks did not get a sense that Rebecca cared very much.

Rebecca had a few more questions that Ms. Hendricks could answer by nodding. "What are you here for today ... uh," Rebecca quickly glanced at the cards as she handed them back, "... Claire?"

Today's visit was for a CT-guided biopsy of a lung nodule to rule out the possibility of recurrence of her cancer.

Ms. Hendricks pantomimed with her hands what she thought a scan of her chest would be like, but Rebecca thought Ms. Hendricks was pushing air into her lap. Then Ms. Hendricks tried to mime tumors on her lungs, but Rebecca thought she was signaling that she had spilled her Cheerios this morning.

Rebecca had a mixture of boredom and annoyance on her face. "Says here you're supposed to have a CAT scan. That right?" Ms. Hendricks nodded gratefully. "Okay, third door down on the left. The nurse in CT has more questions for you." Rebecca seemed to be dismissing her, but Julia had not gotten back from parking the car yet.

Ms. Hendricks had lost some weight lately and was a little frail. She was not used to walking a lot. Julia had put her in the chair as a precaution, kidding her by saying, "Don't worry, Gramma, no one's gonna think you're old just 'cause you're in

Meaningful health care doesn't just happen; it takes a little bit of effort on our part. Humility, compassion, and respect cannot be conveyed in a slogan or a rehearsed line.

a wheelchair." But now, without Julia, Ms. Hendricks felt very old, and the chair felt cumbersome. It took too much effort.

Ms. Hendricks had kicked away from the registration window and managed to wriggle the chair a short distance when she heard Rebecca bark, "You need some help?" Rebecca did not wait for an answer but turned around, yelling, "Hey, get a volunteer to wheel this ol' lady here to radiology. And tell 'em she can't talk, too." Ms. Hendricks flushed with embarrassment. She hated being an old lady. And she hated people thinking she couldn't talk.

Soon a young volunteer sprang up to Ms. Hendricks. Her nametag said, "Ask Me! My name is Tamara! I care!" and Tamara launched into nonstop chatter.

Tamara said, "This your first trip here? I know, it can be scary, what with the noises and faces and smells, especially the smells, like, I remember my first time here, I was eight, and I was climbing a tree, out by the old playground, and I cut my knee and the nurses and doctors were great, and I told myself, Yup, I said, I want to be just like them when I grow up and be a doctor or a nurse, and y'know what? I am gonna be just like them, a real ER nurse or doctor, yup, I'm doing my science classes now and when I finish school, I'm gonna decide if I'm gonna be a doctor or nurse or maybe a paramedic, and I can't wait till I can get right in there and save lives and stop bleeding and do all those neat things that real nurses do, not this dumb stuff, like just wheel people around. Well this is radiology, have a nice visit here, and maybe I'll see you in the ER one day!" And, completing her mission, Tamara was gone.

Ms. Hendricks thought that perhaps Tamara cared too much. But only about Tamara.

The radiology waiting area was cold and lifeless. A TV in the corner blared a soap opera. There was a sign on the wall matching the nametags, announcing, "We care!"

In a few minutes a door swung open and a woman in scrubs appeared.

"You must be Mrs. Hendricks, correct? Hi, I'm Terry, and I'll be starting your IV and helping you out today. Do you have any questions?" Ms. Hendricks was relieved to hear a warm, friendly voice. She needed some comforting.

Ms. Hendricks pointed to her tracheotomy scar, and was mouthing something.

Terry sniped, her soft voice turning to broken glass, "Aw, for Crissake, you can't talk? How are we gonna ...? Don't you have one of those electric thingies?" Ms. Hendricks pointed to the door, hoping to see Julia, and pantomimed that she had one, but it was not here. Her effort was lost on Terry, who appeared quite frustrated. Her comforting magic had vanished.

Terry said, "OK, wait here," as she disappeared through the doors.

Ms. Hendricks could hear her from down the hall. Terry was saying, "Yeah, she's here but she can't talk! Jesus Christ, no, she doesn't have one. Oh, crap, all right, I'll stick her, but whatever we do, it's a waste of time. She's so old; she looks like she's ready to kick off any minute."

At that moment, Ms. Hendricks wished she would just kick off.

Terry returned. Some of the honey was back in her voice. "Okay, now, Mrs. Hendricks, we'll get you taken care of. Don't worry about a thing. All I need to do is start your IV and get you on the table. Have you ever had one of these tests before?"

Ms. Hendricks nodded yes. But, she thought to herself, this is my last one.

How was Ms. Hendricks's care today? Would you have treated her any differently? You might say, "Whoa, these people are out of control! How could anyone be so callous? I'd never behave like that!" But sometimes, in our monotonous yet busy lives, we might behave like Rebecca or Tamara or Terry. We're not intentionally mean or cold. But sometimes we miss the chance to give our best to our patients.

What can we do to assure we always give our very best to our patients?

First, we can act with compassion.
The cornerstone of compassion is empathy.

We must always imagine what life is like for the other person. Empathy is a learnable skill. It's like starting IVs or typing or singing; it takes practice. Empathy is not just a feeling. It is

> Empathy is a learnable skill. It's like starting IVs or typing or singing; it takes practice.

making sure the other person knows we can imagine what life must be like for them.

How do we display empathy? We stop what we are doing, just for a second, and look at the person in front of us. We look at the expression on his or her face. Then we make that same facial expression. Even our patients who cannot speak will know that we can feel their pain when we share a meaningful smile or frown or grimace with them.

If we were caring for Ms. Hendricks, we might also offer some words of comfort. We could say, "I know it must be hard for you without your voice ..." or "I admire you for doing this alone ..." or "We realize it can be confusing here, but don't worry, someone will guide you all the way ..." The inclusion of a few comforting words whenever we start to speak to our patients goes a long way toward showing compassion.

Second, we must respect our patients. The linchpin of respect is validation.

When we validate someone, we recognize their efforts. We praise their accomplishments. We are proud of the work they have done. And we safeguard them from any experience of embarrassment, foolishness or shame. No matter how mistaken, erroneous or "noncompliant" our patients may be, we can never make them feel foolish or embarrassed. Shame and embarrassment are some of the worst feelings we can create, and are worse still coming from those who are supposed to be comforting and nurturing.

Please, please don't ever let your patients feel foolish!

If we were caring for Ms. Hendricks, we might have offered her a pad to write with, saying, "Oh, you forgot your voice box? That's okay; we all forget things now and then. It's no big deal." Or we could say, "Are you alone? That's no problem. Would you rather wait till your family gets here, or shall we forge ahead? It's fine with me, either way!"

The clear affirmation that someone is okay just as he or she is, is one of the nicest gifts we can give to anyone.

The clear affirmation that someone is okay just as he or she is, is one of the nicest gifts we can give to anyone.

A third virtue, which distinguishes great health care workers from average ones, is humility.

While we are with our patients, they are most important. Our schedules, our issues, our concerns and our baggage must be secondary to our patients and their immediate needs and concerns.

How can we display humility? Two ways:

1. *For the first few seconds of every encounter with a patient, focus all of your energies on her. Look at her. Let her be the center of all of your attention. This refocusing will work wonders for you. It's quick and easy and it doesn't take much time. (During these few seconds, you can also be empathizing; this will strengthen your bond with your patient.)*

2. *Translate. We must never use our special, complex medical/health care language when talking to our patients unless we also immediately define what we are saying. Even simple acronyms like CAT scan, which we assume everyone understands, can invoke fear and confusion in lay people. Every medical term you use must be defined by you when you use it.*

When you add these three keys together, compassion + respect + humility, you create an expression of love. Agape love—our unconditional love for all humanity. When we practice our jobs in health care with agape, we make life a little better for all of our patients. And for ourselves. No matter what our role is in the health care setting, we have a huge impact on any patient's experience.

"But," you might argue, "the registration clerk and volunteer are not really providers. They are outside of our department. We have no control over them!"

Sorry. There are no excuses for rude, cold or degrading behaviors. Every employee that patients meet, from the time they drive onto the hospital property until they drive off, is a care giver. We all must be singing from the same hymnal. With sincerity. And conviction. If you are caring for a patient who has had a negative experience elsewhere in your facility, you are responsible for attending to their distress by:

For the first few seconds of every encounter with a patient, focus all of your energies on them. Look at them. Let them be the center of all of your attention. This refocusing will work wonders for you.

1. *apologizing,*

2. *validating the patient's or family member's distress and*

3. *taking appropriate action to resolve the situation.*

There are lots of ways we could improve on the care that was provided by Rebecca and Tamara and Terry. I am sure you can list more than I can. Let's discuss a few of the things these care givers could have said and done to improve Ms. Hendricks's experience.

What might we do differently if we were Rebecca? First, any nametags, buttons or signs proclaiming "We care!" or "Compassion comes first" must have our words and actions to back them up. Without that backup, the words stand as a mockery and detract from any believability or credibility our institution might seek.

Therefore, if we were Rebecca, we might extend our hand in greeting, smile and offer a warm "Hello, my name is Rebecca. I'll be helping you with registration today." We'd never call Ms. Hendricks by her first name unless Ms. Hendricks invited us to do so. And we certainly would never show any displeasure at the additional work someone's infirmity may cause us. If we were Rebecca, we'd remember to always be as polite as possible when discussing our patient with someone else.

Now, if we were Tamara, we might ask Ms. Hendricks some questions about herself. When we discovered that she could not speak, we might simply give a simple tour of the hospital. Or we'd ask only yes and no questions. Or we'd share a simple story about our life. (Tamara's story about her childhood knee laceration is fine; however, anything we say about us is with the goal of making our patient's experience better. It's never really about us.) Tamara's egocentric rambling seems harmless. Yet it is actually a verbal and emotional barrier. Her words distance her from her patients. Tamara seems to confuse talking *at* her patient with talking *with* her patient.

I find Terry's actions to be the most troubling of all. She is insincere. Her pleasant façade deteriorates when she is faced with a challenging patient. Her lack of sincerity, her offstage tantrums and her duplicity (her two-facedness) all convey that

> Any nametags, buttons or signs proclaiming "We care!" or "Compassion comes first," must have our words and actions to back them up.

> Anything we say about us is with the goal of making our patient's experience better. It's never really about us.

she is not to be trusted. And if we can't trust her, can we trust the radiology department? Can we trust the whole hospital?

If we were in Terry's shoes, how might we behave differently? Certainly, we would never be two-faced. We would honestly admit the limitations Ms. Hendricks's forgetfulness might cause us: "Hmm, since you cannot talk, we'll have to do this all in writing. It'll take us a few extra minutes, but we'll get it done, don't worry."

Even during a time of our busiest maelstrom, with critical patients and whining doctors and demanding families, we'd be honest:

"I need to attend to this critical patient here for a few minutes. Please be patient. I'll be back shortly."

Or:

"May I ask you to be patient with us while we take care of some serious problems? I want to give you my undivided attention, and I cannot do that at this moment."

We'd be warm and courteous both in front of our patient and behind the scenes. We'd make sure that our patient's extenuating problem, be it mutism, obesity, lack of education, or whatever, is never a problem for us. We'd be proud to take care of our patient. And we'd humbly defend our patient's right to compassion and respect to every care giver with whom we discuss our patient.

Meaningful health care doesn't just happen; it takes a little bit of effort on our part. Humility, compassion and respect cannot be conveyed in a slogan or a rehearsed line. Compassionate, respectful health care comes from our hearts. It comes through mindfulness, good habits, loving actions and sincere expressions of compassion and respect and humility. It comes from unconditional love—agape love.

Self-Knowing and Self-Care: A Determinate of the Quality of Our Relationship with Others

—Susan Edstrom and Mary Koloroutis

A person must decide to take the journey.
The path has infinite patience.
It will always be there for those who decide to travel it.

—The Sacred Tree

Self-knowing and self-care are fundamental to establishing healthy relationships with patients, families and members of the health care team. Jean Watson's research in human caring supports this basic assumption. Watson writes that in order to enter into a therapeutic relationship with a patient, to be emotionally present and to monitor and safeguard the needs of patients and families, the fundamental first step for care givers is to know themselves:

> *Our knowledge of and relationship with our self determines the quality of all of our relationships.*

> *I emphasize that it is possible to read, study, learn about, even teach and research caring theory; however, to truly "get it," one has to personally experience it. ... This is both an invitation and an opportunity to interact with the ideas, experiment with and grow within the philosophy, and live it out in one's personal/professional life. ... Each one is also asked, if not enticed to examine and explore the critical intersection between the personal and the professional; be able to translate their unique talents, interests, and gifts into human service of caring and healing, for self and others.*

> *(Watson, 1988)*

Reigniting the Spirit of Caring (*RSC*) has been a useful forum for self-exploration. The workshop encourages self-reflection and exploration of the "critical intersection between the personal and the professional." Participants explore their caring practices through individual reflection and through interaction with colleagues. The value of listening and silence is explored as a means to deeper self-knowing. Participants discover and express feelings and thoughts about their care-giving practices through reflective journaling and storytelling. The telling of stories provides the opportunity to share something of meaning and to experience the power of mutual vulnerability. Storytelling moves us from the cognitive realm of learning to an emotional/spiritual realm. We discover meaning that may otherwise have been inaccessible.

> The telling of stories provides the opportunity to share meaning and to experience the power of authentic vulnerability.

The power of intention is developed throughout the *RSC* workshop. Individual ownership for learning and gaining value in any experience is emphasized by establishing intentions for each day of the experience. Intentions help the participants focus on what is uniquely theirs to own and clarify how they can gain the most benefit from each day. The practice of consciously setting intention for self-care and care for others may assist care givers in the practice setting to balance their work and expectations in a more realistic and conscious way.

In *RSC*, the participants also learn about the importance of attending to the body, mind and spirit as essential for personal growth, health, healing and self-knowing. The following ideas are presented and explored:

Caring for our body includes sound nutrition, exercise and health monitoring. It also includes learning to respect and enjoy our body. It calls us to be responsible for our own health.

Caring for our mind means being aware of and attending to our thoughts, attitudes, beliefs and values. Our minds enable us to gather wisdom and experience from the world around us. Our mind can bring us great joy and discernment or be the major source of worry and pain.

Caring for our spirit includes appreciating and developing our emotional self through connecting with our inner-self and with our greater source of spiritual power. Developing this dimension of ourselves allows us to feel the depth and breadth of human experience and find meaning and fulfillment in ourselves.

The following body, mind, spirit assessment provides insight into personal balance:

Assess your personal well-being and balance in Body, Mind and Spirit by completing the following brief questionnaire. Rate yourself on a scale of 1-4 with 1 being "rarely" and 4 being "most of the time." Upon completion, review your strengths and areas for growth and identify one or two actions you can take to improve your Body, Mind and Spirit Balance.

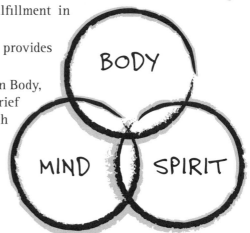

BODY

_____ I eat to maximize my health.

_____ I get enough sleep (at least 7 hours per night) and feel generally rested.

_____ I have a high level of physical energy throughout my workday.

_____ I am open to and use humor; I find reasons to laugh every day.

_____ I apply breathing principles and physical stretching techniques to manage stress and refresh my body.

_____ I practice meditation and/or prayer; I understand it is healthy for my body.

_____ **Total Score**
_____ **Average Score (Total/7)**

MIND

_____ I find my work mentally stimulating.

_____ I know what helps me to focus, and I take the required actions to achieve focus.

_____ I have a positive mindset and am generally content with my life.

_____ I identify choices and act on them during periods of stress and/or discontent.

_____ I maintain hope and perspective in most situations.

_____ I know my core values and beliefs, and I act on them.

_____ I do what it takes to work through complex or difficult situations.

_____ I am able to discern my own sphere of influence.

_____ I am able to let go of the "small stuff."

_____ I can make the decision to mentally detach and leave my work problems at work.

_____ **Total Score**
_____ **Average Score (Total/10)**

SPIRIT

_____ I know my purpose in life.

_____ I generally feel confident and competent.

_____ I make it a practice to prioritize time for personal renewal.

_____ I participate in spiritual practices that are meaningful and fulfilling to me.

_____ I let go of those things that are beyond my control.

_____ I share my thoughts and feelings with other trusted people in my life.

_____ I generally allow myself to be vulnerable and open to others.

_____ I experience and express gratitude.

_____ I use my personal "failures" as an opportunity to grow and learn.

_____ I am aware of and responsible for my own mistakes.

_____ I am able to forgive others and myself.

_____ I accept others and myself as imperfect.

_____ I listen.

_____ **Total Score**
_____ **Average Score (Total/13)**

Ask yourself these questions:

- *"What are some key priorities or issues for me?"*

- *"What are my areas of strength? What choices do I make to create these areas of strength?"*

- *"What are areas of imbalance? What would it take to bring things into balance?"*

- *Periodically do a self-check by coming back and completing these questions and asking yourself, "What is my balance of Body, Mind, Spirit at this point in time?"*

- *"What has changed or what am I doing differently?" Consider keeping a log or journal for self-reflection.*

We know we cannot be in an optimum position to care and extend to others if we are not caring for ourselves.

References: Four Worlds International Institute. (1984). *The sacred tree: Reflections on Native American spirituality.* Lotus Light Publications.

Koloroutis, M. (Ed.). (2004). *Relationship-based care: A model for transforming practice.* Minneapolis, MN: Creative Health Care Management.

Watson, J. (1988). New dimensions of human caring theory. *Nursing Science Quarterly,* 1(4), 175-181.

Taking Charge of Your Health

—Mary Jo Kreitzer

> When decisions about life and work are based on your gifts and passions, the power of purpose emerges, bringing alignment, energy, flow and aliveness. What gets you up in the morning?

Few of us in health care would argue with the idea that "taking charge of your health" is important. In caring for patients, we are proactive in educating our patients about health promotion and disease prevention as well as how to better manage their chronic conditions. The unfortunate reality is that we do a much better job of taking care of patients than taking care of ourselves. If we are honest with ourselves, as individuals and as professionals, we have not generally made "living a healthy lifestyle" a priority. In our work environments, there are few positive rewards or incentives for healthy behaviors and many opportunities to slip into a pattern of unhealthy behaviors.

There is abundant evidence that positive health choices, such as regular exercise, eating nutritious foods, managing stress and avoiding toxic substances like tobacco can improve your overall health and well-being. And there is compelling evidence that working in the health care field is inherently stressful and that many of our colleagues in health professions struggle with health issues that are directly related to unhealthy patterns. In the large, longitudinal Nurses' Health Study (http://www.channing.harvard.edu/nhs/), investigators examined how well nurses met five good-health criteria: a healthy weight, nonsmoker, at least 30 minutes of moderate to vigorous activity daily, a healthy diet and a moderate use of alcohol. A healthy diet was defined as being a high-fiber diet low in saturated and trans fats with limited sweets and refined grains. Only 3% of the nurses in the study met all of the criteria and those who did had far better health. The women who did not meet the criteria developed almost five times more heart problems and ten times more diabetes than the women who did meet the criteria.

A first step in taking charge of your health is to assume more personal responsibility for lifestyle choices and health habits. My Health Planner was designed to help you reflect on various aspects of your health and to:

- *identify your strengths and areas for improvement,*
- *set goals,*
- *recognize challenges,*
- *assess readiness for change, and*
- *identify action steps that you plan to take.*

My Health Planner was developed at the University of Minnesota, and is offered on-line as a free assessment tool. It includes information on eight domains that contribute to health and wellness. Thinking about your own life and health goals, you may choose to work within one domain, or all eight.

The following descriptions give you a sample of information to consider as you reflect on how well you are doing in each domain.

My Health Planner

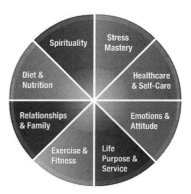

Copyright, University of Minnesota, 2006

Diet and Nutrition:

Americans are becoming increasingly overweight and obese at an alarming rate. Being overweight is associated with many diseases, including Type 2 diabetes, stroke, osteoarthritis, respiratory problems, heart disease, gallbladder disease, sleep apnea and breast cancer. There are many fad diets, and new research is emerging daily on what constitutes a healthy diet. Study after study shows that good food choices have a positive impact on health and poor diets have negative long-term effects. What are your eating habits and how have they changed over time?

> **Diet and Nutrition Health Tips**
>
> - Eat more fruits, vegetables and whole grains.
> - Get enough calcium-rich foods.
> - Eat foods low in saturated and trans fats.
> - Restrict sugar and salt.
> - Eat moderate portions.
> - Use alcohol in moderation.

Exercise and Fitness:

As we move into our adult years, there is a dramatic decrease in physical activity. Many of us lead very sedentary lifestyles and yet there is strong evidence that a lack of physical activity is associated with increased risk of obesity, anxiety, stress, depression, high blood pressure, coronary artery disease, diabetes and osteoporosis. It is no secret that physical activity is essential to improving physical and mental health and in preventing and reducing the risk of disease. Are you knowledgeable about the current guidelines for physical activity?

> **Exercise and Fitness Health Tips**
>
> - Do 30 minutes of moderate exercise daily.
> - For greater benefits, engage in more vigorous physical activity for about 60 minutes a day.
> - Include cardiovascular conditioning, stretching and resistance exercises for muscle strength and endurance.

Stress Mastery:

Stress is a normal part of life. Prolonged stress can be very detrimental to our health and can adversely impact every system of the body. How do you experience stress and do you know when you are at risk for stress? What works to alleviate stress? Learning to master your stress is an ongoing journey that is vital to improving your health and well-being.

> **Stress Mastery Health Tips**
> - Practice meditation or other quiet reflection.
> - Take minibreaks during the day.
> - Engage in expressive therapies such as art, music or dance.
> - Talk with people you trust.
> - Ask for and accept help.
> - Choose not to worry about things you cannot control.
> - Have fun through sports, hobbies or social activities.

Spirituality:

The search for meaning and connection is universal and transcends age, gender and culture. There is a growing body of evidence indicating that spiritual practices, such as prayer or meditation, are connected with better health outcomes. Spiritual practices include journaling, reflection, prayer, meditation and connecting with nature. What experiences in your daily life are fulfilling and life giving?

> **Spirituality Health Tips**
> - Spend time each day in contemplative practices—reflection, journaling or meditation.
> - Develop and maintain meaningful relationships.
> - Become connected with a community.

Relationships and Family:

The health risks from being alone or isolated are comparable in magnitude to the risks associated with cigarette smoking, high blood pressure and obesity. Family and support networks are an essential component of a person's overall health. Are you making time for important people in your life?

> ### *Relationships and Family Health Tips*
> - Prioritize time with family and friends.
> - Volunteer.
> - Join a cause.
> - Work out at a gym with a partner.
> - Find others who share a hobby.

Emotions and Attitudes:

Feelings may be triggered by an experience or a memory. Emotions are how we experience those feelings and are largely shaped by our attitudes, judgments and expectations. Our attitude has a tremendous impact on how we view life and the world around us. When we are emotionally well, we have a healthy self-esteem and are able to express the full range of emotions that occur in the human experience. Are you aware of your attitudes, beliefs and emotions and how they impact the choices you make?

> ### *Emotions and Attitudes Health Tips*
> - Be aware of all your emotions.
> - Accept emotions without judgment.
> - Recognize that you control your attitudes and behaviors.
> - Express true emotions.
> - Shift negative emotions consciously.

Life Purpose and Service:

Enjoying a fully alive life is learning to reframe important life questions, letting go of what's no longer relevant and taking on new questions guided by an evolving life purpose. When decisions about life and work are based on your gifts and passions, the power of purpose emerges, bringing alignment, energy, flow and aliveness. What gets you up in the morning?

Life Purpose and Service Tips

- Discover solitude.
- Keep a journal.
- Talk with others.
- Go on a retreat.
- Pay attention to dreams.

Health Care and Self-Care:

We are often far more concerned about caring for others than caring for ourselves. It is up to you to be informed about your health and health care options, intentional about what you want, and involved in decision making. Do you consider yourself a vital member of your own health care team? Do you get regular checkups and screenings, use safety equipment and know how to access up-to-date health information?

Health Care and Self-Care Tips

- Choose a provider or clinic where you can get your needs met.
- Be prepared to discuss the reason for your visit clearly.
- Ask questions.
- Understand the outcomes and goals of your recommended treatment.
- Research the health information you need.
- Ask for what you want.

In reality, you are the only person who can really manage your health and health care. We teach and coach our patients and families on how to care for themselves. It is time to ask the tough question "Are we modeling healthy behaviors in our own lives?" Our health care system needs to shift from focusing primarily on illness and disease to also addressing health promotion and disease prevention. Primary care begins at home—with us. It's time that we role model the change that we want to see and provide leadership on "taking charge of our health." My Health Planner is a tool that can help you get started. While it is designed to be used by individuals, it is also being used by small groups who choose to meet over a period of eight weeks, going through one health domain each week. Using My Health Planner in a group setting adds both the dimension of group support and personal accountability.

If you are interested in more in-depth information or tracking your progress online, go to www.csh.umn.edu and click on My Health Planner. It is free!

Living the Four Agreements

—Mary Koloroutis

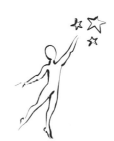

In his best-selling book, *The Four Agreements*, Don Miguel Ruiz offers four pieces of timeless wisdom. When practiced in our daily lives, each helps free us from thoughts that rob us of joy and create needless suffering. While the Four Agreements are meant as a guide for everyday living, I have mined them here for the wisdom I believe to be of specific benefit to those of us in health care.

Ruiz's Four Agreements are:

- *Be Impeccable with Your Word*
- *Don't Take Anything Personally*
- *Don't Make Assumptions*
- *Always Do Your Best*

To **be impeccable with your word** means to speak with integrity. Say what you mean, and act in alignment with what you say. It means to speak with kindness and respect.

When leading change, it is important that you "walk your talk" in a way that is conscious, visible and consistent. Ruiz sets a high bar with this agreement. To be "impeccable" (having no flaws, perfect) requires an awareness of the power of the word, the ability to speak with intention, and an understanding that every interaction is an opportunity for a leader to inspire or discourage, to inform or deny, to heal or to hurt.

The agreement **"Don't take anything personally"** is a big challenge for most of us. Ruiz reminds us that words that originate with others can never really be about us. However, when someone merely implies that we are "out of touch" it can cut us to the quick.

In truth, nothing others do or say is really because of us. What others say and do is a projection of their own worldview. Mental and emotional immunity to the actions and opinions of others frees us from a tremendous amount of needless suffering. It also allows us to stay open and responsive to the ideas and experiences of others. We are able to respond with compassion and wisdom if we remember that "it's not about me; this is this person's response to the situation." A patient's anger may be an expression of fear, powerlessness or vulnerability. The wise care giver understands that and does not personalize it.

The trick is to be conscious of doing our best within our current reality.

If we **don't make assumptions**, what is left to us is to ask about the things we don't understand. We sometimes make assumptions because we are too afraid or impatient to ask questions. And we also make assumptions simply because it is our habit to do so. If we think of ourselves as adept judges of what is going on around us, we are likely to habitually jump to conclusions about what we perceive.

The importance of this agreement was driven home for me when I was nursing director in an acute care hospital and one of my areas of responsibility was the emergency department. I arrived unannounced early one morning to check in with the staff members in the department. We'd been having problems with patient relations in this particular department, and I had been working very closely with the staff to turn that around. When I arrived, the department was quiet. One lone nurse was sitting at the front desk playing solitaire. This particular nurse had a history of inappropriate interactions with the public, and I was less than pleased to see her in public view playing solitaire. Rather than jumping to the assumption that was running through my mind, (divine guidance?) I asked her how she was and what was going on. She told me she was "numb" and "shell shocked." That night, a 30-year-old man had been admitted to the ER following an accident. He had been walking along the road when a car hit him and took off his right leg almost to the hip. The ER team worked for hours stabilizing him and getting him to surgery. She had just finished cleaning up all of the blood in the room, the ER docs had gone to lie down, and she was trying to hold on. She then collapsed into my arms, sobbing. What would have happened if I had simply assumed that she was being "inappropriate" and focused on the solitaire?

To **always do your best** sounds so simple. Those of us who value our own work also value doing our best. But our best can be different from one moment to the next. The reality of health care is that sometimes so much comes at us all at once that we end up "doing our best just to get by." Still, at other times we do what we consider "our very best work." The trick is to *be conscious of* doing our best within our current reality.

Resource-driven practice is a norm in health care today. Now more than ever, we are being asked to do the best we can with the finite resources available to us. As we find ourselves the careful custodians of people, time and materials, we have a prime opportunity to practice this fourth agreement. To do our best requires that we deliberately pay attention to what we *can accomplish* instead of what we can't get to today.

To do our best, we must be realistic about what we have to work with, prioritize what is important, and focus our energy and creativity into accomplishing all that we are able with the resources at hand.

Ruiz's framework is a mental model that helps us to navigate the very real challenges of living and leading. Consistently practicing even one of these agreements will be life altering. Taking on all four will remove a lot of needless difficulty from our lives and work—putting us on a path to living as more conscious and creative leaders.

Reference: Ruiz, D. M. (1997). *The four agreements: A practical guide to personal freedom.* San Rafael, CA: Amber-Allen.

Change the World

—Sharon E. Melberg

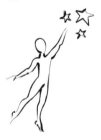

If not you, who?
If not now, when?
If not here, where?
If not for good, why?
If not justly, how?
Do it by hand.
Do it by heart.
Do it from memory.
Do it with imagination.
Do it for hope.
What is good? or is not?
What can be is up to you
 —and to me.

PART

III

Infrastructure

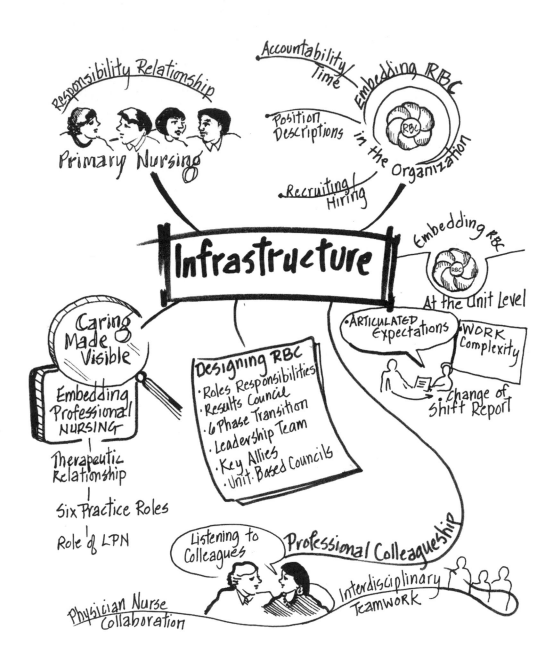

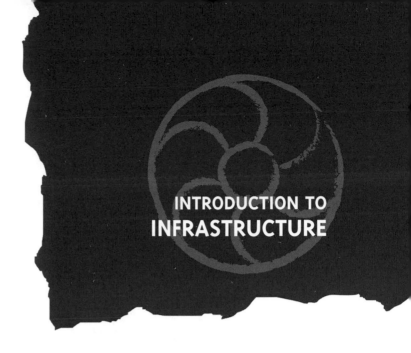

INTRODUCTION TO INFRASTRUCTURE

A well-designed *infrastructure* brings Relationship-Based Care (RBC) to life within the organizational culture and within the practice of individual leaders, clinicians and staff. The focus on a well-designed infrastructure is one of the factors that differentiates Relationship-Based Care from other initiatives which often end up referenced by disillusioned staff members as just another "flavor of the month." Infrastructure refers to the roles, systems, practices, processes and behaviors employed by every group and individual at every level in the organization. *Infrastructure* clarifies the responsibility, authority and accountability at all levels of the organization. Infrastructure brings empowerment to life. When an organization decides to take on RBC's way of *being*, the leaders then take a thorough look at all of the ways they currently do things.

In organizations in which Relationship-Based Care thrives:

- *the physical environment supports care delivery and the well-being and healing of patients, families and staff members,*

- *there is clarity of role responsibility for caring and clinical competencies for each member of the clinical professional disciplines and nonclinical support staff,*

- *staff scheduling is built upon continuity of patient/ care giver relationships as a conscious and high priority,*

- *teamwork and communications systems are structured to advance professional relationships and care delivery, within the nursing team and across disciplines and departments,*

- *therapeutic relationships with patients and families are regarded as essential to quality care, and*

- *leaders expect (and model) that compassion, respect and healthy interactions are the norm in all relationships.*

During the planning and design phases that precede RBC implementation, roles, systems, policies, processes and behaviors at every level are assessed for the degree to which they support a culture of humane care and continuity of patient/ care giver relationships. While this may sound dauntingly comprehensive, an appreciative assessment (see page 96) of practices already in place will invariably reveal that an organization is already doing a great deal to advance, safeguard and/or protect the sanctity of patient/care giver relationships. Much of what we do in integrating RBC into the infrastructure of the organization is to formalize what is already working well and to identify actions to continue to build on those identified strengths. Those aspects of the infrastructure found not to advance a relationship-based culture and the organization's desired vision are eliminated or redesigned.

Part III addresses the specific aspects of infrastructure that must be in place in order for RBC to take hold in an organization, as well as ways to help people embrace these structures. In this section we describe concrete actions, behaviors and attitudes that make RBC come alive in the organizational culture, in individual leaders, in the way priorities are established, in the way systems and processes are designed, and in the way relationships with patients and their families are established to maximize compassionate quality care. Most notably, the nurse-patient relationship is highlighted as a fundamental component of Relationship-Based Care delivery, and tools and suggestions to improve health care team communication and collaboration are provided.

You will notice in this section that we address the same topics and issues from slightly different vantage points. This is intentional to assist readers in considering and applying each component to their own organizations. Redundancy is intentional as we hope the different perspectives will be valuable in assisting readers in addressing their unique questions.

CHAPTER FIVE
Designing and Organizing Relationship-Based Care for Your Organization

Getting Started: The Six-Phase Transition to Relationship-Based Care

—Jayne A. Felgen, Colleen Person, and Susan Wessel

We believe people are in health care because they want to be in relationship with the patients and families they serve, whether directly or indirectly. Actively advancing the patient/care giver relationship requires not only getting back in touch with the very essence and meaning of our work, but seeing to it that every structure and relationship that exists within our organizations serves that relationship.

There are six phases to the design and implementation of Relationship-Based Care (RBC). As every organization has a unique history and culture, the design and implementation of RBC works best when the strengths of the organization and its members are leveraged into a new, shared vision for customizing RBC within their culture. In addition to using the best that we find within an organization, we also put some of our own time-tested methods into place that have proven vital to the functioning and sustenance of Relationship-Based Care. In transitioning to RBC we maintain a balance between building on the best that exists in an organization and intentionally guiding organizations into what will be for them a sustainable, fully integrated cultural change.

The preparation phase begins with an organizational assessment using Appreciative Inquiry (AI) (see page 96). In the spirit of appreciation, we seek to understand those areas of practice that already reflect the principles and values of Relationship-Based Care. We use AI in these assessments because highlighting positive, lived experiences helps people to realize that their past successes have positioned them well for even greater success in the future. The assessment brings forth amazing, touching stories of care in which the ownership and compassion of hospital staff made a profound difference in the patient's experience of healing. We invariably hear stories of exceptional teamwork in which interdependence, cooperation, and healthy communication prevailed. Stories emerge that reflect the deep values, beliefs and commitment of the organization's staff and physicians and the dedication and vision of its executive leaders. These stories of human connection and compassionate leadership further inspire the organization's commitment to relationships, to human compassion, to clinical excellence and to productive and effective teamwork. These stories lift up organizations' principles and create the foundation for moving forward with a new and compelling shared vision for intentional caring relationships.

Stories emerge that reflect the deep values, beliefs and commitment of the organization's staff and physicians and the dedication and vision of its executive leaders.

In this phase, leaders and stakeholders at the strategic, operational, tactical and individual levels are identified and then educated about what it will take to transform their existing culture to one in which every individual consciously expresses the principles of Relationship-Based Care in his or her professional practice. The RBC leadership team typically consists of an executive sponsor (the executive leader who brought RBC to the organization), an executive nurse leader, an executive medical leader, a human resource executive, a board champion and an RBC Project Leader.

A multidisciplinary Results Council is formed to oversee the implementation of RBC throughout the organization (see page 208). The initial work of this group is to organize the change process, create a shared vision for change, understand and support the RBC principles developed by the nursing executive team, and establish desired outcomes, measurable goals, and a timetable for accomplishing results. This diverse group of leaders has the important and immensely satisfying task of answering questions like:

- *What are we calling for as an organization?*
- *How can we best serve our patients and their families?*
- *How can we best serve our community, our staff and our physicians?*
- *What will it take to achieve our shared vision?*
- *How will we measure our success in accomplishing our vision?*

A high-priority task in the preparation phase is to determine what the scope of the RBC implementation will be within the organization. Will RBC be implemented hospital-wide or within the nursing department only? Will it begin with the nursing department and then eventually include other departments and areas? These are important decisions, best based on the vision of each individual organization.

No matter what the eventual scope of RBC is to be in an organization, however, RBC cannot be successfully achieved on all clinical units within the organization at the same time. Successful implementation occurs in stages that we call "waves." Only three or four clinical units can launch their plans at any one time. This allows for monitoring of progress and for units scheduled for implementation in subsequent waves to learn from the experience of the units they follow.

When managers and staff leaders from units in the first wave are identified, they establish Unit Practice Councils (UPCs) to accomplish the work of planning and implementing RBC in their work areas (see page 214). It is essential that leaders be identified from all levels of the organization and that the Unit Practice Councils are broadly inclusive in their membership. It is critically important for Unit Practice Council members to be selected by their peers. These council members are specifically chosen because they are highly respected for *already living RBC values,* and because their peers want them to lead the change process on their unit. Thoughtful peer selec-

A high-priority task in the preparation phase is to determine what the scope of the RBC implementation will be within the organization. Will RBC be implemented hospital wide or within the nursing department only?

tion reduces issues and barriers down the line. It is essential for peers to select the colleagues who will represent them. This selection strengthens the process and promotes ownership of the change.

Throughout the preparation phase, it is natural for leaders both established and previously unrecognized to emerge. Behind every success at every level, there is a person who has the potential to lead change either as a mentor or as a council member. It takes the commitment and participation of everyone in the organization to embody and sustain Relationship-Based Care.

The final step in the preparatory phase is called "Getting Smarter" (see page 473). In this important step, leaders immerse themselves fully into the concepts of Relationship-Based Care. This includes reading recommended books and articles, and viewing and discussing related videos and DVDs in order to become completely familiar with the concepts of Relationship-Based Care. The RBC Leader Practicum is offered frequently through by Creative Health Care Management so that leaders also have the option of learning with leaders from other organizations (see page 468).

The structure phase has a direct and pragmatic focus. In this phase, council chairs, co-chairs and recorders are selected for the Results Council, the group that oversees the entire transformation process. Similarly, leadership roles are determined by the Unit Practice Councils, the groups that oversee the transformation of individual units. Meeting times are established and mutual agreements are defined for all councils. Responsibility, authority and accountability are defined for each council, as is the scope of leadership roles. Each council goes through a process of articulating expectations between leaders and members, and a communication network is set up between the Results and Unit Practice Councils and between council members and their stakeholders. A critical factor for success is to establish effective communication between all unit staff members. Regular meeting times are determined as is the approach to taking meeting minutes and disseminating the minutes for information sharing and progress reporting.

**Phase II:
Structure**

In this phase, a conversation takes place in the councils regarding who should be given "strategic invitations" to the Results Council and/or the Unit Practice Councils. These "key allies" may include physicians, board members and influential managers. The purpose is to form key alliances that will enhance the organization's ability to achieve the transformation to RBC and live its values at all levels of the organization (see page 221).

A crucial step within the structure phase is for the Results Council to affirm a set of principles for Relationship-Based Care. These principles serve as the blueprint for all Unit Practice Councils as they determine how Relationship-Based Care will be implemented on their units.

Phase III: Planning

The planning phase focuses on action planning. The Results Council develops a 12 to 18 month plan to support the Unit Practice Councils' efforts via specific functional responsibilities.

The Results Council is charged with:

- *integrating RBC with other organizational initiatives, such as customer service, Joint Commission, or Magnet designation*

- *communicating the vision and influencing others to support it,*

- *integrating RBC principles into the organization's strategic vision and plans and into its day-to-day operations,*

- *defining both process and outcomes measures to monitor results,*

- *providing educational support specific to Relationship-Based Care,*

- *securing the involvement and support of physicians,*

- *establishing and/or refining a caring and healing environment, and*

- *diminishing barriers in work processes.*

Concurrently, the Unit Practice Councils develop 12 to 18 month plans for the implementation of RBC on their individual units and present their plans to the Results Council for discussion, refinement and encouragement.

To create their plan, the Unit Practice Councils review RBC principles received from the Results Council and assess the extent to which their units are already working in alignment with the principles. The UPC members respond to a comprehensive set of questions specific to each principle and identify areas of strength and areas for change. They then reach consensus about how to design their patient care delivery to honor the RBC principles, prioritize areas for action and develop their plans for change.

Each Council's planning also includes helping peers learn about RBC, engaging all colleagues in the move toward RBC, inspiring colleagues to create a common network of support for the change, and outlining a plan for monitoring and evaluating progress at the unit and individual levels. In this phase, organizational indicators are identified along with unit-specific indicators as a means of monitoring progress and evaluating results (see page 590 for organization-specific and unit-specific indicators).

Concurrently, the Results Council will develop plans for supporting the RBC implementation. The plans will include strategies and actions specific to each of the functional areas of responsibility held by the Results Council, as well as provide communication links to kcy stakcholders.

These functional areas are initially important in order to deal with the reality of our complicated, chaotic organizational environment. Frustration with real or perceived barriers will arise; the best intentions for effective communication will sometimes fail. The Results Council needs to help ease the frustration by leading, staying the course and maintaining a constancy of purpose. As each area of responsibility is addressed and owned, the chance of getting sidetracked with the latest "organizational crisis" is diminished.

This is a unique phase in which all planning is reviewed before it is implemented. It is the phase in which plans are assessed for their degree of alignment with the mission and vision of the organization, their degree of alignment with RBC principles, and their overall feasibility. As always, the plans are

**Phase IV:
Review and Support**

assessed using Appreciative Inquiry, so this phase tends to be especially inspiring. This is a time to share best practices, to think creatively, and to articulate expectations (see page 255 for articulated expectations) for all members of the organization. Because it is a review of all that has been done so far to bring RBC to life in the organization, this phase also allows for conscious commitment to the implementation that will follow it.

During this time, meetings, presentations and discussions are held to determine how each plan for change can be refined to best engage every stakeholder in the transition to Relationship-Based Care. The Results Council reviews the plans devised by each of the Unit Practice Councils, finds each plan's greatest strengths and helps the Unit Practice Councils determine how best to build on those strengths. At the same gathering, the Results Council presents to the Unit Practice Councils the Result Council's plan for preparing the organization and community for Relationship-Based Care. The Results Council will share their plans for communication, education, coordination, integration, healing/caring practices, service support, physician relationships and engagement of all stakeholders (see page 217).

Phase V: Implementation

We work from the assumption that "we get what we pay attention to," so we continually pay attention to even the smallest of our successes.

In this phase, the action plans are put into operation. We recommend adopting a spirit of learning in which organizations consider a 6-month "settling in" period. During this period, working with change is challenging to old habits. As people learn to work differently, there can be a tendency to want to slip back into old patterns. A commitment of six months allows sufficient time to work out any structural and emotional glitches that might keep people from doing what it takes to make RBC a reality in their organization. A persistent focus on what changes are working and a commitment to increase their frequency models the Appreciative Inquiry (AI) approach and encourages long-term success.

During this phase, predetermined review times (typically twice a month) allow for ongoing monitoring and course correction. Orientation and continuing education support the implementation. In this implementation phase, we use reflection, affirmation and celebration to make successes visible. This is accomplished through practicing AI and sharing exemplar stories. We work from the assumption that "we get what we pay attention to," so we continually pay attention to even the smallest of our successes. Stories of RBC progress are integrated into leadership meetings, board reports, medical staff meetings, rounds, unit shift reports and staff meetings. Successful implementation must be encouraged, reinforced and continually and appreciatively refined.

This phase is ongoing. It is what keeps RBC evolving and what sustains the gains. In this phase, members of the health care team work together to remove barriers to quality care and simplify work processes. Their goal is always to improve care and service to patients and families. The entire team safeguards the care giver's relationship with the patient and family by continually monitoring the extent to which everything that goes on in the organization advances that relationship.

A strategy for "sustaining the gains" through continuous improvement needs to be defined. This would ideally include ongoing monitoring of progress and consistency in focus on achieving the specified goals and outcomes. Continuous learning is a key aspect of this phase; therefore educational assessment and ongoing development is critical to success. This is also where diligent utilization of the I_2E_2 formula for leading sustainable change—with its systematic addressing of the Inspiration, Infrastructure, Education and Evidence aspects of the implementation—will have its greatest impact.

Relationship-Based Care becomes "hardwired" into organizations with the focus on patients and families as the core for all relationships and decision making. Reflection on RBC is integrated into all meetings, processes of care are addressed, competency monitors are developed and evidence informs practice at all levels. The Results Council continues to provide leadership or is integrated into existing structures, but the focus continues. Other Shared Governance Councils may evolve. The Unit Practice Councils sustain the continued development by renewing and refreshing membership and by continually reflecting on practice, affirming and enhancing.

Phase VI: Continuous Improvement

The entire team safeguards the care giver's relationship with the patient and family by continually monitoring the extent to which everything that goes on in the organization advances that relationship.

Key Allies: Engaging Patients, Trustees, Physicians, Community Leaders and Health Care Faculty

—Jayne A. Felgen

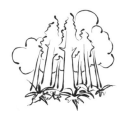

The Relationship-Based Care (RBC) implementation process actively engages many diverse and interested groups of individuals who will all play a strategic role in the longevity of RBC in the organization.

Many of our organizations have secured the active involvement of physicians or trustees, and sometimes have invited patients to play key RBC leadership roles on Results Councils. However, one organization stands out as successfully engaging not only all of these constituents but also community leaders and school of nursing faculty. This particular organization (Faxton-St. Luke's, Utica, NY) is a model for thoughtfully recruiting leaders from their extended "family" to contribute to the implementation in both short-term and long-term efforts. Their Results Council includes active leaders from the units all the way to the board and beyond.

Inviting a patient onto this oversight team sends a strong message to everyone in this organization that there is substance to their commitment to focus all energy on making the patient and family experience an outstanding one. Not surprisingly, council members report that they perform at a higher level when the ultimate recipient of their care is seated with them at the table. Including patients in shaping of the organization's practice in meaningful ways also embodies the intention of Joint Commission, Magnet and Baldrige standards.

Inviting and expecting full participation by medical staff leaders is crucial to the living collaboration that lies at the heart of Relationship-Based Care. Physicians may not have time available to regularly attend meetings during the day, but interested and committed doctors and council members have discovered ways to be fully participative without being physically present at all times. For example, in some cases physicians have read all preliminary RBC reference materials and all subsequent meeting minutes. In addition, before each meeting one council member and the physician would talk together about their responses to readings or previous minutes and make recommendations so the physicians' voices would be represented at the council meeting. This practice is often replicated at the unit level so that several doctors have important roles to play and all physicians have a mechanism to become involved.

At one organization a physician became so involved in the change process that he took a day off from his patient practice to join the Unit Practice Council in making its presentations to the Results Council and the executive team. Another medical leader joined his executive team members and attended a 5-day *Relationship-Based Care Leader Practicum* so that he was fully informed and a full partner in leading his organization's transformation to Relationship-Based Care. Including physicians in RBC implementation is an act of respect for what they alone bring to the patient experience. We must find ways to involve them and partner with them. Our patients deserve nothing less.

Most hospital boards have quality committees through which trustees have involvement in reviewing the clinical and fiscal outcomes of the organization for which they have volunteered their leadership. Many organizations are fortunate to have highly committed and visible trustees who take their fiduciary responsibility quite seriously. In these facilities it would be routine to see board members making monthly "rounds" on the patient care units in order to learn firsthand from providers of care what excites them most about their work and what patient or family outcome makes them most proud.

When a board member is also the dean of the school of nursing for affiliated students, one board member fills two roles for an even better effect. Engaging this trustee in the implementation as a member of the Results Council ensures

> Including physicians in RBC implementation is an act of respect for what they alone bring to the patient experience. We must find ways to involve them and partner with them. Our patients deserve nothing less.

that the RBC concepts are deeply understood and valued, and that the future nursing curriculum includes these concepts. The underlying theories of RBC are more likely to become integrated into the core curriculum if there is faculty involvement in Results Councils and/or Unit Practice Councils. When RBC gets integrated into the curriculum, faculty members become more conversant and supportive of practices. New graduates have less trouble acclimating to their work environment.

Hospital board members are actively recruited from leaders in the community; involving them in more than just reviewing a progress report assists the organization in spreading the word throughout the community about the real mission of the organization. Concepts become real to community members, most of whom have no clinical experience except as a patient or family member.

Another hospital board put sharing an "RBC moment" in a prominent place on the trustee agenda—before any fiscal reports. A compelling story of RBC practice happening right in their own organization helped members consciously focus each board meeting on improving the experiences of patients and their families.

Another hospital made RBC the focus of the annual board retreat. Every board member was given the RBC book, as well as a summary of each chapter and related assessment questions. Board members were asked to read the introduction to the book and the summaries and complete the assessment questions before the retreat. Since the assessment questions required information about what was really going on in units and departments throughout the organization, each board member was asked to interview a member of the executive team, a leader at the point of care, and an active member of one of the Unit Practice Councils in order to arrive at the retreat prepared to participate fully. Thus, the assessment of the current status of that dimension of RBC was evaluated through the eyes of leaders from the bedside to the boardroom.

Imagining, planning, recruiting and assigning meaningful work is both an art and a science. It takes creativity, resourcefulness and diplomacy to persuade busy people to become even busier. It also takes thoughtful, measured wis-

A compelling story of RBC practice happening right in their own organization helps board members consciously focus meetings on improving the experiences of patients and their families.

dom to align talented and influential human resources with practical functions that require expert performance and emotional commitment. Engaging these individuals redefines the boundaries of a partnership model and allows for many more stakeholders in the organization to more fully experience the rewards of their commitment.

Organizing Roles and Responsibilities for a Successful Implementation of Relationship-Based Care

—Susan Wessel and Jayne A. Felgen

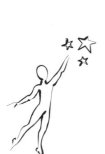

Experience has shown us that there are three important elements for the successful design and implementation of Relationship-Based Care (RBC):

- *committing to the course of the transformational change over time,*

- *setting up clear roles and responsibilities at all levels, from administration to the point of care, and*

- *fostering a culture in which extensive open communication is expected and appreciated.*

Relationship-Based Care must be planned and implemented by the staff, and at the same time leaders at all levels should prepare the organization and also coach and support the staff councils. The key leader in the executive team (often the CNO) needs to organize the effort carefully, using the existing shared governance or committee structure when appropriate, and linking groups through overlapping membership and ongoing communication mechanisms.

Regardless of the scope of the RBC implementation (nursing department only or organization-wide) it is crucial that an infrastructure be put in place to provide clarity about the roles and contributions of each individual, so everyone feels the freedom to focus on his or her primary role. Everyone in the organization has an important role in making the implementation of this complexity a success. In order for RBC to become embedded in the organization—to become the culture of the organization—it is important that each individual at every level of the organization knows how to actualize his or her role and contribution.

Figure 1 depicts the roles and responsibilities in a structure where everyone's role is valued. As administration, Results Council, managers and staff members carry out their respective roles for this major change, they must attend to all four essential components of successful change: inspiration, infrastructure, education and evidence. These elements should be repeated across time to sustain the momentum. (See page 25.)

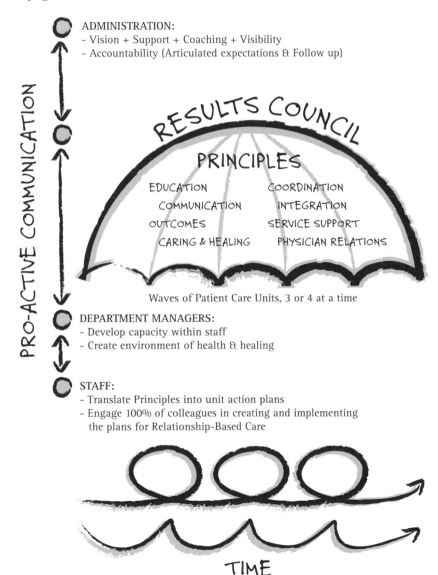

ADMINISTRATION:
- Vision + Support + Coaching + Visibility
- Accountability (Articulated expectations & Follow up)

PRO-ACTIVE COMMUNICATION

RESULTS COUNCIL

PRINCIPLES

EDUCATION   COORDINATION
COMMUNICATION   INTEGRATION
OUTCOMES   SERVICE SUPPORT
CARING & HEALING PHYSICIAN RELATIONS

Waves of Patient Care Units, 3 or 4 at a time

DEPARTMENT MANAGERS:
- Develop capacity within staff
- Create environment of health & healing

STAFF:
- Translate Principles into unit action plans
- Engage 100% of colleagues in creating and implementing the plans for Relationship-Based Care

TIME

Figure 1

Administration establishes the vision for Relationship-Based Care and articulates its connection to the organizational mission, strategic goals and desired outcomes. Executives understand that the expression of this vision in the day-to-day operations must come from those who provide the care and those who support the care givers. They also model the way by living RBC concepts and values. They coach their leaders and visibly support them by framing the RBC implementation as an investment in their future.

The Results Council (steering or oversight team) serves a key role in leading the transformation to Relationship-Based Care. This council is charged with bringing the vision set forth by administration to life. Council members coordinate the effort, integrate with other initiatives and pave the way for the staff's success through communication, education and solving system problems that impact patient care. Their work begins with the important role of establishing and endorsing a set of principles for Relationship-Based Care. These RBC Principles describe their expectations for the care delivery model and the culture of Relationship-Based Care and are developed in the following areas:

- *Caring and Healing Environments*
- *Responsibility for Relationship and Decision Making*
- *Work Allocation, Schedules and Patient Assignments*
- *Communication With the Health Care Team*
- *Leadership and Management*
- *Process Improvement*

The principles are given to staff councils at the unit/department level (Unit Practice Councils) and serve as the framework, or blueprint, from which the staff make their unique plan for RBC on their unit.

Additional and equally important responsibilities of the Results Council—which are best done through functional sub-group assignments—include:

- *devising a 12 to 18 month communication plan that reaches the hospital and surrounding community constituents;*
- *establishing a 12 to 18 month education plan for the organization;*

- *inviting key ancillary department leaders to help by working on one or two areas where support services could be improved to have a big impact on patient care;*

- *establishing a team to become experts in evidence-based caring and healing practices and to guide the councils in adopting these practices for patients and families;*

- *developing a partnership with the medical staff to strengthen relationships and encourage and expect their involvement in key areas of the implementation;*

- *integrating key decisions with human resources and other operational departments so that planned changes toward RBC are imbedded in appropriate job descriptions, hiring practices or performance standards, and operations functions; and*

- *planning the RBC outcome and process indicators that will be used to measure the impact of Relationship-Based Care.*

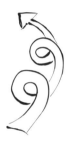

The Results Council attends to all four essential components of successful change: Inspiration, Infrastructure, Education and Evidence (I_2E_2). These elements are repeated through time such that the momentum of the change builds upon itself, and successes along the way serve as fresh inspiration for all participants.

Department managers involved in the implementation should serve on the Results Council and support the work of their Unit Practice Councils (UPCs) in multiple ways. This may include:

- *articulating expectations for RBC on the unit;*

- *leading and coaching staff in an empowering, decentralized fashion;*

- *freeing staff members from the patient care schedule for council meetings;*

- *helping the council to develop as a team and to learn effective meeting management;*

- *supporting and encouraging communication between UPC members and the rest of the staff through the established communication network; and*

- *providing public and individual recognition for making progress and meeting goals.*

The manager not only handles roadblocks experienced by the UPC, but he or she also has a key role in sponsoring and facilitating changes on the unit that would transform the environment into one that is more conducive to caring and healing for staff and patients.

The ultimate role of the manager is to develop their staff members to be the best they can be in service to their patients and families. These managers understand that their greatest achievement is the professional nurturing of their staff through the creation of a healthy work environment, where lifelong learning and innovation are highly valued.

The Staff, through their role on Unit Practice Councils, are responsible for leading their colleagues in the development of action plans in which the RBC Principles are applied to their unique patient population and unit culture. This representative group accomplishes this by utilizing a proactive communication network such that all staff members have influence in the decision-making process. The chairs of these UPCs may also be members of the Results Council and keep the Results Council updated on the status of their UPCs' progress.

Communication in all directions is essential to the success of this change process. Minutes should be taken at all meetings. Results Council meeting minutes should be shared with Unit Practice Councils and administration. Unit Practice Council minutes should be distributed to all staff on the unit and to the Results Council and Department Manager. Conversations should occur before and after each meeting to fully involve all key stakeholders on their communication network list. Communication about RBC should occur at board meetings and medical staff meetings, in newsletters, at open employee meetings, at unit staff meetings and at all types of management meetings.

It may be useful to consider a typical course of events for an organization as it implements Relationship-Based Care. In reality, these events rarely fall in such an organized pathway, but all components are attended to at some time in the process.

Typical Implementation of RBC

Literature is searched for professional practice models and ways to improve patient care.

Relationship-Based Care selected as the means to achieve the vision and mission.

RBC leadership team educated via books, articles, seminars, videos, *Relationship-Based Care Leader Practicum*, etc.

Appreciative assessment of patient care and team relationships conducted; this facilitates the discovery of elements of RBC currently in the culture. Develop a shared vision for RBC, taking care to the next level of excellence.

Design: Scope of implementation determined; roles and responsibilities for implementation by adapting existing councils or committees established. New expectations for council roles for Relationship-Based Care articulated.

Executives, managers and unit leaders attend workshop, *Leading an Empowered Organization* (*LEO*).

Results Council is formed and oriented, becomes educated about RBC and develops/endorses Principles for RBC within the organization. Functional subgroups begin their work intended to support work of Unit Practice Councils.

Initial 3 to 4 units selected for first wave of implementation; Unit Practice Councils are formed.

Members of Unit Practice Councils attend inspirational/educational programs, watch videos, and read books and articles to gain knowledge of the science of caring and team building.

Education for Unit Practice Councils in Principles of RBC, group process, communication and expectations of role including timetable.

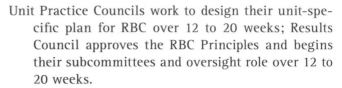

Unit Practice Councils work to design their unit-specific plan for RBC over 12 to 20 weeks; Results Council approves the RBC Principles and begins their subcommittees and oversight role over 12 to 20 weeks.

Manager provides ongoing support and encouragement to Unit Practice Council; Project Leader meets with them for status check meetings.

Final presentations of plans by Unit Practice Councils and Results Council to each other and other key leaders.

Implementation begins with much support and celebration from the organization.

Unit Practice Councils and Results Council continue to meet monthly to review outcome and process measures and to promote continuous improvement.

Second group of units (Wave 2) may be initiated three quarters of the way through this first cycle by the Results Council.

Subsequent waves are initiated in a staged and orderly manner.

Implementing Relationship-Based Care requires sustained focus and effort over 2 to 3 years or more. Maintaining that effort is not easy with so many competing priorities, but with clear allocation of time and resources it is possible. Utilizing the I_2E_2 formula for assessing progress and planning next steps will help keep this task manageable.

The most successful organizations see RBC as the overarching "way of being" in the organization, aligning and integrating all initiatives.

It's important to find sources of inspiration to keep the momentum, whether through patient rounds, stories of success or the satisfaction of seeing the outcome measures improve. Part I of this field guide provides many inspiring stories and creative ways you can capture your own successes and create your own inspiration.

Your RBC Leadership Team— From Formation to Function

Jayne A. Felgen and Susan Wessel

In the most successful Relationship-Based Care (RBC) implementations, there are at least four leaders of the project, each with interdependent and complementary roles:

- *one executive sponsor,*
- *two co-leaders of the Results Council, and*
- *one or two internal project leader(s).*

Executive Sponsor

The role of administration is to prepare the organization and community for Relationship-Based Care and visibly support all the groups involved in this cultural transformation. This starts by developing a shared vision for Relationship-Based Care and articulating that vision throughout the process. That vision will take shape as others are engaged in personalizing it.

There will be one (or occasionally two) Executive Sponsors of Relationship-Based Care implementation. The sponsor's role is to keep the entire senior team informed and to involve them in communication with key stakeholders.

Senior leaders coach and support other leaders and managers as they lead the implementation efforts. This support may take the form of understanding the nonproductive time and dollars involved in staff councils as an investment in the future. It also means holding themselves and those who report to them equally accountable for completing their respective assignments in service to this implementation—particularly the Results Council functional groups. Each level and group must do its fair share. In addition, some executive team members "adopt" individual Unit Practice Councils (UPCs) and visibly support their progress by serving as an additional coach and resource.

Executive Sponsor Qualifications

The executive sponsor is typically the Chief Nursing Officer or the Vice President of Patient Care, though the position is not limited to individuals in these roles.

Two key concepts must be embedded in the consciousness of the CEO and the entire senior team.

The only way substantive change in practice will occur is when the entire organization owns the process.

They must understand RBC and the profound impact it will have on both patients and employees.

This insight can be gained in a number of ways. Commonly used methods are attending workshops including the *Relationship-Based Care Leader Practicum*, reading *Relationship-Based Care: A Model for Transforming Practice*, listening to stories from patients having experienced RBC principles in their care, and engaging in conversations with fellow executives at organizations having implemented Relationship-Based Care.

They must believe in and endorse RBC as the best method or pathway to achieving the mission and vision for excellence in patient care and employee recruitment and retention.

Members of administration should be able to articulate to their many stakeholders how RBC supports the mission, vision and values. It's also helpful to organize the effort so that resources can be integrated with other initiatives, such as quality programs, and designations such as Magnet designation or Malcolm Baldrige.

Responsibilities of Executive Sponsor

The senior leader sponsor of RBC has overall responsibility, authority and accountability for shepherding the culture change and involving senior colleagues. The sponsor's role will include things such as:

- *Understanding RBC in all its dimensions and how it supports the organization's strategic plan, mission and financial and quality outcomes.*

- *Determining the best strategy and timetable for implementation.*

- *Educating the entire senior team about RBC and submitting a proposal for consultative assistance.*

- *Leading the senior team in developing a shared vision for RBC including its linkage to corporate mission, vision and values.*

- *Representing RBC to all constituents. Inviting hospital leaders to the RBC workshop.*

- *Using the existing shared governance structures when possible and incorporating RBC implementation into their scope and functions.*

- *Recruiting membership for the Results Council.*

- *Appointing one or two Project Leaders from within the organization.*

- *Communicating with all patient care employees about RBC and their future involvement. This should include multiple communication channels.*

- *Discussing with the senior team options for communication with the medical staff, board, community and employees at large.*

- *Attending Results Council meetings and supporting and encouraging all groups in their work.*

- *Meeting regularly with Project Leaders, relieving some of their regular duties as needed to ensure that they have adequate time to focus on Relationship-Based Care.*

- *Incorporating the developmental phases of RBC into the nursing strategic plan.*

- *Sustaining their vision and focus on RBC even with other competing priorities and crises.*

- *Keeping inspired through activities such as hearing the plans of staff councils, attending the Reigniting the Spirit of Caring workshop, attending the Relationship-Based Care Leader Practicum, and conducting patient rounds following implementation.*

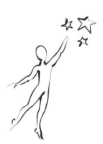

> • *Leading, supporting, encouraging and celebrating progress along the way.*

The success of RBC is a direct result of the enthusiasm and support of the senior leadership team. Although it is possible to implement RBC on a smaller scale quite successfully, the full impact on patients is best felt with the full involvement and support of all senior and mid-level leaders throughout the organization.

Results Council Leaders

Savvy and sound leadership of the Results Council (RC) is critical to the successful management of the change process. Selecting two additional leaders from within the organization distributes the related workload and diminishes the chance of overload and burnout. It also creates an opportunity to showcase internal talent and engage other "stars" in the organization in a meaningful way.

Often, those most successful as Results Council Leaders are mature in their roles, committed to excellence, and have superior organization, coordination, diplomacy and facilitation skills. Increasingly, these leaders represent nonclinical service support, allied health professionals and clinical professional departments. Complementary skills and a commitment to contribute individual talents have resulted in very dynamic leadership and implementation results.

Results Council Leader Qualifications

Results Council Leaders are key leaders who are respected by their peers for their values and commitment to patient and family care. Ideally these leaders are:

- *dedicated to patient and family care,*
- *passionate and knowledgeable about Relationship-Based Care,*
- *possessed of highly developed interpersonal skills,*
- *skilled in organizing events and the efforts or others,*
- *well versed in quality improvement, and*
- *interdisciplinary department heads and/or human resources leaders.*

Responsibilities of the Results Council Leaders

It's important to emphasize that the Results Council Leaders need to guard against doing too much. Having two RC Leaders to share the coordination role ensures that forward movement occurs even when one RC Leader may need to be away.

The most vital role of the Results Council Leaders is to establish a communication network between the RC and 100% of the organization's management and physician leaders. The only way substantive change in practice will occur is when the entire organization owns the process. Department heads, senior leaders and physician leaders must be informed, involved and confident that they are listened to and that their input matters.

While ultimate accountability for dissemination of information falls to the RC Leaders, each Results Council member is responsible for sharing information, asking questions, getting input from other leaders and using that input in making decisions. Members are also responsible for giving information about team actions, plans and decisions. The communication network is the framework for meeting this responsibility. Face-to-face dialogue is preferable to surveys and notes for generating ideas and involving all of the staff.

The only way substantive change in practice will occur is when the entire organization owns the process.

Project Leaders

One or two experienced and respected leaders are designated by the organization to serve as internal Project Leaders for implementation of Relationship-Based Care. They serve as the eyes, ears and hands of the organization and coordinate all activities related to implementation. In most organizations—especially those that are larger or more complex—it's optimal to have two individuals serving as co-Project Leaders. This not only spreads out the additional responsibilities, but also provides an important source of support and inspiration for both leaders.

Project Leader Qualifications

The ideal Project Leader will have the following qualities:

- *highly regarded in the organization with recognized values consistent with Relationship-Based Care*
- *already in an operational position of authority*

- *strong background in patient care leadership (some line-management experience is a plus but not essential)*
- *in-depth knowledge of the organization including its culture and structures*
- *reputation as an effective leader, coordinator and facilitator*
- *excellent relationships with staff, managers and executives*
- *someone who can "make it happen!"*

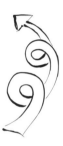

The internal Project Leader serves as liaison to the groups within the organization's infrastructure, advising them of all needs and problems during the entire project. In order to fulfill this role, Project Leaders need to be in regular contact with Unit Practice Councils and the Executive Sponsor. The Project Leaders will be called upon to explain RBC to multiple audiences and to maintain a constant flow of communication throughout implementation.

Responsibilities of the Project Leader

Successful Project Leaders will generally carry out most of the responsibilities listed below. Since every organization presents its own unique challenges, Project Leaders should demonstrate creativity and autonomy in finding additional ways to keep up the momentum and coordinate all efforts.

- *Become well educated on Relationship-Based Care.*
- *Assist the executive sponsor to organize the RBC infrastructure including Results Council and Unit Practice Councils to integrate existing initiatives and groups (e.g., shared governance, customer service initiatives).*
- *Link RBC with the organization's mission, vision and strategic goals, working closely with the executive sponsor, the Results Council and consultant.*
- *Support the success of Unit Practice Councils:*
  a) *facilitating the process for councils to seek support in facilitating meetings and resolving*

> *meeting conflict (often there are internal experts on group facilitation)*
>
> b) *visiting meetings on a regular basis for encouragement and updates*
>
> c) *gathering unit council chairs periodically for coaching, mutual support and idea sharing*
>
> • *Keep the CNO informed with regular communication. Advise the CNO and other executives when their presence or encouragement is needed.*
>
> • *Coordinate the activities or RBC implementation with internal infrastructure and external consultants.*

One of the biggest challenges for Project Leaders is to stay focused and sustain their efforts over the months and years necessary for this cultural transformation. Project Leaders need regular contact with colleagues who are positive and excited about Relationship-Based Care. Using continuous improvement strategies to share successes through data and stories will help maintain this focus.

Leaders Inside and Out

Relationship-Based Care is more than an innovative transformation model to achieve what is best for patients, families and employees. Relationship-Based Care is also a model for successful leadership in life. One CEO described RBC to a peer about to begin implementing it in his own organization as "the single most important contribution you will make in your entire career." This CEO understands and lives the principles of RBC each and every day, at work, at home and in the community. All positional RBC leaders are both pledged and committed to embody the principles of RBC in all walks of life, and these leaders confirm for us again and again that "living RBC '24/7'" makes a positive impact not only on their organizations but on their lives as a whole.

One of the biggest challenges for Project Leaders is to stay focused and sustain their efforts over the months and years necessary for this cultural transformation. Project Leaders need regular contact with colleagues who are positive and excited about Relationship-Based Care.

Results Councils

—Jayne A. Felgen

The Results Council (RC) is the leadership body, the steering team, which oversees the entire Relationship-Based Care (RBC) implementation process. While each organization will determine the personnel mix of its Results Council, these councils function best when they are multidisciplinary—comprising individuals from a variety of disciplines, primarily of leaders with positional authority and also staff leaders of the units/work areas directly involved in the RBC implementation.

> **The Results Council must be perceived by the larger organization as a group with the accountability for its mission and strategic plan.**

The Results Council must be perceived by the larger organization as a group with the responsibility, authority and accountability for its mission and strategic plan. The work of the RC is the means and method of achieving strategic goals. Consequently, this group must consistently demonstrate that it is "in touch" with what is already happening in the organization as well as what is realistically possible for the organization's transformation. Results Councils can be anywhere from 12 to 35 members, depending upon the size of the organization. Expert organization skills and clearly articulated expectations overcome the traditional ineffectiveness associated with large work groups. In fact, embracing an enthusiasm for inclusivity over exclusivity has had very favorable effects on members' ownership and widespread organizational support.

The first step when planning an RBC implementation is to identify individuals within the organization who already demonstrate an inclination toward relationship-based practice and principles. Leaders with positional authority who are respected by their peers for their values around patient and family care are ideal recruits for key RBC leadership roles. These four roles include RBC project leader, executive sponsor, and Results Council chair and co-chair (see page 201).

The Results Council membership will include:

- *senior executives*
- *medical staff*
- *board members*
- *department heads responsible for human resources, community relations, quality outcomes, organizational and staff development*
- *allied health professionals*
- *managers and staff leaders on each of the units in the first "wave" of implementation*
- *a community representative (optional)*

Physician participation in the Results Council is especially important to facilitate interdisciplinary partnership vital to the achievement of positive patient and family outcomes. One specific goal of RBC is to assure that each attending physician is provided pertinent patient information from the Primary Nurse. Strong, collaborative working relationships among RNs and physicians positively affect patient outcomes. Physician participation in the Results Council helps bring the RBC principles and philosophy into the community of physicians within the organization.

In most cases, 4 to 6 weeks are allowed for the initial talent search and recruitment, and the establishment and orientation of the Results Council. Once identified, these individuals are invited to attend an all-day meeting in which RBC concepts and the roles and responsibilities of the Results Council are discussed. Those invited may be asked to review *Relationship-Based Care: A Model for Transforming Practice* prior to the meeting so they have a clearer notion of the new direction the organization intends to take with their help. Some may attend Creative Health Care Management's *Relationship-Based Care Leader Practicum* (see 468).

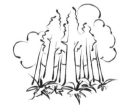

The Results Council champions the entire change process. This council owns the responsibility, authority and accountability for the design; integration with mission, values, vision; implementation; periodic evaluation of impact; and ongoing support necessary to implement and sustain the actualization of all RBC principles throughout the organization. The council has Level 3 authority over this process (see 486).

In order to coordinate this comprehensive multidisciplinary effort, functional subgroups are formed to develop action plans specific to their areas of expertise. These groups present their draft plans to the Results Council to gain consensus endorsement, and later report their progress monthly and lead discussions for course enhancements or celebration as appropriate (see below). All subgroups address areas that are critical to the success of implementing and sustaining Relationship-Based Care.

Results Council	Subgroup Functions
PRINCIPLES	The chief nurse and the executive nursing leadership team are responsible for developing clearly defined principles for nursing that will guide the implementation of Relationship-Based Care throughout the facility, regardless of clinical settings. Principles for other clinical professions, allied health services and support staff are developed by the appropriate RC members. These principles serve as the blueprint for a consistent approach to care with the expectation that their translation into unit design, allied health and service support departments will be as unique as the clinical settings in which RBC will be experienced.
COMMUNICATION	A 12 to 18 month communication plan is needed that includes all stakeholder groups impacted by this change process to create a sense of excitement and relevance to the facility's core mission. Thus, it is likely that messages regarding the launch and achievements of the RBC initiative will be integrated into meeting agendas, annual reports, and newsletters to the community, board of trustees, medical staff, executive team, managers and staff.
EDUCATION	A 12 to 18 month educational plan that meets the needs of all stakeholder groups that are involved in this process is essential. This will likely include leadership and management skills, caring relationships, critical/creative thinking, and relationship management skill building for everyone. Implications for staff recruitment, hiring, orientation and continuing education should be considered in order to sustain the model over time.

SERVICE SUPPORT

Two or three department heads responsible for the provision of support services to patients and families may serve as a team. Their role is to assess, design and implement strategies that will assure that patients, families, and nurses and staff have what they need when they need it. It is assumed that these efforts will include input from the patient care unit representatives and front-line staff in these service areas. Their goal will be to eliminate the barriers to care that are most common.

CARING/HEALING

A small group of colleagues interested in caring/healing modalities will have the responsibility to research caring/healing practices that have been success-fully launched in traditional health care facilities, and to inform the RC and Unit Practice Councils (UPCs) of their findings. This responsibility includes the engagement of all disciplines in this process including the educational subgroup so that the core values of RBC are introduced and sustained, again over a 12 to 18 month period initially.

PHYSICIAN COLLABORATION

This group's goal is to develop a 12 to 18 month plan to implement or enhance strategies that will fully engage the physicians in support of the RC and UPC efforts to achieve positive patient and family outcomes. It will also focus on the creation of healthy work environments for physicians. One RBC principle is to ensure that each attending physician is provided key, pertinent patient information from the Primary Nurse. A partnership model with RN, physician and patient managing the patient's care is expected to favorably impact patient outcomes. This relationship will require mutual respect and trust.

INTEGRATION

The chief nurse or vice president of nursing and human resource executives typically form this subgroup to ensure that all good ideas and changes made at all levels of the organization are translated into the daily fabric of the organiza-tion (e.g., management protocols and language, job descriptions, performance evaluations, staffing patterns and physical environment).

OUTCOMES

This group is responsible for drafting a plan to measure key outcome and pro-cess indicators known to be related to work redesign (human resource, patient cost of care, clinical quality, perceptual quality, patient and staff satisfaction), and those specific to Relationship-Based Care. Baseline and periodic measures should be included in a report-card format and shared at all levels of the orga-nization. Unit Practice Council members will anticipate guidance and support in developing unit-based measures specific to their implementation.

COORDINATION	A Relationship-Based Care project leader serves as "air traffic controller" for this comprehensive transformational process. The project leader ensures that the scheduled activities are possible and communicated using a 12 to 18 month plan as the template initially and over time to monitor progress. This person is the chief liaison with the chief nurse and the Creative Health Care Management consultants, and serves in support of the RC leaders and members.
OTHER	There are often preexisting work groups actively developing plans for related activities (i.e., Joint Commission preparedness, Magnet designation application process, healthy workforce initiatives and schools of nursing). Inviting representative leadership to participate as full members or as periodic ad hoc reporters enhances the integration functions.

Working with Results Councils is immensely satisfying. My biggest "take-aways" when working closely with these councils have been:

The relationship between the ultimate success of the implementation and the clear, visible support of the CEO and other executives is compelling.

1. The relationship between the ultimate success of the implementation and the clear, visible support of the CEO and other executives is compelling. In organizations that have successfully embedded the RBC principles into their fabric, the CEO and senior executives have held each other and each council member responsible for full participation in the work of the council and integration into their departmental functioning and reporting. Relationship-Based Care is not just another project, but rather is viewed as the "ultimate work of the organization and contribution of their careers."

2. The shared leadership among the executive sponsor, the project leader, the chair and co-chair allows a depth and breadth of leadership engagement that plays to their talents, strengthens the overall effort and diminishes the possibilities of overloading any one person. This partnership model effectively reinforces RBC concepts. Joint attendance of

these RBC leaders at the *Relationship-Based Care Leadership Practicum* has provided a solid foundation, strengthened their work as a team and facilitated both a shared vision and a strategy for success.

3. Immersion of RBC leaders and Results Council members in RBC books, videos and related reference materials is vital to grounding for future action planning and decision making. This grounding dramatically eases implementation. Time spent preparing is absolutely critical to clear understanding of RBC and what RBC means to them and others in their organization. Staging these efforts leads in the end to a more effective and efficient implementation. Relationship-Based Care is about deep and lasting transformation—it is "a marathon, not a sprint."

4. Engaging patients, families, community leaders and professional communities in the RBC implementation has successfully broadened the impact of organizational efforts. This has established RBC organizations as leaders in their geographic and professional communities.

Clear and strong leadership by the entire Results Council will engage all stakeholders to commit to an RBC environment and will reinforce the vision for this care delivery transformation, resulting in extraordinary benefits to the patients, their families, all staff and physicians!

Clear and strong leadership by the entire Results Council will engage all stakeholders to commit to an RBC environment

Unit Practice Councils

—Colleen Person

Editors' note: *The term Unit Practice Council (UPC) typically refers to clinical nursing units. The term Area Practice Council (APC) may be used for councils comprising members from clinical disciplines, allied health and/or support service departments.*

The Unit Practice Council (UPC) has the responsibility, authority (Level 3) and accountability to plan, implement and continuously improve their unit-specific Relationship-Based Care (RBC) (see page 486). The plans are based on the principles and macro outcome measures selected by the Results Council (RC). The principles and desired outcomes are typically derived from findings that emerged through an Appreciative Inquiry assessment of the organization. Consistent with Level 3 authority, unit-specific plans will be discussed with the Results Council prior to implementation. Continuous evaluation and performance improvement are integral parts of the process.

The members of the Unit Practice Council are chosen by their peers to represent them. Each staff member notes who they want to represent them through a sociometric methodology designed to select the formal and informal leaders on the unit. The UPC is responsible for designing the unit-specific plan through a consensus-based decision-making process that includes two-way communication with 100% of the staff. Unit Practice Council members promote healthy interpersonal relationships with peers.

The work of the Unit Practice Council unfolds in the following six phases (see page 182):

- *preparation,*
- *structure,*
- *planning,*
- *review,*
- *implementation, and*
- *continuous improvement.*

Unit Practice Councils are provided with information, education and, when an implementation is supported by Creative Health Care Management, a customized *Relationship-Based Care Implementation Guide* to focus their activities throughout the six phases. An *Implementation Guide* provides focus, describes the sequencing of activities critical to success, and contains questions to guide the development of Relationship-Based Care (RBC) at the practice level. As council members answer the questions specific to each principle, their unit-specific plan begins to take form.

Phases I and II include the preparation and structure of the Unit Practice Council. Phase III is the planning phase for the unit-specific plans. A set of principles, grounded in Appreciative Inquiry findings and approved by the Results Council, is used as the guiding framework for the plan (see example 224).

Unit Practice Council members develop plans through a consensus-based decision-making process. In order to assure unit-wide involvement and ownership of the plan, the UPC members establish a communication network so that they may provide information to 100% of their staff colleagues and solicit input from them throughout the planning process. The unit plans are shared with the Results Council in Phase IV and after discussion and support, the plans are implemented in Phase V. Phase VI, continuous process improvement, is ongoing and based upon identified outcome measures at both the unit and organizational level.

The work of the Unit Practice Councils typically provides the essential foundation for the development of a Shared Governance Model to support Professional Practice. Staff members develop as decision makers and become clearer about their scope of responsibility relative to their relationships with patients, their roles as team members, and the care delivery model that organizes their daily work. The experience of planning, making decisions and implementing their ideas at the unit level establishes a foundation for the evolution of organization-wide shared governance councils with areas of focus such as leadership, quality improvement, professional practice and education.

Staff members develop as decision-makers and become clearer about their scope of responsibility relative to their relationships with patients, their roles as team members, and the care delivery model that organizes their daily work.

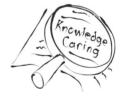

Directors and managers provide direction, and they support and promote the growth and development of the UPC and other staff at the unit level. These leaders articulate expectations for the unit, clarify the boundaries (including the level of responsibility, authority and accountability of the UPC), provide assistance in managing resources, help the council problem-solve and eliminate barriers to the implementation of their plan. Unit Practice Councils turn vision and principle into action. The leadership team provides an essential link with the Results Council and the UPC throughout the process.

The Results Council is responsible for the overall design and implementation of Relationship-Based Care Delivery (see page 208). The members (comprising executive leaders, managers and staff council leaders) design the organizational framework, principles and outcomes measures. They provide inspiration, direction and support for the initiative. Members of senior administration support the Council through their specific operational duties.

An Internal Project Leader for Relationship-Based Care assists with communication, resources, facilitation, and coordination of activities to support the implementation. Consultants from Creative Health Care Management are available to provide education and consultation to facilitate the work of the UPCs, the leadership team and the Results Council. The members of the Interdisciplinary Team, including physicians and support/service departments, are welcomed as essential colleagues and contributors to the success of Relationship-Based Care.

In a decentralized approach to the development and/or enhancement of care delivery and professional practice, each council has clearly defined roles and responsibility, authority and accountability. Furthermore there are clearly defined communication networks so that every voice is heard and all ideas listened to before consensus-based decisions are made—all essential for caring in every relationship to become a reality.

In a decentralized approach to the development and/or enhancement of care delivery and professional practice each council has clearly defined roles and responsibility, authority and accountability.

Status Checks: Monitoring and Encouraging the Progress of Unit Practice Councils

—Susan Wessel and Jayne A. Felgen

An important role of the Project Leader for Relationship-Based Care (RBC) is to support, coach and monitor the progress of the Unit Practice Councils (UPCs) as they plan how to implement Relationship-Based Care. Unit Practice Councils typically meet for between 16 and 20 weeks to plan their implementations. Their manager should check in with them regularly to support and encourage them. A second and equally important source of support comes from the Project Leader in the form of status check meetings during the planning phase. The frequency is determined by the needs of the groups. When Creative Health Care Management (CHCM) consultants are assisting with RBC implementation, we perform these status check meetings at 4 to 6 week and 14 to 16 week checkpoints, the second meeting falling about 4 weeks prior to expected presentations. The primary goal of this last meeting is to assure that the UPC has stuck to the chief principles of RBC, and that members are clear about what they will do, not just what they want to do, to change their practice. A secondary purpose of this last meeting is to help the staff prepare for their final presentation to the Results Council and the other Unit Practice Councils.

It's helpful if these status checks have a positive tone overall—meeting the staff where they are, celebrating the work done so far, and coaching them as needed. We have used the two tools shared below to help us and the Unit Practice Councils prepare for both the status check meetings and the final presentations. It's helpful to give the agenda to councils before the status check meeting to assist them with preparation.

Unit Practice Council Status Check Agenda

Objectives

- *To reflect on progress to date*
- *To celebrate progress*
- *To develop specific action plans to sustain momentum and prepare for presentation to Results Council and subsequent RBC implementation*

Agenda

1. Celebration: What are you most proud of accomplishing since the last visit?

2. Organization and Structure: Who is the leader, co-leader, recorder, facilitator, executive sponsor?

3. Membership: How many UPC members are there and how were they selected?

4. Communication Network: How many contacts does each member have? Who are they? Who are the additional ally contacts (physicians, other departments)? How many meaningful conversations have taken place?

5. Meetings: How many times has the UPC met? How long are the meetings? Have they gone well? Has everyone completed the "get smarter" assignments? Which event has been most inspiring so far?

6. Review plans specific to the RBC principles.

7. Lessons learned: What has been learned about RBC and leading a change process with peers? What have been the individual and group *Aha*'s?

8. What have you determined will be your greatest challenge? What will it take to overcome that challenge?

9. Needs: What support do you need from UPC colleagues, peers, managers, administrators and/or CHCM to be successful?

> **Reflection and Expectations**
> 1. Review the schedule and agenda for the next check—or for the final presentation
> 2. Questions and discussion

Relationship-Based Care Implementation Plans Presentations

Presentations should involve all UPC members and will showcase how RBC principles will be uniquely implemented on their unit. One hour and fifteen minutes may be allocated for each UPC and for the Results Council. This allows for a 45-minute presentation followed by a 15-minute Q&A session. A 15-minute break following each group will allow the next group time to set up. Each group deserves undivided attention. Handouts are recommended.

All UPCs attend all presentations along with nurse managers, Results Council members, executives, CEO and selected medical staff. Community relations or a photographer should be invited in anticipation of newsletter publications.

The Results Council should consider presenting last. Their purpose is to describe the status of each of their functional work groups and how they will support and measure the efforts of the UPCs.

Presentations

Presentations should creatively reflect each group and include at least the following topics:

- *Introduction of UPC members*
- *Description of unit and patient populations served (Patient and Practitioner Profile)*
- *Communication network and methods used to share information, engage their peers and achieve "buy-in"*
- *How RBC Principles will be visible on their unit, particularly the accountability relationship between the RN or care giver and each patient. Consider organizing presentation by the six elements of RBC Principles*

- *Unit-based quality outcome measures selected to measure the impact on patients, families, physicians and colleagues*

- *What their immediate next steps are, and support requested before implementation date*

- *Summary*

- *Question and Answer*

- *Affirmation and Celebration*

The spirit of the questions should be affirmative and encouraging. When staff members experience this type of feedback it serves to reinspire them for the next stage of their work while at the same time achieving the type of follow-up that fosters accountability for results.

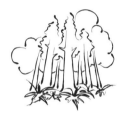

Adapting Relationship-Based Care Principles for Your Organization

—Susan Wessel and Colleen Person

The RBC Principles represent the heart and soul of Relationship-Based Care (RBC). The RBC Principles provide the overarching framework for every department to plan their own unique RBC design—customized to their own services or specialty. During the planning and implementation phases, the RBC Principles guide the development of definitive plans at the unit and department levels so that RBC can be *lived* in every relationship throughout the organization.

When designing Relationship-Based Care and the principles of the care delivery model (whether the organization intends for RBC to be interdisciplinary or "nursing only")—organizations have two options: 1) they may adopt Creative Health Care Management's (CHCM's) classic RBC Principles, or 2) they may customize the principles to their own organization. Many organizations find that CHCM's RBC Principles (which have been refined over 20 some years of experience in working with hospitals of all sizes) fit their culture and values well.

The essential values of Relationship-Based Care are embedded into CHCM's RBC Principles as they apply to each of the six elements of a care delivery model:

1) *caring and healing environment*

2) *responsibility for individualized relationship and plan of care*

3) *work allocation, schedules and assignments*

4) *communication*

5) *leadership*

6) *process improvement*

Customization of RBC Principles

While organizations should take great care not to change the essence of the RBC Principles, they may find language for the principles that more closely aligns with their own vision and culture. In this way they connect their own organizational vision with desired outcomes. The results of the organization's Appreciative Inquiry (AI) assessment (see page 96) can be used to infuse findings from the "discovery phase"—those reflecting the best of what is—into the articulation of the organization's RBC Principles. In addition, the AI assessment's "dream phase" provides a shared vision for the ideal future which can also be integrated into RBC Principles.

For example, when the themes from stories of outstanding patient care reflect that patients and staff have a more meaningful experience when they are in an individualized relationship with one another over time, this supports building a Primary Nursing role principle into the first element of the care delivery model. The registered nurse (Primary Nurse) is responsible for establishing a therapeutic relationship and an individualized plan of care with the patient and family for their length of stay.

If the visioning results in a desire for a smooth and seamless continuum of care during patient transitions, this will be reflected even more prominently in principles. One hospital added a principle saying:

The Primary Nurse takes into consideration the continuum of care, being attentive to aspects of the patient's care prior to this experience and to transitioning the plan of care to the next setting.

As another example, if an organization prides itself on family-centered care, this too will appear in the principles.

We have seen organizations customize their RBC Principles by:

- *emphasizing elements from the vision for patient care,*

- *including terms from the organization's customer service initiative,*

- *using terminology suited to their culture ("Attending Nurse" rather than "Primary Nurse" for nursing or*

"*Primary Contact" rather than "Lead" for clinical disciplines),*

- *incorporating language from a specific nursing theory embraced by the organization, and*

- *specifying that a partnership model of Primary Nursing will be used.*

While organizations should make RBC Principles their own, it's very important to minimize changes to the principles as much as possible. The heart of Relationship-Based Care is:

Preserving the Essence of Relationship-Based Care

- *The registered nurse has full authority for determining the kind and amount of nursing care a patient will receive, the work that care requires, how much of that work requires the attention and time of the registered nurse, and how much can be delegated to other care givers.*

- *Patient assignments are based on continuity of relationships, complexity of care required, and the skills and knowledge of the care giver.*

- *The manager creates an environment supportive of professional nursing practice where registered nurses are autonomous decision makers and creative problem solvers.*

RBC Principles provide the framework for the consistency of what RBC will look like across the organization. They guide the development of the unique plans of each unit and department. Relationship-Based Care comes alive when all staff members make behavioral choices in their practice to behave in a manner that is consistent with the RBC Principles.

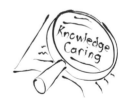

Exemplar: Primary Nursing Principles from University of California–Davis Medical Center

—Katherine Smith

The following principles were adopted by the University of California-Davis Medical Center (UCDMC) in November of 2003 to be the guiding principles for the implementation and continued development of our Primary Nursing Care Delivery Model. The principles flowed from Appreciative Inquiry sessions conducted with nursing staff and were affirmed by the Nursing leadership team.

Nurse Practice Councils on each of the units at the academic medical center were engaged in developing unit-specific plans and actions based on these principles. The councils are currently engaged in continuous sustained improvement of the model.

Professional Nursing Practice

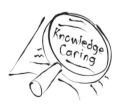

The foundation of the Professional Nursing Practice Model is the UCDMC Nursing Philosophy.

Professional Nursing Practice is relationship-based with a therapeutic presence.

Professional Nursing Practice is autonomous, evidence-based, and collaborative.

The principles of the UCDMC Professional Nursing Practice Model in each of the four elements of a defined nursing care delivery model are:

Element	Principles
Element #1: *Responsibility for Relationship and Decision Making*	1. The Primary Nurse is responsible for establishing a therapeutic relationship and an individualized plan of care that is to be in effect for the duration of the patient's experience on the unit or setting of care. 2. The Primary Nurse has unwavering commitment to establishing, implementing, communicating and revising the individualized plan of care. 3. The Primary Nurse takes into consideration the continuum of care by involving the patient and family, noting the biopsychosocial aspects of care prior to this hospitalization and coordinating the plan of care at the time of transfer to the next setting of care. 4. The patient and family know what to expect of the Primary Nurse relationship.
Element #2: *Work Allocation and Assignments*	1. Staff scheduling, assignments and delegation are driven by continuity of care and consistency of relationships of Primary Nurses and practice partners with the patient and family. 2. Assignments are congruent with patient needs and care giver competence, and provide educational opportunities for further growth and development.
Element #3: *Communication with the Health Care Team*	1. The Primary Nurse is responsible for communicating, integrating and coordinating the nursing plan of care with the interdisciplinary plan of care. 2. Representing the "voice of the patient," the Primary Nurse facilitates direct, effective communication amongst the patient/family, the nursing team and the interdisciplinary team across shifts and settings of care. 3. The Primary Nurse collaborates with the physician on rounds and with the interdisciplinary team.

Element	Principles
Element #4: *Leadership*	1. Leaders and staff create a shared vision for the unit in conjunction with the mission and vision of the Medical Center. 2. Leaders articulate goals and anticipated outcomes, using resources efficiently. Leaders achieve results by role-modeling, affirmation and a commitment to mutual problem solving of barriers to effective care and related systems issues. 3. Leaders recognize that the Primary Nurse functions in a leadership role. 4. Leaders take responsibility for their own growth and development. 5. Leaders promote professional competency development.

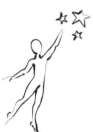

The principles and plans have guided the Nurse Practice Councils since early 2004 and serve as the focus for continued reflection and development.

Successful Change = Empowerment; Empowerment= Successful Change

—A Marie Manthey classic

There are only two kinds of change: successful and unsuccessful. Successful change has one consistent dynamic; it empowers people. Changes that don't empower people may initially appear successful, but sooner or later the "change" will dissipate and the new state will be worse then the old one. Or if the new initiative will be sabotaged or it will fail "suddenly" for no apparent reason, or the agent of change will leave—voluntarily or otherwise, but either way, his or her leaving signals a return to the prechange conditions.

For change to be truly successful, the people involved need to change the way they think about things, not merely the way they do things. This ultimately requires willingness on the part of the 'changee,' without which the change comes through coercion rather than through the agreement and commitment of those involved. Coercive changes, no matter how great the power base, seldom last.

People are empowered when responsibility, authority, and accountability are meted out in equal measure.

- **Responsibility** *is the clear allocation and acceptance of assignment so that everyone knows who will do what and when it will be done. The clear assignment of responsibility must be visible within the organization.*

- **Authority** *consists of the right to act in the area for which one has and holds responsibility. Authority must be commensurate with that responsibility, and it must be exercised or it is lost.*

- **Accountability** *involves the retroactive review of decisions made and actions taken to determine*

Originally published in Nursing Management, *20(6), in 1989. Used with permission.*

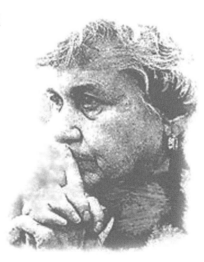

whether or not they were appropriate. If they were not, corrective (not punitive) action must be taken.

For change to be truly successful, the people involved need to change the way they think about things, not merely the way they do things.

Once responsibility is accepted, a person becomes keenly aware of the authority necessary to carry out that responsibility. Many innovations are defeated by staff and managers who effectively resist them, before the innovations even get off the ground. They refuse to accept responsibility, which results in the rejection of authority. This in turn creates a victim mindset that is exacerbated by a feeling of powerlessness over change, which is then reinforced by the refusal to accept responsibility, which reinforces a victim mindset—and on and on and on. Only by accepting responsibility and authority can we break this cycle. In this case, the process is as important as the outcome—or maybe more accurately, the process is an outcome in itself.

Experience is the best teacher. A well-designed and carefully supported change process can provide more quality education than months or even years of traditional staff development. The key experience in successful change is decision making. Management must believe that the people who perform the work know more about the work than anyone else; therefore, they are the right people to make decisions about how the work should be done. Thus, a fundamental aspect of an effective change process is to involve the people doing the work in the change decisions about the work.

A well-designed change process is founded on four points:

1. Informal leaders—those who will lead by benefit of their ability to influence others without being in positional leadership roles—should be identified and included on the team that designs the change. It may come as a surprise to many that it is important to have both the negative attitude as well as the positive attitude leaders on the team. The best way to identify informal leaders is to ask every group member to identify the people they would like to see as members on the design team other than the manager (a formal leader). For true empowerment to be achieved, managers should practice their leadership and "cheerleading" skills (not their directional/control techniques) when dealing directly with the change.

2. Establish a healthy group process based on open communication, mutual respect, and at least a functional level of trust. Clear, consistent response to group members' needs and requests begins the process. Sometimes a person skilled in facilitating groups can be used to develop a healthy group process. If the group process falters, or a few individuals dominate, the quality of the group's decision making will drop.

3. The group must have the authority to make final decisions about the way their own work is handled and the way their own units operate. Consensus decision making can be achieved using several techniques, but "voting" generally is not desirable because it often polarizes a group. Consensus is a negotiated agreement, achieved through the use of process skills to be learned if not already in place.

4. Finally, a formal communication network must be established between every member of the design team and every member of the staff. It is crucial that the design team's considerations and activities not become—or even be *perceived* as—a "secret." Every staff member needs access to both the information available and the decision-making process.

When these four key steps are carefully followed as the basis for a change/empowerment process, the right decisions will be made. No one knows more about how work should be organized than those who are doing it every day. As the attitudes of the design team begin to change—as open communication, trust, and respect become the norm for the informal leaders who comprise it—those "process changes" are transmitted to the rest of the staff via the communication network. In this way empowerment is to change as change is to empowerment. When the change process itself includes those who will be working the change every day, everyone involved becomes empowered. This empowerment, in turn, makes the change successful. And successful change—designed by those who will bring it to life—empowers all involved.

> No one knows more about how work should be organized than those who are doing it every day.

> Changes that don't empower people may initially appear successful, but sooner or later the "change" will dissipate and the new state will be worse then the old one.

229

CHAPTER SIX

Embedding Relationship-Based Care Into the Organizational Structure

Creating a Culture of Caring, Commitment and Creativity

—Colleen Person

Editor's note: *An earlier version of this article appeared in* CHCM News, *5(1), in 2001.*

Those of us involved in providing the care in health care often feel like we're living the old Chinese proverb/curse: "May you live in interesting times." These interesting times are indeed filled with challenges as we learn to balance increasing demands with limited resources. In meeting these challenges, a few key elements consistently emerge among those most successful in providing the care in health care. It becomes clearer each day that our success depends upon our ability to create and nurture cultures of caring, commitment and creativity.

As consultants we are honored to be invited into organizations across the world, and it is our experience that you can actually feel the difference in those that are committed to the human dimensions of caring as well as to the clinical and technical dimensions. We are seeing the reexamination of current mindsets about the use of time and staff resources. We see a difference in the way leaders model a balanced approach to their work and personal lives. We see it in the way staff members relate to patients and to one another; they consistently tell us that they value their current level of connection and that they want to experience even more connection in the future.

We've identified three dimensions of commitment in health care:

- *The first is the leaders' commitment to valuing the contributions of individual employees to the success of the whole. This helps staff members at all levels of the organization to take pride in what their individual work means to patients, their families and the community.*

- *The second is a shared commitment among leaders and staff to the vision and values of the organization. Clinical staff consistently demonstrate extraordinary efforts in meeting the needs of patients, but these efforts can only take place in an environment that values empowerment and teamwork.*

- *The third dimension of commitment is a personal one—it is the individual commitment to the caring relationship. When individuals feel that their contributions make a difference, they experience far more satisfaction in their work.*

Creativity

In recent years, newspapers and trade journals have been filled with stories about companies providing educational experiences—with some even creating corporate learning universities—to meet employee demands for new skills and opportunities. In the mission statements of companies across the globe, an increasing number are including an emphasis on employee development at all levels, and are reflecting this in their budgets by expanding dollars for training.

The changing nature of work requires rethinking how we can do our work more efficiently and effectively; it requires thinking creatively and critically with a perception of the big picture and a vision for the future. In her book *The Creativity Force in Education, Business and Beyond*, Dr. Berenice Bleedorn underscores the need for creativity and innovation, the need for involving employees in decision making to develop their sense of ownership, and the need for recognizing that human capital is a constant, vital resource to be recognized, cultivated and rewarded (Bleedorn, 1998). Effective teaching of creativity demands reflection and direct, experiential involvement in new ways of thinking—and it requires recognition on the part of the organization of the need to devote time to learning. It's a win-win situation when employers expand the ability of their workforce to meet the very real challenges they face. But to do so requires that leaders attend to the quintessential paradox of meeting the staffing requirements of "today" and legitimizing time and money to invest in the development of staff members as the organization's most valued resources.

Creating, enhancing and sustaining a culture of caring, commitment and creativity in our health care organizations is one of the many strengths of Relationship-Based Care. Relationship-Based Care organizations affirm successes; rethink and balance present work in light of current realities.

Reference: Bleedorn, B. (1998). *The creativity force in education, business and beyond.* Lakeville, MN: Glade Press.

Cultivating Leaders at Every Level

—Mary Koloroutis and Colleen Person

One of the hallmarks of Relationship-Based Care (RBC) is that it fosters a culture of empowerment. This empowerment typically reaches beyond shared governance structures and gives nurses the authority to make more decisions for their patients at the point of care delivery.

Power is "the ability to act or do." Traditionally we have thought of power as positional, embedded in defined leadership roles. Meg Wheatley in her mindset-changing book *Leadership and the New Science* states, "A leader is anyone who wants to make a difference at this time." In this new mindset—one completely consistent with the RBC mindset—power is personal as well as positional. In RBC's culture of empowerment, leaders make a difference by empowering care givers at the point of care to make their own decisions about how to "act or do" in the way that best serves their patients and families.

In a culture of true empowerment, positional leaders clarify the responsibility, authority and accountability of defined roles and committees. These leaders then actively seek out individuals at all levels of the organization and encourage them to enhance their own personal power and influence at the point of care as well as elsewhere in the organization. Great ideas are everywhere. Great contributions are everywhere. Models of integrity and admirable work ethics are everywhere. Great leaders mine their entire organizations for the leadership necessary to continually grow and improve the organization.

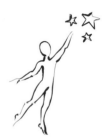

In a true culture of empowerment, no one in the organization is ever "justa" manager or "justa" nurse or "justa" transporter. "Justa" doesn't respect an individual's personhood, and "justa" backs people away from individual ownership and responsibility. Conscious recognition of employees as people means structuring our organizations to recognize that leaders

In a true culture of empowerment, no one in the organization is ever "justa" manager or "justa" a nurse or "justa" transporter.

can and do emerge at every level of the organization again and again. We find leaders at all levels by *looking for leaders at all levels.* We find out who has what skills by asking and observing, and by making it our business to know the strengths of those who work with us.

In the early phases of transition to RBC, staff members emerge who could be tapped for leadership within the new culture—perhaps those who have been working within the principles of RBC intuitively or those who have come to the organization with strong knowledge and values of professional nursing practice. It is often helpful to bring these individuals into the transition plans as positional leaders, either as members of Unit Practice Councils (see page 214) or as clinical managers if they have the requisite qualifications and experience and there are management positions to fill. Tapping these individuals for leadership brings a positive new influence into the existing management team as the entire group learns together what it will take to adopt the principles, practices and philosophies of Relationship-Based Care.

Still, the most pivotal role of positional leaders in RBC is to empower individuals at the point of care to make decisions for the patients and families they care for within established standards of care. While positional leaders will also have "management duties" such as devising budgets and schedules, it is fundamental to the success of RBC that all leaders recognize themselves as leaders rather than managers, and that they are working with people rather than tasks. Respect for each individual and his or her contribution regardless of position is essential to the successful integration of Relationship-Based Care.

At her speech at the 2004 American Nurses Credentialing Center (ANCC) Magnet Conference, Marie Manthey spoke of the importance of the role of positional leaders in empowering nurses when she said, "It's up to people in leadership positions to find that voice and to begin to speak the truth about nursing ... to [talk about] how smart we are—that nurses are smart enough and tough enough to save lives." The most important arena in which to find and express the "voice" Manthey refers to is at the point of care itself. It begins with our own recognition that the work of all point-of-care care givers is the most important work that happens in any health care organization.

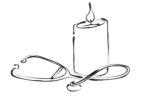

Respect for each individual and his or her contribution regardless of position is essential to the successful integration of Relationship-Based Care.

Within a culture of empowerment, individuals are called upon to work in less conventional ways. If individuals limit their thinking, initiative or voice to their own perception of a circumscribed role, they're less likely to step into new possibilities of relationship-based practice. Later in her ANCC speech Manthey says, "We discovered that the roles that people are in pretty much determine the way they behave. It was an amazing revelation to me to understand that when you give people authority for decision making, they become decision makers; and if they don't have the authority to make decisions, they don't make them." What is really happening in a hospital is happening where hands touch patients. Perhaps when people don't "go the extra mile," it's because they perceive they have no authority to do so.

This thinking is new for many, and it is essential to reinforce a "leader at all levels" mindset through validation, reflection and inquiry. When care givers make effective decisions at the bedside it is important for managers to initiate non-threatening, reflective discussions on the actions taken. Ask other team members what decisions they have made in similar situations—or what decisions they might make next time. The questions themselves reinforce the notion that critical thinking and decision making—an act of leadership—is one of the most vital things individuals are empowered to do in the care of patients. The discussion could go something like:

> *When you cared for Mrs. Jones, I noticed how you identified that she was anxious about her daughter's visit. It was a subtle cue and may have been missed—in fact you may have just as easily misinterpreted it as inappropriate anger directed at you. When you validated what was underneath her distress, she was able to open up to you and express her fears. I believe your intervention will help her cope with this daunting situation and the implications for her family. Your care raises some important questions that I think are valuable to reflect on with the rest of the team so that we can learn from your exemplary care.*

The cultivation of leaders at all levels of the organization is an act of enlightened self-interest.

The team reflection on the care could focus on these questions:

- *What did you notice that helped you indentify anxiety?*

- *How did you stay focused on Mrs. Jones rather than taking her agitation personally?*

- *What do you think would improve our care of Mrs. Jones?*

- *How can we help the other members of the team stay tuned in and supportive — especially when Mrs. Jones becomes afraid and may be seen as "difficult?"*

- *What are some key insights for us to take away from this experience?*

When front-line care givers are invited by their manager to discuss their practices in an open, nonjudging culture of reflection and learning, they begin to recognize their own leadership. They become leaders at the point of care through their actions alone, but they don't always realize they are leaders until it is validated through reflection and discussion. Front-line care givers have always made decisions that shape the patient's and family's experience more than anyone else. Too often, however, they have not been empowered to make decisions that differed much from "the way we've always done it." In an RBC culture care givers are encouraged and empowered to shape the patient/family experience through critical thinking and leadership.

An RBC culture invites conversation and initiative, and it counts on the fact that each of us has (or is willing and able to develop) the personal leadership and courage to know how to influence others. We don't check our personhood at the door. Relationship-Based Care challenges us, more than any other mode of practice, to "show up" as full human beings. In RBC organizations we don't hear, "That's not my job!" We hear, "I am the one who will help you."

The cultivation of leaders at all levels of the organization is an act of enlightened self-interest. If we intend to keep our most capable people, we must tap into the full range of their capabilities, help each person maximize his or her personal contribution, and create a culture of continued growth and development. If we hope to achieve excellence, we must cultivate expansive thinking and encourage people to use their unique gifts and abilities—we must help them to access the leader within—in order to bring the shared vision of Relationship-Based Care to life.

If we hope to achieve excellence, we must cultivate expansive thinking and encourage people to use their unique gifts and abilities

Recruiting and Hiring: Integrating and Modeling Relationship-Based Care

—Mary Koloroutis

Putting together a staff that works harmoniously as a team is one of the most significant actions a manager takes. In the context of the myriad demands made upon middle managers, it is understandable that one may see the process of hiring and recruiting as a "task to get done," thereby losing perspective on the broad and far-reaching implications of each hiring decision.

It is important for managers to be constantly mindful that the recruitment and hiring of new staff is a fundamental building block in positioning their units to offer the best care possible to patients and their families. It is also an opportunity for individuals involved in the hiring and recruiting processes to model the values and principles of Relationship-Based Care (RBC) for those having their first real exposure to the organization.

Since people are our number one asset, even during the bleakest staff shortages, it's not enough to find a "willing and warm body" to fill a position. We always want to find the most talented and best people to add to the unit—people who share the values of the unit, who have solid clinical and interpersonal skills, and who have a passion for caring and learning.

It also bears noting that one of the important foundations for successfully recruiting and hiring new staff is to treat existing staff members with respect every minute of every day. Good people want to work in organizations where they know they will be treated well, and this knowledge comes through observation of and interaction with existing staff.

It is important for managers to be constantly mindful that the recruitment and hiring of new staff is a fundamental building block in positioning their units to offer the best care possible to patients and their families.

Recruitment

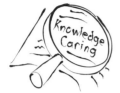

Relationship-Based Care organizations tend to attract clinicians and managers who strive for excellence in patient care and value healthy team relationships. Once RBC implementation has begun, recruiting materials should be assessed for their current level of alignment with RBC values and principles. Nursing students in particular are drawn by the quality of nursing and medical care in an organization and are always looking for indicators of the degree to which an organization will allow them to express what they went into nursing to do in the first place. If your organization promotes its commitment to treating nurses and other clinicians as empowered leaders at the point of care, it will attract nurses and clinicians who are ready to make a positive difference for patients and their families.

Because it is essential that anything an organization promotes in its recruitment materials is congruent with what is actually happening in the organization, revision of recruitment materials to reflect RBC works best as an ongoing process. If RBC is used as a recruitment strategy before the experience of RBC has become visibly integrated into the organization's culture, there will be a backlash. People who are promised a culture of empowerment and caring and then hired into a culture that falls short of that promise will likely feel betrayed.

Hiring

Candidates believe that the way they are handled through the hiring process parallels the way they will be treated as employees.

A fundamental guideline is for the hiring process to be as respectful and welcoming for people being interviewed as the organization's admissions process is for new patients. If our commitment to respectful care means that we wouldn't keep a patient waiting or fail to return a family member's phone call, that same commitment should be the basis for all other interactions as well.

Candidates believe that the way they are handled through the hiring process parallels the way they will be treated as employees. It only makes sense that we would want people in our organizations who notice whether human interactions and processes are respectful or not. The hiring process is a way to demonstrate to compassionate, self-aware candidates that we are an organizational match to their way of being. This means keeping appointments as promised, returning phone calls promptly and following up exactly as we say we will.

It is in the hiring process that candidates reach their first conclusions about the organization. Examine your current hiring practices with RBC principles in mind:

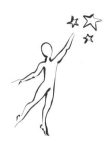

- *How would candidates rate the intake process on a scale of 1 to 10? (10 being very personal and friendly; 1 being very impersonal and not friendly)*

- *What practices/standards do you have in place regarding welcoming and establishing rapport with candidates for hire?*

- *Are calls returned promptly?*

- *Are requests handled in a timely manner?*

- *Is it obvious that new candidates are considered to be a valued part of the organization?*

- *How is this value conveyed?*

- *How would candidates rate the follow-up process on a scale of 1 to 10? (10 being timely, respectful, as promised; 1 being not timely, not respectful, nonexistent)*

- *Are candidates treated with respect in every step of the process whether they are hired or not?*

The Interview Process

In an RBC organization, success is based on the formation of solid, meaningful relationships, and the organization's value of these relationships should be visible in the interview process. For this reason it is helpful to include some standard questions designed to draw information about the candidate's current knowledge including both clinical expertise and his or her understanding and valuing of professional practice and relationship-based patient care. Inquiry regarding caring behaviors and healthy interpersonal relationships will elicit responses about what individual candidates value and expect in their practice and in the work environment. Questions can also be designed to elicit information about commitment, teamwork, judgment, decision making and values. Some sample questions for an interview for a clinical staff nurse position follow:

1) Professional Practice	• Why did you choose to become a nurse? • What inspires you to continue in the nursing profession? • How do you feel about your work/practice? • What draws you to work in this unit?—with this particular patient population? • What journals do you read to stay current in your practice? What are ways you continue to learn and remain current in the field?
2) Caring and Compassion	• Knowledge-based caring is extremely important in our practice here. Describe a time in which you cared for a patient/family when you knew your caring actions made a positive difference in their experience. • Describe the way you establish a therapeutic relationship with a patient and family. What is most challenging? Most rewarding?
3) Team Relationships	• What are two qualities your colleagues would use to describe you? • Describe a time you experienced extraordinary teamwork and what made it possible. • Describe a time you experienced a difficult situation or conflict with a colleague, manager or physician. How did you work toward resolution? What did you learn?
4) Commitment	• Describe a dilemma you have experienced in your practice and what steps you took to resolve it. • Describe a significant change you have been involved in and how you worked with and/or adapted to the change.

Questions like these get to the heart of what we really want to know about each candidate while also demonstrating the organization's focus on what behaviors it values most.

It is important for key staff members to be involved in the interview process for new staff members. Team relationships are vitally important to the successful delivery of quality care, and care givers already working on the unit are aware of what candidates would be the best fit. Interviews that include other staff members also establish early relationships and allow the candidates to get important information about the life of the unit through the experience of their peers. All individuals involved in the interviews need to be coached on the expected tone, the nature of the interaction and the specific objectives of the interview. These coaching sessions then become a very effective way for the peer interviewers to review what is important for their unit together with their manager, strengthen their own experience of team relationships and learn from each other.

It is important for key staff members to be involved in the interview process for new staff members.

In RBC practice, a promise to a patient is sacred. Because RBC has its greatest impact when it is thoroughly integrated into the organization, every promise we make to anyone is equally sacred. In the hiring process, it is important that you do what you say you will do. It erodes trust to do otherwise, and keeping a promise is an opportunity to model and reinforce caring behaviors. Each promise is an opportunity to demonstrate integrity and the importance of respect and follow-through that we hope to express in our interactions with patients and families.

Follow-Up Procedures

The entire follow-up process is an opportunity to model working in the way you'll want team members to work when they are a part of the organization. Even when you decide not to hire a candidate, handle it respectfully. While it is true that you may want a candidate later and that he or she may also talk to peers in the field, the real reason to handle it respectfully is that respect for human dignity is fundamental to the organization you represent.

Nurse Recruitment:
A Relationship-Based Approach

—Beth Ware

> "We are a community of compassionate and skilled care givers devoted to meeting the physical, spiritual and emotional needs of those we serve."
>
> —Eliza Coffee Memorial Hospital
> Mission Statement

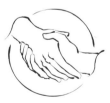

Eliza Coffee Memorial (ECM) Hospital is a not-for-profit regional medical center located in northwest Alabama. For many years we were financially strong and had little competition for employees or patients. However, the combination of a stagnant economy, a more mobile society and significant changes in health care reimbursement brought about a financial crisis of major proportions which required some drastic measures, including cutting long-established programs and personnel. This time of intense change and uncertainty left our nursing leadership and staff feeling somewhat helpless. We had lost faith in ourselves.

In May 2004, we began to work with Colleen Person from Creative Health Care Management. Through the process of Appreciative Inquiry our nursing leadership and staff looked into our hearts to chart our course for the future. We envisioned working as a team to achieve excellence in health care at ECM, and we identified as one of our top priorities for achieving this vision the development of a professional practice model. We agreed that changing our nursing staff skill mix by adding more RNs would be an initial step toward developing a more professional practice. We knew that nurse recruiting would be difficult at best and that our financial limitations meant that we would have to be creative and focused in our approach. But we also believed that we were up to the challenge.

Eliza Coffee Memorial is fortunate to provide educational experiences for both a BSN and an ADN nursing program which graduates a total of about 140 new nurses each year. But we had not been successful in the past in recruiting very many of the new graduates. Through introspection we recognized that we had never focused on establishing relationships with the students and instructors who came to our hospital. In being very honest with ourselves, we had to admit that we had often been cold, appeared to be noncaring, and at times even treated them as if they were a burden.

We began by implementing *relationship-based recruiting principles*. We first had to heal our broken relationships with the faculty of the nursing schools. Our nursing leadership team attended their faculty meetings and discussed our change in focus and told them of our desire to partner with them to educate their students. Since then we have worked creatively to provide additional clinical rotations for the schools. We provide management and clinical preceptor experiences for the nursing students and work with them on research projects. Our patient care managers also stay in close contact with the nursing faculty to make sure that their students' experiences are positive.

We have brought to life our philosophy that recruitment isn't limited to the visits we make to the schools; it is also the experiences we create for the students each time they visit our hospital for a clinical day. Now, instead of our staff viewing providing nursing students educational experiences during their clinical day as a burden, they view the students' presence as a golden opportunity to select a future teammate. Our staff nurses serve as preceptors for students for both clinical and management experiences. Our nurse managers follow up with the students during their clinical rotations to answer any questions that they may have and to make sure that they are having positive experiences. When they are making rounds throughout the hospital, our directors prioritize visiting with the nursing students in order to develop relationships with them early in their educational process. And the result of doing all of these things is that we have been successful in hiring many of our student nurses once they have graduated.

We began by implementing relationship-based recruiting principles.

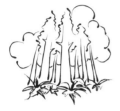

In addition, we are now hiring prenursing and nursing students as Patient Care Technicians. This means that we have had to be flexible in arranging their work hours around their school schedules. We have found that through this process, students become a part of the patient care team and develop trusting relationships with nurses whom they would like to have precept them when they transition from the role of student to registered nurse.

Now when we attend recruiting events at the schools, it is a time of fun and sharing because the relationships have already been established. We take this time to talk with the students one-on-one to determine whether or not they plan to remain in our community after graduation and what their practice area will be when they begin their careers.

Recently a new graduate shared an experience that reaffirmed for us that we were accomplishing our goal of changing our culture. This new graduate nurse had had clinical rotations at our facility while in school and had interviewed for a job with us. She also interviewed for three different positions at another local hospital that has higher entrance-level pay than we do. She shared that she tried to make the other facility feel like home, but it felt so cold and uncaring. She went on to share that at ECM everyone she had worked with was kind and caring and that it just felt like home, so she wanted to join our team despite the lower starting pay. What a joy to see that with intention we are creating what we dreamed of becoming!

Our change in culture to a relationship-based focus for recruiting has allowed us to significantly increase the number of graduate RNs we have hired over the last two years. Our leadership team is committed to helping our new employees, and our established nurses find the areas of practice that bring them joy and fulfillment because we know that this is what will make them want to stay at our hospital. The success we have had in utilizing the power of relationships in recruiting has inspired us to focus with intention on our relationships with our existing nursing staff and to implement Relationship-Based Care as our philosophy of caring for the patients and families we are privileged to serve.

Exemplar: RN Job Description, Karmanos Cancer Center

—JoAnn Maklebust and Kathleen Fedoronko

In January 2005, the Karmanos (Detroit, MI) Cancer Center's Oncology Nurse Practice Committee was given a mission from the Vice President and Chief Nursing Officer to find possible options for a new philosophy of nursing. In August 2005 several members of the Karmanos Cancer Center's leadership team (two clinical nurse specialists, two clinical managers and one director) attended a conference on Nursing Care Delivery Models held in Las Vegas and sponsored by the Forum. Sessions hosted by Jean Watson and Marie Manthey depicting Relationship-Based Care (RBC) were of particular interest to us. We were inspired by the conference and returned home realizing that we needed to inspire others in order to deliver great nursing care.

We presented nursing leadership with our suggestion to adopt Relationship-Based Care at our cancer center.

The chairperson of the Nurse Practice Committee decided to change the focus of our annual nurse practice retreat, which in previous years had reported on nursing unit accomplishments. For the February 2006 nurse practice retreat, the focus would be an introduction of Relationship-Based Care to the nursing staff. Each nursing unit or clinical area was asked to create a team of registered nurses representing all three shifts. Each nursing team was assigned a chapter from *Relationship-Based Care: A Model for Transforming Practice.* The teams were required to read, discuss and develop a PowerPoint presentation highlighting major themes from their chapter. They were asked to choose some of the moments of excellence from the end of their chapter and create discussion points to engage the audience.

Additional retreat presentations included "Patient Satisfaction," "Patterns of Nursing Care Delivery" and

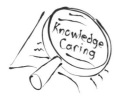

"Implementing Change." The presentation "Putting the Care Back in Healthcare" integrated caring behaviors into the RN's job description. The presentation began with how nursing has the privilege of helping others at times of crisis in patients' and families' lives and how very few professions have that kind of impact. Those in the profession need to recognize the power that it is afforded and accept the responsibilities associated with it. *Relationship-Based Care: A Model for Transforming Practice* was used as a reference for developing and defining the concepts to be incorporated into the hospital's culture. These concepts were translated into behaviors for the actual job description. The staff nurse job description addresses the following:

- *establishing a caring and healing environment;*

- *developing collaborative relationships across the disciplines including the patient and family;*

- *determining the RN's responsibility, authority and accountability when managing a patient's care; and*

- *defining leadership role expectations.*

At the retreat the new job description was presented in a very powerful way. The clinical manager and one of the staff nurses used the job description to role-play the nurse's annual evaluation. The manager read the language from the job description and the staff nurse answered with how she performed that part of the job. This method was very effective in presenting the job description to the audience.

After the nurse practice retreat, all of the nursing department job descriptions were rewritten (RN, LPN, Nursing Assistant, Student Nurse Tech, etc). The job descriptions were discussed and approved by the Oncology Nurse Practice Committee and then sent to Human Resources for grading. The RN job description presented here is in use at Karmanos Cancer Center and is used as the criteria for the annual RN evaluation.

KARMANOS CANCER INSTITUTE
Job Description & Performance Evaluation

Job Title:	*Staff Nurse*

Job Summary:

The Registered Nurse (RN) is a member of the Patient Care Services Team. The Registered Nurse is responsible to set the standards for the level and quality of care. The RN has responsibility, authority and accountability for the provision of nursing care. The RN manages and provides patient care activities for a group of patients and their families through application of independent judgment, communication and collaboration with all team members including ancillary and support services. The role of the Registered Nurse at the KCI encompasses leadership, partnership, collaboration and supervision. The RN establishes and maintains collaborative relationships with physicians, other health care providers, patients, and families, to achieve desired patient outcomes throughout the continuum of care. The RN delegates, assesses, provides and evaluates patient care. The RN assesses, monitors and evaluates patient status by observing the patient, noting data collected by other team members and analyzing this information to independently develop a plan of nursing care which is implemented by the care delivery team under the supervision of the RN. This plan of care has pre-established goals that are determined in conjunction with the patient and family. Psychosocial needs are assessed and prioritized by the patient and the health care team. The RN provides and delegates patient care activities to team members based upon patient needs and team member skills/abilities and supervises the delivery of care by other team members. The RN evaluates patient response to treatment and nursing interventions and if needed, revises the plan of care. The RN monitors patient progress and prepares patient for discharge, utilizing established clinical pathways. The RN reports directly to senior unit management and participates in shared decision-making activities.

Essential Job and Department Specific Functions:	*Does NOT Meet*	*Meets*	*Exceeds*
1. Demonstrates an understanding of and a commitment to customer service values of respect, courtesy, ownership, privacy, professionalism and responsiveness.			
2. Incorporates the KCI mission, vision, values and code of Business Conduct into planning patient care.			
3. Participates in the employment process related to peers and subordinate team members, addresses employee problems, complaints, disputes or requests as the first level of supervision; evaluates their performance post hire; and is authorized to issue work improvement plans to subordinates.			
4. Provides leadership to other members of the team by articulating expected standards of care and encouraging and supporting team members and their contributions.			
5. Establishes a therapeutic relationship and creates a detailed plan of care with the patient and family, mutually determining the aspects of care which are most important.			
6. Evaluates the effectiveness of plans and interventions to promote optimum achievement of established goals.			
7. Initiates and maintains open communication with other members of the team to assure that the patient and family receive the full scope of interdisciplinary expertise and services with a coordinated and integrated plan of care.			
8. Communicates with patients, families, subordinate staff and peers to ensure that plans and associated interventions are understood, operationalized and revised, as appropriate.			

Essential Job and Department Specific Functions:	*Does NOT Meet*	*Meets*	*Exceeds*
9. Assigns, delegates, and supervises other employees and intervenes as appropriate to ensure that the plan of care is carried out, continuity of care is provided and that established outcomes are achieved through availability and appropriate utilization of human, material and financial resources.			
10. Provides supervision, including guidance, counseling and mentoring, to targeted peers and subordinates to enhance learning experiences and improve the professional practice environment within the designated work setting.			
11. Participates in process improvement activities with an emphasis on increasing continuity in the nurse to patient relationship minimizing rework, redundancies.			
12. Demonstrates a commitment to improving the work environment through participation in meetings, timely and effective communication and an embracement of cultural diversity.			
13. Completes mandatory education and training that includes review of age-specific needs, caring behaviors, and interpersonal skills, as defined by KCI.			
14. Maintains a safe working environment through compliance with established policies and procedures and timely reporting of safety variances.			
15. Adhere to all KCI policies and procedures.			

Department Specific Functions:

1.

2.

3.

Rating: 1.0 through 4.0 _____ (transfer score to Performance Evaluation worksheet)

      Comments:

Core Competencies:	*Does NOT Meet*	*Meets*	*Exceeds*
1. Ability to establish and maintain positive, caring relationships with executives, managers, physicians, non-physician providers, patients/families other departments and staff.			
2. Ability to work productively and effectively within a complex environment, handle multiple/changing priorities and specialized equipment.			
3. Critical thinking, analytical and problem solving abilities required as related to various aspects of patient care.			
4. Good reading, writing, mathematical and comprehension skills.			
5. Good clinical judgment.			

Copyright Karmanos Cancer Institute, 2005

Core Competencies:	Does NOT Meet	Meets	Exceeds
6. Mobility and visual/manual dexterity.			
7. Critical thinking skills necessary to exercise and to lead others in application of the nursing process.			

Rating: 1.0 through 4.0 _____(transfer score to Performance Evaluation worksheet)

       Comments:

Behavioral Competencies:	Does NOT Meet	Meets	Exceeds

1. **Customer Focus:** Contribution of patient, family and/or customer satisfaction
   • Conveys a positive image of the Barbara Ann Karmanos Cancer Institute
   • Respects and protects the dignity of each person. Conveys kindness and compassion. Assists customers to maintain a control and feel valued.
   • Treats customers with courtesy at all times.
   • Takes pride in his/her work environment. Recognizes every customer as his/her responsibility at all times.
   • Ensures customers' rights to privacy and modesty. Maintains a secure and trusting environment.
   • Maintains professional behavior and dress to build customer confidence.
   • Puts the needs of customers first. Provides service in a prompt and timely manner.			

2. **Team Work:** Work as part of a group to achieve results
   • Helps create and maintain a positive environment.
   • Shares equally in the department's success and failures.
   • Works effectively and constructively to find mutually beneficial solutions for all concerned parties.
   • Shares knowledge and expertise with others to ensure the success of the team and individual efforts.
   • Asks for input and participation from others.
   • Supports co-workers by maintaining attendance requirements.			

3. **Adaptability:** Demonstrates creativity, innovation, flexibility and willing to accept challenges
   • Demonstrates willingness to adapt to change, both individual and institutional roles, needs and environment.
   • Exhibits a problem-solving attitude; constantly seeks ways to improve processes, increase efficiency, find solutions to current situations or to develop new methods and procedures.
   • Demonstrates attention to diverse populations.			

Behavioral Competencies:	Does NOT Meet	Meets	Exceeds
4. **Responsibility:** Accepting responsibility in all matters • Accepts accountability for actions, choices and outcomes; assumes nothing; answers for own conduct and obligations. • Manages his/her own work activities.			
5. **Commitment to Excellence:** Striving to do the best every day • Consistently provides quality product/service. • Commits to the principle of continuous improvement in the workplace. • Projects pride in their work as exhibited in day-to-day interactions with staff, coworkers, patients and all those they come in contact with.			

Rating: 1.0 through 4.0_____ (transfer score to Performance Evaluation worksheet)

Comments:

Physical Activities and Working Conditions:	Does NOT Meet	Meets	Exceeds
1. Physical stamina for frequent walking, standing, lifting and positioning of patients. **Supervision:** Reports directly to the Clinical Manger, Patient Services, or the Manager, Ambulatory Operations or the Executive Director, Radiation Oncology. **Working Relationships:** Internal: Contact with all employees of Karmanos Cancer Institute. External: Contact with patients, their families, and other outside parties.			

Qualifications:

1. Graduation from an accredited school of nursing.

2. BSN preferred.

3. Oncology experience preferred.

4. Licensed to practice as a registered nurse by the state of Michigan.

This job description is intended to reflect the types of responsibilities typically required of this position. However, this description does not limit or in any way modify the right of any supervisor to assign, direct, or control the work of the employee assigned to this position. The use of any particular statement describing responsibilities shall not be held to exclude other duties or responsibilities not mentioned that might be of a similar type or level.

Scoring:	Exceptional	Commendable	Meets Expectations	Needs Improvement
	4.0-3.6	3.5-2.6	2.5-1.9	1.8-1.0

Definitions:

Exceptional: Consistently meets and often exceeds all relevant performance standards. Provides leadership, fosters teamwork, is highly productive, innovative, responsive and generates top quality work. Active in industry-related professional and/or community groups.

Commendable: Consistently meets and sometimes exceeds all relevant performance standards. Shows initiative and versatility, works collaboratively, has strong technical and interpersonal skills or has achieved significant improvement in these areas.

Meets Expectations: Meets all relevant performance standards. Seldom exceeds or falls short of desired results. At times, still learning the scope of the job.

Needs improvement: Consistently falls short of performance standards.

Exemplar: Nurse Management Performance Development, North Shore–Long Island Jewish Health System

–Karen McGlynn

North Shore University Hospital (NSUH) is an 850-bed tertiary care hospital located in Manhasset, New York. The nursing leadership team at NSUH is committed to the delivery of high-quality, outcome-driven, service-based care. In an effort to continuously improve nursing practice, the model of care delivery has been transformed to one that promotes Relationship-Based Care (RBC).

Philosophy

Our philosophy of patient care is centered on the principle of caring for the patient as a whole being in a healing environment, within the context of the family and community. The nurse-patient relationship is the cornerstone of our professional nursing practice.

We believe that evidence-based nursing practice involves the integration of education and research into nursing practice. Critical and creative thinking is the foundation of our professional practice.

The blending of the nursing art of caring, data collection and application of science enables the nurse to coordinate care to provide the opportunity for patients to achieve the best possible outcomes and to advance the practice of nursing.

Vision

Our vision is the delivery of exceptional nursing care to patients and their families, by a highly competent, well-educated staff, in a safe and healing environment.

Guiding Principles

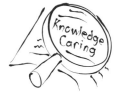

The patient and family are the central focus of our work.

- *The relationship between the nurse and the patient is vitally important and must be safeguarded.*

- *Healthy interpersonal relationships are highly valued and are based on trust, mutual respect, consistent and visible support, consideration of cultural diversity, and open and honest communication.*

- *Our nursing care is deeply respectful of the dignity and cultural diversity of each person, is attentive to mind, body and spirit, and promotes the healing power of relationships.*

Our staff is entitled to ongoing feedback and guidance to continually improve their practice, as well as to feel valued and appreciated. North Shore University Hospital has long used a 1–5 Likert-like scale (*does not meet standard* to *exceeds standard*) in evaluating the performance of its staff. This system is not only tedious, but also meaningless as the staff member focuses only on his or her "score" and not on the content of the performance appraisal. It was our desire to make the evaluation process more meaningful, professional and encompassing of Relationship-Based Care.

A task force was convened and Individual Performance Development Plans were developed for the nurse manager, the assistant nurse manager and the staff nurse. The principles and dimensions of Relationship-Based Care are threaded throughout the performance appraisal. The performance appraisal process is a highly interactive one that requires the nurse to come prepared to discuss the performance of the past year by providing evidence of how each goal was met. Any goal that was not met would require an Individual Development Plan (IDP) and timeline, which would be mutually set and agreed upon by the nurse and the evaluator.

This process of self-evaluation encourages the professionalism that Relationship-Based Care fosters. The Individual Performance Development Plan that follows is for the nurse manager.

The Individual Performance Development Plans were developed by: Karen McGlynn, MSN, RN, CNA, BC; Cecilia Maceda, BSN, RN; Lillian Diaz, BSN, RN; Debra McElligott, RN, ANP, HNP; Margaret Cooper, BSN, RN; Denise Josephs, RN; Susan Ferraro, BSN, RN-BC; Elizabeth Connors, BSN, RN; and Linda Tessier, BSN, RN.

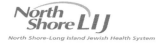

Individual Performance Development Plan

It is the policy of the North Shore-Long Island Jewish Health System (NSLIJHS), as part of its performance management program, to conduct ongoing performance appraisals for all employees.

Employee Name:	Department Name:
Job Title: **Nurse Manager**　　　Title Code: **2335**	Dept. #:
Date Employed:	Reports To:
Last Competency Assessment (if clinical):	Evaluation Due Date:
Evaluation Period - From: January, 2006	To: December, 2006

POSITION SUMMARY: As a key leader at the point of care delivery, the Nurse Manager creates the relationship-based culture of healthy interpersonal relationships so that caring and healing practices flourish. Assists the Director in assuming 24-hour responsibility for the overall assessment, planning, implementation and evaluation of patient care on the unit. Carries out the Hospital and Patient Care Services mission and vision for overall strategic planning, clinical management, patient care, budgeting and quality management on the unit. Responsible for promoting the customer service standards, creating a patient focused caring environment while addressing and meeting the individual needs of the patient and staff.

Instructions: Rate the individual on attainment of goals.

Department or Business Related Goals (see attached for examples)	Does not Meet	Meets	Exceeds
1. To create relationship-based culture of healthy interpersonal relationships	≤	≤	≤
2. To improve patient satisfaction and to increase %ile rank in Service Excellence	≤	≤	≤
3. To articulate clear expectations for staff performance **4. To engage staff in applying principles of critical and creative thinking** **5. To participate in professional self-development and education** **6. To lead with a purpose** **7. To effectively manage financial responsibilities of my unit** **8. To improve staff morale and staff satisfaction** **9. To establish a relationship-based culture in which colleagues are respectful of one another's feelings and opinions**	≤ ＜ ≤ ≤ ≤ ≤	≤ ＜ ≤ ≤ ≤ ≤	≤ ＜ ≤ ≤ ≤ ≤

Instructions: Rate the individual on meeting expectations.

Competencies for Excellence	Does not Meet	Meets	Exceeds
Accountability/Ownership (Takes responsibility for resolving problems)	≤	≤	≤
Adaptability (Changes based on unit needs)	≤	≤	≤
Caring (Shows compassion to others)	≤	≤	≤
Customer Focus (Exceeds customer expectations)	≤	≤	≤
Energy Level (Has passion for the job)	≤	≤	≤
Engagement (Shows up on time, ready to work)	≤	≤	≤
Execution (Completes all work accurately)	≤	≤	≤
Innovation (Brings new ideas to the job)	≤	≤	≤

Annual Performance Appraisal (Rev. 10/06)

	Does not Meet	Meets	Exceeds
Integrity (Acts honestly and respects others)	≤	≤	≤
Teamwork (Works well with others)	≤	≤	≤
Technical Skill (Performs responsibilities of Registered Nurse)	≤	≤	≤
Urgency (Acts quickly to meet deadlines)	≤	≤	≤

Instructions: Rate the individual overall on meeting expectations for the below categories.

Overview	Does not Meet	Meets	Exceeds
1. Organizational Goals	≤	≤	≤
2. Competencies for Excellence	≤	≤	≤
3. Overall Ratings	≤	≤	≤

"DOES NOT MEET" RATING REQUIRES ACTION PLAN AND TIMELINE TO ADDRESS ISSUES IMMEDIATELY.
Instructions: *Identify steps the individual can take to help achieve organizational goals, increase competencies and grow personally and professionally. Schedule classes at CLI (Center for Learning and Innovation), outside courses, work assignments, supervisory tasks or coaching. The IDP goals can be mutually set by the manager and individual.*

INDIVIDUAL DEVELOPMENT PLAN (IDP)	Target Date
1.	
2.	
3.	
4.	

SUMMARY STATEMENT OF EMPLOYEE'S OVERALL PERFORMANCE (include key strengths and development areas):

_____
_____
_____
_____
_____

EMPLOYEE'S COMMENTS OF THE EVALUATION AND DISCUSSION:

_____
_____
_____
_____
_____

EMPLOYEE NAME (PLEASE PRINT)_____   **DATE DELIVERED:** _____

SIGNATURE: _____

REVIEWER'S NAME (PLEASE PRINT) DATE DELIVERED: _____

SIGNATURE: _____   **DATE DELIVERED:** _____

Send the completed evaluation to your site's Human Resources Department. Retain a copy in Department files.

Annual Performance Appraisal (Rev. 10/06)

CHAPTER SEVEN

Embedding Relationship-Based Care at the Unit Level: Practical Considerations

Articulated Expectations: An Essential Tool for Clinical Managers

—Mary Koloroutis

Articulated expectations shape the culture of a work area by clearly defining behaviors and norms for teamwork, individual accountability and performance, and the care of patients and families. Articulating expectations involves assessing what staff members need to be successful. By providing for the growth and development of the staff, clinical managers help staff members meet the articulated expectations. This requires two-way communications between managers and team members.

We recommend managers articulate expectations in group settings. When all team members hear the expectations at the same time, it allows them to engage in conversation with each other and their manager. These conversations maximize clarity, minimize misinterpretation and build group ownership of the expectations.

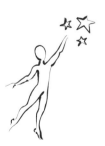

The development of articulated expectations is simple. Sit down with the intention to compile as complete a list of your clinical and behavioral expectations as possible. Then on a blank sheet of paper, write:

"I expect ..." and start your list. Your list of expectations need not be long; however, it should address all major clinical and interpersonal behaviors necessary to achieve the vision for excellence in patient care and healthy team relationships. Some examples of articulated expectations follow:

Examples of Clinical Expectations for a Relationship-Based Care Nursing Unit

I expect:

- *every patient and/or family member to know the name and role of their Primary Nurse within twenty-four hours of admission,*

- *appropriate information directing the care of each patient to be written and accessible to all who care for the patient,*

- *the professional registered nurse to determine the amount and type of nursing care patients will receive based on available resources, and*

- *continuity of relationships to be a major priority in determining patient care assignments.*

Examples of Appropriate Interpersonal Behavior Expectations for a Relationship-Based Care Nursing Unit

I expect:

- *each member of the staff to establish and maintain healthy relationships—those characterized by open communication, trust and respect—with other members of the staff,*

- *each member of the staff to take responsibility for identifying and working with others to resolve problems that affect patient care and/or the operations of the unit, and*

- *each staff member to be on time for work.*

To provide people with what they need to fulfill the expectations, the manager needs to assess any new competency requirements. For example, in order for members to work directly with each other to resolve problems, they may need skills in non-defensive communication, or they may need someone who is willing to coach and role-play with them before a difficult conversation.

Once expectations have been articulated and new skills provided for, it is essential that the manager assume responsibility for consistently managing the unit according to the articulated expectations. For example, if when making rounds a manager determines that a patient or patients do not know the name and role of their Primary Nurse, the manager is responsible for speaking with those involved to define the problem and identify actions for resolution. Perhaps even more important, where a manager determines expectations are being met, he or she recognizes and celebrates the achievement.

Articulated expectations promote mutual learning and create the playing field within which people can function safely and with appropriate levels of autonomy. Expectations delineate clearly what are and what are not acceptable practice standards and behaviors in the work area. Articulating expectations is about providing information and developing and supporting staff members for the purpose of living the shared vision every day within a unit culture. Articulating expectations is about taking what may have been "unwritten rules" for practice within a culture and making them explicit, accessible and achievable.

> Articulated expectations promote mutual learning and create the playing field within which people can function safely and with appropriate levels of autonomy.

Reference: Madden, M., and Manthey, M. (1987). *Manual for nurse managers*. Minneapolis, MN: Creative Health Care Nursing Management.

Morale Building for Managers

—A Marie Manthey classic

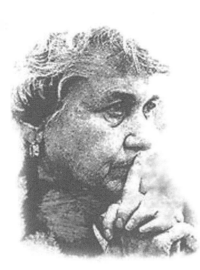

Originally published in CHCM News, (7)2, May 2003.

One of the toughest jobs in health care today is front-line manager. Clinical nurse managers, in particular, stand at a vortex of change, experiencing an unending swirl of forces pulling and pushing them to respond to the powerful demands of stakeholders throughout the complex health care system. They are expected to recruit and retain enough nurses to care for an unpredictable volume of patients, while at the same time keeping salary expenses down, morale up and physicians happy. "Oh, and could you keep your Press Ganey or Picker scores in the 95th to 99th percentiles too, please?"

During the 1990s the audit accounting firms, besides reducing RN ratios to cut salary expenses, left a legacy of multiple-unit assignments to front-line managers. Of course, when the units are very small or very similar, it can make sense to combine them under one strong leader. But what often happened was large, complex units were combined and often assigned to inexperienced nurse managers who didn't have even basic management skills, let alone leadership skills.

Managers, more than anyone else, directly impact the morale of the staff—which directly impacts the quality of patient care on a unit. We all tend to forget how important the nurse manager is to the Staff Nurse, not only as a person with great power over schedules and assignments, but also as a role model, mentor and career coach. Demoralized nurse managers have a profoundly negative impact on how a unit operates, how staff treat each other, and how patients are treated on the unit.

In the same way, nurse executives (and their direct reports) have a strong impact on the morale of the nurse manager. Again, they act as model, mentor and coach. One of the most important lessons nurses, especially those of us in leadership roles, must learn is to discern what is ours to own and what is not. It is very important for us to accept the fact that, more often than not, nursing didn't create the problems and nothing nursing does will solve the problems.

Conversely, we must own our *responses* to these problems. Managing our responses to life and work circumstances is the opposite of victim thinking. Self-management is the key to maintaining personal and professional balance in this time of constant whitewater. The following are key areas where leaders at all levels can model healthy self-management behaviors:

Manage Your Relationships	Nurse executives need to model the ability to communicate openly about sensitive and difficult issues, to exhibit appropriate "functional trust," and to respect everyone regardless of status, race, gender, education etc.
Manage Your Response to Problems	Some problems you can solve, some you can't. Deciding how to respond to those you can't solve is a powerful manifestation of self-management. Often the wisest choice you can make is to live with problems you can't solve without letting them spoil your work experience.
Manage Your Time	This is especially important for nurse executives, because the modeling you do here will ultimately trickle down through the nurse manager to the staff nurse. If you are constantly allowing yourself to be buffeted by others' demands and are unable to exercise even "little choices," you will manifest a victim-like mentality about time use. A couple of time management tricks are: • Establish office hours. Block off in advance 1 to 2 hours a couple of times a week when the staff members know they can find you in the office if they want to touch base with you. (In between visits, you will find this is a great time for paperwork!) • Take half an hour each day for yourself. Again, block off this time in advance. Visit a unit. Grab a cup of coffee in the coffee shop. Go for a walk around the block. Buy yourself an ice-cream cone. Don't just think about it. Do it.

It has been my experience that these "little choices" have a powerful effect on how much control we feel we have over our most valuable resource—our time.

The Caring Model

—Diane K. Bradley

The Caring Model (TCM) takes us back to basics, and uniquely supports creating a caring, healing environment. The model was developed by Sharon Dingman, based on her personal experience while hospitalized. The model is grounded in the research of Watson, Leininger and Swanson. The five Caring Behaviors identified by Dingman are:

- *Introduce yourself to the patient/family and explain your role in their care/service.*

- *Call the patient by his/her preferred name.*

- *Use touch appropriately: handshake, a touch on the arm, holding a hand, a thank-you.*

- *Direct care givers: Sit at the bedside for at least 5 minutes each shift to plan and review care and desired outcomes. Nondirect care givers: Sit, if possible, or be at eye level, to review procedures, tests, processes and service involved in attaining desired outcomes.*

- *Use the mission, vision and values statements in planning care or service.*

When patients feel cared for by an organization, they are more likely to return to that organization for further care and service. The model helps care givers look at themselves and their behavior and identify respectful and caring behaviors toward those being cared for.

Often the model is viewed as too simplistic because the general impression is that "everyone does these things; it's common courtesy." If that were true, all organizations would experience patient and family loyalty. Staff satisfaction, recruitment and retention would not be an issue.

> When patients feel cared for by an organization, they are more likely to return to that organization for further care and service.

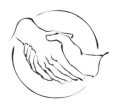

TCM also creates a professional practice environment, an atmosphere of accountability which facilitates sustainability of the model.

The Caring Model provides an orderly framework of infrastructure and education that promotes the incorporation of the five caring behaviors into the daily practice of all clinical and nonclinical staff. Unit and/or Area Teams may be responsible for integrating The Caring Model into their departments. Through increased awareness of the importance of these behaviors to patients and families, staff can be more attentive and intentional.

The Caring Model celebrates the stories of caring from care givers and encourages reflection on why people continue to choose to stay in health care. Care givers discuss how to make a difference for the patient and family. Research has proven TCM improves satisfaction; however, it is not a quick fix. The model must be "lived" throughout an organization and in every relationship with every patient in order to assure success and sustain the results.

The Caring Model also creates a professional practice environment, an atmosphere of accountability which facilitates sustainability of the model. Development of an infrastructure to support the model is critical to success. Critical junctures are explored and become the framework for the unit/department to begin to work on the patient, resident, client, family, employee and physician satisfaction indicators that are being evaluated within the organization's satisfaction surveys specific to their service.

The Caring Model is NOT an addition to what the staff is already doing.

The Caring Model is *not* an addition to what the staff is already doing. It is not a quick fix for patient or employee satisfaction or a solution to all problems. It is not a self-sustaining initiative or a "stand alone" process or a "flavor of the month". The Caring Model *is* the way we do things, not more. The model helps us make the most of time spent with patients, residents, clients and families. It is a way of relating which creates an emotional connection, and it is a proven method for improving patient/family, employee and physician satisfaction.

Work Complexity Assessment:
A Tool for Structuring the Work of a Patient Care Unit

—Leah Kinnaird

Creative Health Care Management's *Work Complexity Assessment* (*WCA*) is an assessment of the complexity and uniqueness of the work of care givers on a patient care unit for the purpose of determining how direct care giver relationships would be best structured on the unit. Every *WCA* unfolds differently, because every patient care unit is different; each *WCA* study group (usually the Unit Practice Council) is different; and the outcomes of each *WCA* are different. And yet, the end result is always the same: a knowledge-based approach to decision making about practice.

When Relationship-Based Care (RBC) is brought to an organization, changes in roles and infrastructure are inevitable. The *WCA* gives a clear, comprehensive picture of how everything works within the unit so that changes in policies, processes, and procedures can be reworked or enhanced to actively advance RBC practice. The consultant facilitating the *WCA* integrates the findings of the *WCA* for the specific organization (along with Creative Health Care Management's own tried and true processes which have proven successful in other organizations) in order to create a plan for change that is customized for the organization.

Four typical steps of a *Work Complexity Assessment* are outlined below:

Step I

A telephone interview is conducted with the nurse manager to determine the goals for the unit and to complete a Nursing Management Minimum Data Set (NMMDS) and Nursing Minimum Data Set (NMDS).

WCA engages staff to understand the unique knowledge-work of nursing practice.

The NMMDS (Huber & Delaney, 1999) provides the information about the unit in a structured format that gives a "snapshot" of the unit at that point in time, for example:

- *the nurse resources (demographics and education about the manager and the staff, number of staff, shifts, part-time and full-time status, etc.), and*

- *the financial resources (payer type, budget, etc.).*

The NMDS provides the information about patient care, for example:

- *patient diagnoses,*

- *patient interventions,*

- *patient outcomes,*

- *length of stay, and*

- *age of patients.*

Answering these questions sometimes stretches the knowledge and experience of the nurse manager, and thus raises the awareness of what is expected in terms of essential data for unit management.

When the Unit Practice Council (UPC) gathers to participate in *WCA*, members are usually surprised by the intensity of the assessment, and they leave amazed at the amount of learning that occurs. I remember a nurse from a hospital in Maryland who said, "I've been a nurse for fifteen years, and now I really understand my practice." Staff Nurses have rarely heard of the NMMDS, which is reviewed with them to have them add to and validate their manager's description. They take pride in describing their unit, and facilitators always learn as much as the study group.

Step II

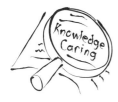

The next step is to introduce a comprehensive definition and description of Professional Nursing Practice that begins to guide them from what is often a task-based way of working to knowledge-based practice.

This involves the introduction of standardized nursing language so that *Nursing Interventions Classification (NIC)* (Dochterman & Bulecheck, 2004) can be used to describe their work. Nursing interventions are part of the Patient Care category of the NMDS. Since there are 514 interventions in the fourth edition of the *NIC* book, this can be an imposing task. We take it on with ferocity until each person knows how to use and refer to the book with ease before the *WCA* ends.

Step III

Once the group has a full understanding of *NIC*, they are ready to take a critical look at the knowledge and skill that is required to carry out the interventions that are appropriate to their unit. A standarized tool is used as the basis for the critical analysis by staff members.

They organize the interventions into mind maps (see page 412) as a way of visualizing and structuring their work on paper. Although the NIC book includes lists of interventions that have been identified by professional nursing organizations, the work of a unit is broader than any one professional nursing organization's list. The completed mind maps provide the structure for planning future educational programs, orientations, implementation of the electronic medical record, and practice improvements.

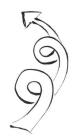

Step IV

Finally, the data collection involves a second set of questions about the amount of work the RN can delegate to other care givers, based on the knowledge and skill required to do the work.

Once the group has determined how time is spent on each domain of nursing interventions, there is a set of numbers that can be put into a spreadsheet to determine the percentage of work that can be delegated to LPNs and unlicensed staff. This spreadsheet becomes a guide for decision making.

The dialogue during *WCA* allows staff to talk about how relationships can be structured for delivering patient care. They are able to answer these questions:

- *Is it better to assign nursing assistants to the full unit or to pair them with RNs and patients?*

- *What will it take to create consistent relationships so that RNs are taking care of the same patients?*

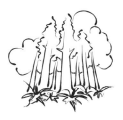

- *What can be done to distinguish the roles of RNs and LPNs (especially on units where LPNs take full assignments just as RNs do and then ask RNs to do those tasks that are not within the LPN's scope of practice)?*

- *What will it take for admission to be a meaningful process and a chance to practice RBC and not just a time to complete a form that is rarely referred to again?*

- *How can shift report be improved so that care is coordinated and seamless?*

- *Who can best care for patients while others are in shift report?*

The list of questions about the roles, the knowledge required, the delegation potential and the structure of patient care that can be raised from WCA is almost endless. When the WCA is completed, a report is prepared by Creative Health Care Management that provides a summary of the WCA session and recommendations for the UPC to undertake to improve practice on their unit.

The Work Complexity Assessment engages staff to understand the unique *knowledge work* of nursing practice. Consequently, they are prepared as individuals and as a UPC team to exercise autonomous judgment in how their unit provides RBC and to work interdependently with individuals on the nursing team and all disciplines. They know the basics of standardized language that they can put to use immediately. They are better prepared for the Electronic Health Record (EHR) and can be more engaged in the "design and build" process when their organization takes that step. Most importantly, the Staff Nurses leave with a keener sense of the value of their work and how every day they are making significant differences in the lives of patients and their loved ones.

References: Dochterman, J. C., & Bulecheck, G. M. (2004). *Nursing interventions classifications.* (4th ed.). St. Louis, MO: Mosby.

Huber, D., & Delaney, C. (1999). *Nursing Management Minimum Data Set©.* NMMDS Research Team. Contact delaney@umn.edu for more information.

Organizing Great Ideas:
Concrete Solutions for Improving Care Now

—Jayne A. Felgen

Relationship-Based Care (RBC) can only live within the context of a caring, healing environment. Any and all fundamental changes within the care delivery system must fit within this context if the changes themselves are to be substantive and meaningful. The values of caring and healing bind individual healers in a collective web of care. It is within this caring and healing culture that the dimensions of RBC can become concrete and live in day-to-day practice.

Principles of caring have an opportunity to blossom:

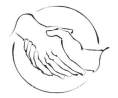

- *in leaders and leadership practices*

- *as expressions of teamwork and collaboration*

- *as the philosophical framework of the professional practice model*

- *as standards and practices in the care delivery system*

- *as compassionate informants in the judicious use of existing resources*

- *as guides to measuring what matters most to patient and family outcomes*

Unleashing an organization full of caring staff and leaders who have become inspired to practice in new ways can be as overwhelming as it is liberating. The question is always asked: "I am so inspired – am I really free to leave this room right now and change my practice?" Absolutely! Any change that involves only your individual practice and that falls within the overall scope of practice consistent with one's license or role

"What Can I Do Now?"

can be acted upon immediately. For example, an RN may want to start the practice of sitting with patients every day for a few minutes to review their plan of care, or to stop at the patient's door and consciously breathe for a few moments while refocusing his or her attention directly on this particular patient.

If, however, an individual becomes inspired to make changes in practice that would have to be performed by all RNs for all patients, then a plan to reach consensus must be created and mobilized.

Collecting Great Ideas

Once staff members become excited about possibilities they could achieve for patients and their colleagues, it's difficult to stop the innovations from flowing.

One simple way I've found to manage a plethora of great ideas without getting overwhelmed (or worse, forgetting them) is to create a file system for bright ideas. The three major file folders include Practitioners, Practice and Physical Environment.

1. The Practitioner File

All suggestions or action plans that support individuals caring for themselves, renewing their commitment to serve or balancing mind, body and spirit fall within the Practitioner file. All ideas for strengthening collegial relationships by nurturing our teammates personally and professionally are also filed here. Recording "best practice" scenarios to share with others is an effective way of legitimizing these practices and encouraging others to embrace caring behaviors at home and at work.

2. The Practice File

The Practice folder has two subfiles: one which includes *actual practices* that touch the patient directly, and another which includes the infrastructure that impacts the patient but is more *structural* in nature. In the first instance, innovations may include consistently answering call bells in 60 seconds, or a one-hour "quiet time-out" for all patients every afternoon during which no therapies, consultations or personal visits

> *Once staff becomes excited about possibilities they could achieve for patients and their colleagues, it's difficult to stop the innovations from flowing!*

occur. It may also include evidence-based practice changes involving complementary care practices, aromatherapy, Reiki, guided imagery, etc. The subfile that includes ideas for changing the infrastructure to impact patients may include things like the practice by which each patient is selected by one RN to establish a therapeutic and accountability relationship for the duration of care on that unit, or like a mechanism in shift report being established to ensure that the patient's number one need or issue is communicated to all involved in that patient's care. This folder invariably fills up quickly.

Sharing great ideas also stimulates others to remember their own great ideas and practices.

3. The Physical Environment File

The Physical Environment folder includes enhancement recommendations to the physical plant. While we know that the ultimate "healing space" is the relationship itself between the patient and the healer, we also know that the physical environment can positively (or negatively) affect the speed and comfort of each patient's healing experience. This folder will be filled with ideas about new construction, extensive or simple renovations, and research findings about the impact of color, nature, noise/quiet, music, light, etc., in the healing environment.

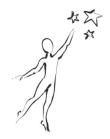

Creating a system to capture and methodically act upon all good ideas is everyone's responsibility, but officially it falls within the role of the Results Council, or to the Unit Practice Councils depending on the scope (or reach) of the idea. This sorting process helps these bodies to respond without becoming overwhelmed to all ideas as they emerge over time. This organizational tool—sorting innovative ideas and actions by these three categories—can also serve as a guide to assess the degree to which innovations are occurring in each of the RBC dimensional efforts. Sharing great ideas also stimulates others to remember their own great ideas and practices. It's a way for all of us to answer the call to continuously share creative and innovative expressions of Relationship-Based Care.

Never be limited by other people's limited imaginations.

Dr. Mae Jemison

Patient Rounds:
A Key Role of Nurse Leaders

—Susan Wessel

A system for making regular patient rounds keeps clinical managers and staff focused on patient care as the top priority and provides invaluable qualitative information. All too often other pressing issues cause rounds to be pushed to the back burner as managers must prioritize an overwhelming list of demands on their time.

In my experience a simple yet organized system of patient rounds, done faithfully, proved to be a powerful mechanism for increasing patient satisfaction and refocusing the time of assistant nurse managers and clinical nursing staff. Rounds resulted in numerous staff compliments and a wonderful opportunity to give positive feedback to individual staff members. Perhaps the awareness that patient feedback was being evaluated also changed behavior. On one unit, the rounding manager uncovered a pattern of patient complaints specific to the night shift. As a result, she began working a few hours on the night shift over the next 6 months. She used this time to talk with staff members, evaluating systems and articulating clear expectations for caring behavior. The response to this was so positive that she has kept this as a regular part of her leadership practice.

Create Systems to Save Time

A short rounds form is effective in setting a positive, appreciative tone for rounds and in capturing and following up on results. This form is particularly useful for nurse managers to reinforce the expectation for rounds with their assistants. The assistant nurse manager (sometimes called team leader or charge nurse) is generally involved in direct patient care and must actively make time for rounds. It's understandably easy to procrastinate when the "crisis of the day" is the focus. A reasonable expectation should be set for the number of patients rounded on each week, maybe 8 to 12. Because of the brevity of the form, one patient visit often takes as little as 3 to 5 minutes. The completed forms should be brought to regular meetings with the manager and discussed. Similarly, expectations should be set for rounds made by the manager and results discussed regularly with his or her immediate supervisor.

A sample rounds form is shown in Figure 1. Notice that the overall tone is positive, and at the same time it gives patients an opportunity to identify any unmet needs. Patients gain a sense of emotional security when they meet the leader of a unit. This reaction can be enhanced by giving business cards and/or telling patients how to reach the manager or supervisor if they have any concerns.

Physician compliments or concerns are sometimes received during rounds. It's helpful to have a system worked out in advance with the Chief Medical Officer or Medical Staff Office for following up on these. Ideally, smaller issues can be handled directly with the physician as a professional colleague rather than creating a paper trail and a complex communication pathway.

Staff Compliments and Recognitions

In an RBC culture, leaders seek to affirm staff contributions through face-to-face interactions whenever possible. Nonetheless managers can save time and still gain the benefits of passing on compliments to individual staff through a simple note system for mailboxes or e-mail. The volume of compliments received by staff makes it unrealistic to remember and pass each one on personally. In addition, a note with a carbon copy allows a record for performance reviews if the carbon is dropped in the employee file on the unit. I used a simple half-page form (most facilities can print these in-house) for "quality of care notes." It was fairly unstructured and could be used both for compliments and the occasional reminder. I had the organization's values printed on the bottom and linked compliments to one of the organizational values when appropriate.

Patients love the opportunity to thank and appreciate their care givers to someone in charge. They also value having a way to resolve issues on the spot. At the same time staff everywhere tend to verbalize that they want more recognition from their managers. The system of patient rounds and staff feedback presented here will accomplish both objectives expeditiously and keep the focus on patient care.

Patient Rounds Record

Instructions: *Introduce yourself by name and title. Ask the patient (or family) if now is a convenient time to visit. Sit at eye level (sitting sends a huge message). Explain that part of your responsibility is the quality of care they receive, and you would appreciate their help by answering a few questions.*

What aspects of your care have been most positive?

_____

_____

_____

How could we make your care even better?

_____

_____

_____

Unit-specific question: (rotate according to need or Quality Improvement (QI) focus, for example pain management, answering call lights, patient education, etc.)

Thank the patient for his or her time, and promise to pass on any compliments and address any areas for improvement. Resolve any concerns immediately if possible, including an apology.

Notes on Follow-up Needed:

_____

_____

_____

Patient Name:

_____

Date: _____   Initials of interviewer: _____

Figure 1

Exemplar: Shift Report at Marion General

—Linda Pullins

Background

In early 2002, Marion General Hospital (Marion, OH) began to work with Ruth Hansten, PhD, RN, of Hansten Healthcare, to implement basic needed changes at the bedside and with unit processes. Leadership of the medical/surgical unit had begun to witness problems with the traditional change-of-shift report. They knew changes needed to happen to improve communication between nurses and improve care planning for all of the patients in these units.

Staff also perceived problems. Change of shift and report were chaotic and noisy, with large amounts of overtime accrual, but little true informational exchange or direct benefit to either the staff or the patient. Staff would often receive detailed, lengthy information about a patient, only to discover a seemingly different patient when they arrived to do an assessment. Shift reports included little to no conversation between RNs, LPNs and NAs. No one asked clarifying questions or sought additional information. Reports would typically start with the traditional reading of each patient's Kardex. Following this reading, various people would report whatever they thought was pertinent information to report. RNs would often spend up to an additional hour post-shift report investigating and seeking out additional information before they were able to start their care.

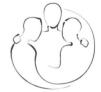

Process

Shift handoff communication was part of an organizational change to outcomes-focused care (Relationship & Results Oriented Healthcare) using coaching practices (see page 118). The first step to improved information exchange was the fundamental action of sitting at the patient's bedside and determining the number one need. Nurses learned to sit at the bedside and use appreciative inquiry in a focused interview with the patient.

The staff used the methodology of the 4 Ps (Purpose, Picture, Plan and Part)in the interview with the patient and/or family:

- *Purpose: Why is this patient here?*

- *Picture: What are the priorities for the hospitalization and for the next shift? What does the next shift need to know to meet those priorities and anticipated results? What is the plan going forward, both short-term and long-term?*

- *Plan: What did or didn't work on my shift?*

- *Part: What part will the next shift play in continuing the focus?*

Finally, they determined if there was any other information necessary to share to provide optimal care.

During the change of shift handoff, nurses used a consistent template for describing the patient situation to the next shift. This enabled the staff to consistently focus on meeting patient needs. Through ongoing, hands-on, real-time work, shift report emphasized not just what tasks needed to be completed, but also what outcomes were desired by both patient and staff. Shift report templates were developed for each unit's specific needs, along with tools for assistive personnel direction and follow-through. Coaches helped refocus communications, asking coaching and clarifying questions that taught the new dialogue and exchange of information.

Results

With a renewed understanding of what shift report should accomplish, it is now viewed as valuable time spent. The plan for the day is more simplified, pertinent and relevant. Staff members feel more in control at the beginning of their shift. Report time has shortened, overtime has decreased and the culture has changed.

Not only did the quality of the information improve, so did assignment making and delegation! The coaches were also able to observe and document firsthand that clinical errors and failure-to-rescue events also decreased. Physicians felt that staff was more prepared with information during rounds, and their overall level of satisfaction with nursing care has continued to improve.

Changing shift report has changed the way all work is organized. Rather than being focused on the Kardex, our work is focused on the needs of patients and families.

Safety Huddles and Walkarounds: Building a Blame-Free Culture of Patient Safety

—Susan Wessel

The Institute for Healthcare Improvement (IHI) has advocated many strategies to help organizations raise staff awareness of safety issues and integrate safety into daily routines. This exemplar will highlight two IHI techniques for developing a culture of patient safety. In both techniques—safety huddles and executive walkarounds—the questions asked are designed specifically to uncover and understand system breakdowns. Unlike most of our questions, they are not "appreciative" in their wording because their specific purpose is to uncover and prevent problems.

Safety Huddles

This intervention is based on Fran Griffin's strategy of "Safety Briefings" presented at an IHI collaborative on Redesigning Culture and Processes in the Medication System (Institute for Healthcare Improvement [IHI], 2002). When this adaptation of Griffin's model was implemented in one organization, nursing and pharmacy staffs responded enthusiastically and a number of changes were made.

The "5-minute safety huddle" is a powerful and easy system to evaluate and enhance the safety of medication systems. During the pilot phase, the VP of nursing and later the nurse manager quickly gathered several people into a huddle once or twice a week, often before or after shift report. The conversation was started by setting a clear goal of spending 5 minutes to learn how to improve medication safety systems (not people). The leader reinforced that the organization was moving toward a nonpunitive environment for errors.

In each safety huddle, three questions were asked:

- *How many people encountered a safety issue or "near misses" related to medications today?*

- *How many of the "almosts" were caught because of our focus on safety or these safety huddles?*

- *Who had patients who asked questions about medications today that may have prevented an error?*

The answers to these questions were used to identify opportunities to prevent medication errors in collaboration with pharmacy.

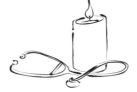

The number of issues brought forward was tracked as a measure of the effectiveness of safety huddles. All changes made were communicated back to staff. The experience of IHI has shown that staff members grow to enjoy safety huddles and miss them if they stop. Bringing forward potential safety issues will eventually become a part of the unit culture. Once this happens, a spontaneous system of notes or index cards dropped in a clearly labeled box can be used for staff to jot down their safety thoughts and suggestions. Active thinking about how to prevent medication errors becomes a part of the staff's collective psyche. Eventually safety huddles can be conducted less often, with the safety idea cards taking over a large part of the system. It's important to continue to share the improvements made as a result of the huddles or cards with the staff.

Executive Medical Safety Walkarounds

A broader intervention targeted at all aspects of patient safety was described by Alan Frankel of the IHI (IHI, 2002). As a nurse executive, I have adapted his technique, the Executive Medical Safety Walkaround, in all departments including support and clinical disciplines.

Executive walkarounds are designed to be shared by senior leaders. The leader takes one hour a week to walk to departments and discuss patient safety in a scripted, well-planned process. Employees see senior leaders carrying the banner of patient safety, and the leaders learn about various safety issues in their organization.

Before beginning, the Quality Improvement Department needs to design a process to follow up on the issues and get back to the senior leader with the outcome. This allows the senior leader to stop back at the department and share the follow-up. Initially the number of safety suggestions and system issues can be overwhelming, but it's hard to imagine a more important task for the quality department and managers to attend to. Executive walkarounds need to be part of the peer review structure in order to legally protect the confidentiality of the information they collect. This can be accomplished through a letter from the Chair of the Quality Committee sanctioning the executive walkarounds as part of the peer review structure.

To implement executive safety walkarounds, the senior leader walks up to any employee and asks if they could have a brief conversation about patient safety. Reassurance is given that everything is confidential. The overall goal to improve safety is described, with the emphasis on the environment and systems, not individual people. The leader should explain that the organization is moving toward a blame-free environment to help uncover ways to improve systems and protect people from the risk of errors. The ground rules on the next page will be helpful to leaders; they may want to choose just two or three questions for each interaction. At the end of the safety conversation, the executive commits to following up on the issues identified, and in return asks that the employee share the concepts discussed with two other people.

Reference: Institute for Healthcare Improvement. (2002). *Quantum leaps in patient safety: Redesigning culture and processes of the medication system.* Learning Session 1, June 25-26, 2001, Atlanta, GA.

Ground Rules and Script For Executive Safety Walkarounds:

Employees should be reassured that all information discussed is strictly confidential.

Opening Statements (use all, preferably in order)

- *We are interested in making the organization safer for patients and staff, so we're moving toward more open communication and a blame-free environment for adverse events.*

- *I'd like to ask you a few questions about our safety systems. We want to focus on the system and not individuals, so no names are necessary.*

- *The discussion I'm having with you is confidential. What we talk about won't go beyond this small group if you don't want it to.*

Questions to be Asked (choose several)

- [ ] *Are you aware that we are actively promoting a blame-free culture for reporting incidents, and focusing on systems rather than individuals?*

- [ ] *Can you think of any events in the past few days that have resulted in prolonged hospitalization for a patient?*

- [ ] *Have there been any "near misses" that almost caused patient harm but didn't?*

- [ ] *Have we harmed any patients recently that you can think of?*

- [ ] *What aspects of the unit environment are likely to lead to the next patient harm?*

- [ ] *Is there anything we could do to prevent the next adverse event?*

- [ ] *Can you think of a way in which the system or your environment fails you on a consistent basis?*

- [ ] *What would make these executive walkarounds more effective?*

Last Comment

We are going to work on the information you've given me. In return I'd like you to tell two other people you work with about the concepts we've discussed in this conversation.

Exemplar: Enhancing Continuity of Care and Nurse Satisfaction with the 7/70 Staffing Mode

—Katie Boyle

Recruiting and retaining qualified nurses is critical for health care providers to maintain a high level of patient care. Nationally, hospitals have a nurse turnover rate of about 18 percent and a vacancy rate of about 13 percent. However, Froedtert Memorial Lutheran Hospital in Wauwatosa, Wisconsin had a nurse turnover rate of only 9.73 % in 2004 and a nurse vacancy rate of just 4.25 %. In 2005 RN turnover was 11.06 % and 3.80 % vacancy rate for RNs. We also have not found it necessary to use outside agency nurses except for a brief period of 12 months in 2001, and then it was only three to eight shifts a day within our over 400 bed tertiary facility. We have been very proud of our ability to recruit and retain nurses.

Editors' note: *Originally published in Health Care* Heroes, *a supplement to* Small Business Times, *December 9, 2005. Used with permission.*

Pamela Maxson-Cooper, CNO and Vice President Patient Care Services at Froedtert, attributes Froedtert's success to its unique 7/70 scheduling plan, in which full-time nurses work 70 hours over seven days and then have seven days off.

"[This] extremely popular scheduling plan has contributed significantly to the recruitment and retention of nurses here," said Maxson-Cooper, who nominated Froedtert for a Health Care Heroes Award. "There is no doubt among administration or the nursing staff that the 7/70 scheduling plan is an important factor in the hospital nursing staff's stability."

The 7/70 scheduling plan originated when Froedtert opened 24 years ago and is based on three overlapping 10-hour shifts for seven consecutive days. During the overlap time, two shifts of nurses are on duty to manage admissions, discharges and transfers during the peak activity times of the day. Patient Care Technicians and Unit Communicators also work the 7/70 schedule, resulting in cohesive A or B Week teams.

Nurses work 25 weeks throughout the year and have one 70-hour week of paid time off. The scheduling plan enables professional nurses to build a strong therapeutic relationship with their patients and families. We opened our doors in 1980 using the Primary Nurse model for patient care delivery. At that time we were able to provide 100% all-RN care delivery model. However, as healthcare costs increased and availability of RNs changed over the years we realized a supportive care delivery team made up of Patient Care Assistants made perfect sense to help meet the timely needs of our patients. As skills and technology evolved, we have grown our supportive Patient Care Assistants into Patient Care Technicians, always focusing with the RNs on patient needs as a team. "The 7/70 scheduling plan promotes continuity of care and contributes to the high quality medical care Froedtert provides," Maxson-Cooper said.

"The traditional schedule is 80 hours in two weeks," she said. "With the 10 hour shifts, seven hours in a row, nurses and patients have the continuity of time which enables the trusting relationship to flourish, which is an advantage over two days on, one day off. Additionally, traditional staffing models have you rotating shifts within a particular month or three month period. This schedule allows nurses to know their schedule for years to come."

There are many other advantages to the 7/70 schedule. Maxson-Cooper said. "On the personal side, they like the predictability of their schedules. They liked the time off because it allows them to pursue other activities—families, education and vacations," she said.

"It offers a lot more flexibility in that you have the week off, and I have two small kids at home," said Susan Moderski, a Staff Nurse at Froedtert. "You have your week on and your week off to be with the kids. Compared to the traditional schedule, my kids feel like I'm home more."

Froedtert's staff surveys also indicate general enthusiasm for the 7/70 system. Seventy percent of staff said they wanted to work at Froedtert because of the scheduling, and 90 percent said they liked the scheduling plan.

"I've been there eight years or so and have worked at other places that don't have it.... It's hard to give up once you get used to it. Most nurses at Froedtert would tell you that it's a big factor in staying because you can't find it anywhere else." Moderski said.

The 7/70 scheduling plan also benefits patients and may be a reason Froedtert can charge less for services than most of its competitors, Maxson-Cooper said.

"The continuity of having the same nursing staff caring for patients for a succession of shifts and days certainly, I believe, would help to impact a decreased length of stay," Maxson-Cooper said. "I think that, plus having registered nurses at the bedside caring directly for patients makes a difference. Every other year we survey our staff to assure ourselves this scheduling plan is still favored by the majority and I'm always amazed at the consistent RN satisfaction with our plan."

Wisdom From a Senior Staff Nurse

—Agnes Cappabianca

Editors' note: This story was told at a Relationship-Based Care Leader Practicum workshop and the participants were delighted by it. Agnes agreed to have it shared in this field guide as it truly is a pearl of wisdom.

The most senior staff nurse on our unit always approaches her day with energy and joy. She floats around the unit addressing all of her patients' needs and always has time to answer doctors' questions, help her colleagues, and support new staff members.

A new graduate nurse stopped her one day and asked, "What is your secret?"

The young nurse expected to hear of some magical formula.

The older nurse responded, "What prayer do you come to work with?"

The new nurse was dumbfounded and didn't respond.

Again, she queried, "What prayer do you come to work with?"

The new nurse was still unsure of how to answer the question.

The senior nurse was now quick to respond for her.

"I know the prayer you come to work with—'Oh God, I hope I have a quiet day!'—and you are always disappointed. My prayer when I walk on the unit is 'God, give me the knowledge and skills to give compassionate care.' And I am never disappointed."

Colleagueship

Background: *The University of California at Irvine is engaged in the implementation of Relationship-Based Care (RBC) in its organization. As part of their inspiration, Unit Practice Council members from the four units that comprise Wave 1 participated in a Reigniting the Spirit of Caring workshop. Upon completion of the "Caring for Colleagues" dimension each of the groups identified and committed to the following behaviors. It is their intention that these behaviors will guide them through the RBC development process.*

As your colleague I will:

Group #1:

- *Come to work with a positive attitude every day*
- *Respect my colleagues' uniqueness*
- *Provide emotional support and praise for a job well done*
- *Allow your frustration in time of your weakness*
- *Respect privacy: yours and mine*
- *Establish teamwork*
- *Make a time to review how the day went*
- *Be open to and accept constructive opinion*
- *Dine out, have pot lucks, and other extracurricular activities*

Group #2:

- *Support and aid my co-workers whenever possible*
- *Actively listen to my co-workers' concerns*
- *Be flexible with the work schedule*
- *Not take it personally when assigned extra work*
- *Validate each other*
- *Just say no to the "3Bs" (Bickering, Backbiting and Blaming) and yes to the "3Cs" (Caring, Committing and Collaborating)!!!*

Group #3:

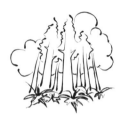

- *Say please and thank you*
- *Speak/request politely in tone and voice*
- *Offer help when others are busy*
- *Offer/provide therapeutic massage*
- *Inform/relate to co-workers' degree of stress*
- *Show/verbalize appreciation for a job well done*
- *Avoid the "3Bs"*
- *Respect individuality*

Group #4:

- *Be supportive to one another*
- *Be polite*
- *Accept the person for who he is*
- *Respect culture differences*
- *Be open to constructive criticism*
- *Do the "3Cs," not the "3Bs"*

CHAPTER EIGHT
Embedding Professional Nursing Practice Into Relationship-Based Care

The Therapeutic Nurse-Patient Relationship, Part I: Ethical Foundation, Nature and Requirements

—Mary Koloroutis

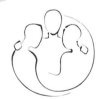

> *When a care provider crosses the threshold of a patient and family's door, he or she crosses a border, moving from the world of practical preparation into that of a personal healing relationship in which everything he or she does is in service to the patient. This border crossing brings care providers into the patient's and family's world—a world about which they know little—and within which they must tread with great humility.*
>
> *—Jayne A. Felgen*

With these words, Jayne Felgen opens the way to understanding the sacred privilege in our relationships with patients and their families (Felgen, 2004). This relationship is like no other. It is a "therapeutic relationship"—one in which the patient's and family's healing is the purpose for the relationship. All interactions within the therapeutic relationship are for the purpose of providing safe and compassionate care to patients and their families.

> All interactions within the therapeutic relationship are for the purpose of providing safe and compassionate care to patients and their families.

The American Nurses Association Code of Ethics outlines the ethical foundation for the therapeutic nurse-patient relationship, the purpose of which is to establish a safe and healing connection between the nurse and the person(s) needing care and service. The template for the therapeutic nurse-patient relationship is captured in Provision 1 of the Code of Ethics for Nurses with Interpretative Statements (American Nurses Association, 2001) which explicitly delineates the moral commitment undergirding the nurses' relationship to patients and their families as well as the ethical imperatives that direct safe and compassionate nursing care.

ANA Code of Ethics for Nurses With Interpretative Statements

Provision 1. The nurse, in all professional relationships, practices with compassion and respect for the inherent dignity, worth and uniqueness of every individual, unrestricted by considerations of social or economic status, personal attributes, or the nature of health problems.

1.1 **Respect for human dignity.** *A fundamental principle that underlies all nursing practice is respect for the inherent worth, dignity, and human rights of every individual. Nurses take into account the needs and values of all persons in all professional relationships.*

1.2 **Relationships to patients.** *The need for health care is universal, transcending all individual differences. The nurse establishes relationships and delivers nursing services with respect for human needs and values, and without prejudice.*

1.3 **The nature of health problems.** *The nurse respects the worth, dignity and rights of all human beings irrespective of the nature of the health problems. The worth of the person is not affected by disease, disability, functional status or proximity to death. The measures nurses take to care for the patient* *enable the patient to live with as much physical, emotional, social and spiritual well-being as possible. Nursing care aims to maximize the values that the patient has treasured in life and extends supportive care to the family and significant others.*

1.4 **The right to self-determination.** *Respect for human dignity requires the recognition of specific patient rights, particularly the right of self-determination. Patients have the moral and legal right to determine what will be done with their own person; to be given accurate, complete, and understandable information in a manner that facilitates an informed judgment; to be assisted with weighing the benefits, burdens and available options in their treatment, including the choice of no treatment; to accept, refuse or terminate treatment without deceit, undue influence, duress, coercion or penalty; and to be given necessary support through the decision-making and treatment process.*

> The therapeutic use of self—the offering of one's self as an instrument of healing—is often referred to as the most important action and responsibility of a professional nurse.

Source: American Nurses Association. (2001). Code of ethics for nurses with interpretive statements. *Silver Springs, MD: ANA, pp. 7-8. Used with Permission.*

This rich ethical foundation provides the context within which nurses form relationships with patients and their families. The nature of this unique relationship and the conditions under which it can be effective are discussed in this first article on therapeutic relationships. It addresses what makes the therapeutic nurse-patient relationship both necessary and possible. This first article will elaborate on the following foundational principles of the therapeutic relationship:

- *The therapeutic relationship is an aspect of independent nursing practice.*

- *Self-knowing is a fundamental requirement for engaging in effective therapeutic relationships.*

- *The nurse's recognition of the inherent imbalance of power in nurse-patient relationships is essential to the creation of an emotionally safe space for patients within therapeutic relationships.*

> • *Professional boundaries must be clearly defined and monitored by the nurse.*

One: The therapeutic relationship is an aspect of independent nursing service.

It is clear that the purpose of the therapeutic nurse-patient relationship is to provide safe, comprehensive, compassionate care to optimize the health and well-being of patients and their families. It is also evident that the therapeutic relationship occurs within the independent realm of nursing practice. In this realm of practice, nurses apply their education and experience to "diagnose and treat the human responses to actual or potential health problems" (American Nurses Association, 2001).

To function in this independent realm, nurses must be knowledgeable about 1) the predictable patterns of human responses that occur for people needing care in particular circumstances, and 2) the unique responses of each individual patient and family. Care circumstances are varied and complex, including preventive and diagnostic services, normal birth and family transitions, chronic and acute illness, life-threatening emergencies, traumatic injuries and death and dying. What is consistent across these varied experiences is that nursing care and service are needed and the individuals needing it are inherently vulnerable.

Gaining knowledge of one's self is a lifelong quest; there is always more to learn and understand in order to be a healing and therapeutic presence to others.

Two: The self-knowing of care givers is a fundamental requirement for engaging in effective therapeutic relationships.

The therapeutic use of self—the offering of one's self as an instrument of healing—is often referred to as the most important action and responsibility of a professional nurse. It is also the most advanced and complex aspect of professional nursing care. Gaining knowledge of one's self is a lifelong quest; there is always more to learn and understand in order to be a healing and therapeutic presence to others.

Confounding this complexity is the fact that there are no adequate task lists or rule books for self-knowing. Self-knowing is built over time through consciousness, patience, maturation, and in many cases, the persistent pursuit of it. It

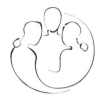

takes curiosity about ourselves and the willingness to inquire of others and to receive feedback in ways that will help us grow. Our individual personalities and life experiences have everything to do with who we are, how we "show up," how we cope with stress, how we learn. In essence, they have a powerful influence on how we will *be* in a therapeutic relationship with others.

Christine Williams and Carol Davis (2005) in their book *Therapeutic Interaction and Nursing* present a practical and comprehensive exploration of Understanding the Self (pp. 3-14) as the basis for the therapeutic nurse-patient relationship. They assert that in order for nurses to form therapeutic relationships with patients, they must have a solid understanding of themselves and conversely that if they lack this understanding it can interfere with their ability to be therapeutic helpers to others. Williams and Davis have identified three areas of inquiry as essential for self-knowing: family of origin, emotional intelligence and level of self esteem. I have added a fourth area: Human Dynamics.

Family of Origin:	Each of us holds a unique worldview that was influenced by our original family. How we respond in the world is affected by our biology, our family system and our sense of self-worth. As adults we need to examine and understand that we are based on where we came from so that we can consciously develop a more accurate view of the world, our relationships and ourselves. Our biases and assumptions about people are rooted in our upbringing.
Emotional Intelligence:	This is the capacity to understand one's own emotional responses and to use that understanding to interact effectively with others (Goleman, 1995). When a nurse has a high degree of emotional intelligence, he or she is more likely to recognize the fear or hurt in a patient's angry outburst and to respond with compassion rather than personalizing the incident. Understanding the dynamics of the range of human responses to stress, illness, trauma, crisis and other life transitions is fundamental to maintaining healthy therapeutic interactions with patients and their families.

Health Professionals' Level of Self-Esteem:	This addresses the notion that people may enter the helping professions to fulfill a need they have within themselves. One fundamental need may be for healing themselves through making life better for others. Other needs include a need to be depended upon, a need to exert control over others, and a need to receive affection or attention. Williams and Davis define self-esteem as the "extent to which we are able and willing to believe in our essential goodness in the face of our own lack of perfection. More than simply self-acceptance, self-esteem includes pride in the promise of ongoing growth and change with maturity and the hope of a richer more peaceful and congruent life as a result of honest day-to-day struggle" (Williams & Davis, 2005).
Human Dynamics:	Developing an understanding of personality dynamics is one of the most valuable mechanisms available for strengthening our own self-awareness and developing a more conscious understanding of others. Human Dynamics teaches us that we each take in information, communicate and learn based on how we are "hardwired" from birth (Seagal & Horne, 1997). Each of us has a primary way of experiencing our lives and the world we live in. Each of us has a primary "way of being or centering." The three primary ways of being are: *mental centering* (logical, linear, thought driven) *emotional centering* (intuitive, integrative, feeling driven) or *physical centering* (concrete, purposeful, practical). Our primary centering determines how we communicate, what we perceive and how we solve problems. Understanding our own dynamic gives us a foundation for fuller self-development, integration and growth. Human Dynamics helps us develop consciousness of ourselves, of others as we relate to them, and of our environment as a whole (see page 396).

Self-awareness and self-differentiation are integral to the concept of self-knowing, as our level of self-knowing determines (among other things) the degree to which we are conscious of where we end and others begin. When we are able to clearly differentiate ourselves from others, we are more able to stay focused on the needs and issues of the "other" rather than becoming distracted by our own issues. As we grow personally and professionally, become more fully competent, and engage others in all of our varied relationships, it is essential to grow also in our capacity to care for individuals and groups with different backgrounds, values and human responses within the therapeutic relationship.

Three: Nurses must understand how the inherent imbalance of power in nurse-patient relationships can create emotional safety issues for patients within the therapeutic relationship.

The balance of power and emotional safety are significant components of the therapeutic nurse-patient relationship. In the nurse-patient relationship, the patient's vulnerability tips the balance of power squarely toward the nurse. The patient's and family's experience of emotional safety is dependent upon a variety of factors including the nurse's ability to assess and understand individual patient and family needs. These needs are based on the individual's unique situation, background, culture, values, beliefs, previous experience in receiving health care services, and the patient's and family's willingness and/or ability to trust.

In the context of the therapeutic relationship, the nurse's power comes from the authority and expertise consistent with his or her:

- *professional role,*
- *knowledge and familiarity with the health care system, and*
- *access to important patient information.*

The patient's and family's power is variable and comes from their individual backgrounds, the degree to which they are debilitated during the episode of care, and their experience with managing the ups and downs of living with the health or illness condition that brought them into the nurse's care. They are nearly always, however, less familiar with the health care system than their care givers are, and are therefore dealing with a stressful event. They are rarely familiar or comfortable with the hospital environment and do not generally have easy access to information.

> In the nurse-patient relationship, the patient's vulnerability tips the balance of power squarely toward the nurse.

I equate the patient experience to being in a foreign country, not speaking the language, and depending on a guide to get you safely and securely where you want to go. In such a vulnerable position, much of your sense of emotional safety would depend upon the degree to which you felt you could trust that your guide had your best interests at heart. Your feeling of confidence that you mattered to your guide would be greatly enhanced if your guide kept you fully informed and assured you that his or her intention was to get you to your destination as planned.

A Closer Look at Powerlessness

I propose that all of these "little things" are really about understanding the importance of power and control and taking actions that protect human dignity and self-determination.

The nursing diagnosis "powerlessness" is defined as "the perception that one's own actions will not significantly affect an outcome; a perceived lack of control over a current situation or immediate happening" (Johnson, Bulechek, McCloskey Dochterman, Maas, Moorhead, Swanson, et al., 2006). I propose that the degree of powerlessness be assessed for most patients and families entering the health care system. The degree of powerlessness could be minimal to great, depending on the circumstances and the patient's or family's capacity to cope with the situation.

In *Reigniting the Spirit of Caring* (see page 524) workshops, patients and families frequently tell stories of feeling powerless. Often their stories are expressions of gratitude for those care givers who bolstered their self-determination in small ways, like remembering that they needed their call light within reach or the tissue box close enough for them to reach when they were recovering from surgery or in some other way limited in mobility. There are stories about the nurse who consistently did what she said she would do and kept the patient and family informed regardless of how busy she may have been. There are stories about care givers immediately putting patients at ease by letting them know that they will check in frequently and that they will make sure someone is there immediately to help them to the bathroom so that they need not fret about it. And there are stories of nurses as translators—those who knew the medical jargon was confusing and patiently clarified what was being said to ensure that the patient and family understood what was going on and what to expect next. These stories are often classified as stories about patients appreciating "the little things." I propose that all of these "little things" are really about understanding the importance of power and control and taking actions that protect human dignity and self-determination.

Emotional safety is closely aligned with perception of self-control or personal power. People experience a sense of emotional safety when they feel cared for, respected, valued as unique persons, and treated with dignity and compassion. When they feel safe, they are able to allow themselves to be vulnerable, open to healing and trusting of those caring for them. One feels emotionally safe when nurses and other care givers:

- *do what they say they will do;*

- *demonstrate caring behaviors and attitudes;*

- *tend to the little things that promote the patient's comfort, security, and sense of personal control;*

- *demonstrate clinical knowledge and competence;*

- *seek to know the patient and family as unique individuals;*

- *demonstrate respect for the dignity and worth of each person;*

- *maintain an attitude of openness and inquiry, suspending both judgment and assumptions;*

- *touch each person with respect and gentleness;*

- *safeguard each person's privacy and confidentiality; and*

- *engage the patient's full participation in decisions affecting their care by providing timely and clear information and by serving as a guide to ensure that the patient is fully informed.*

Four: Professional boundaries must be clearly defined.

Professional boundaries for the therapeutic nurse-patient relationship are a set of expectations that separate therapeutic behaviors from any behaviors that could lessen the benefit of care to the patient and/or family.

The National Council of State Boards of Nursing (2004) created a graphic which I have adapted. It is a helpful way to look at the nature of boundaries and offers valuable guidance for those establishing professional boundaries within therapeutic relationships. The idea that boundaries are violated when we become overinvolved or underinvolved is worth discussion. The authors propose that every nurse-patient relationship can be plotted on this continuum of professional behavior.

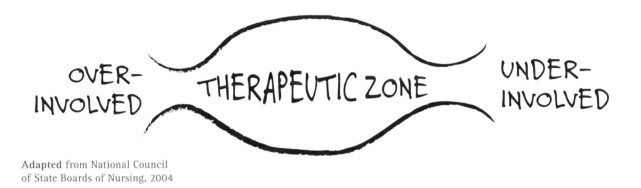

OVER-
INVOLVED

THERAPEUTIC ZONE

UNDER-
INVOLVED

Adapted from National Council
of State Boards of Nursing, 2004

We are at risk of violating boundaries when our own needs or issues become more significant than the patient's.

We have established that the therapeutic relationship is one of a kind and differs significantly from the social relationship in that the needs of the patient/family always come before the needs of the care giver. This places the nurse in a sacred and privileged position of holding the patient's trust in his or her hands. Managing this relationship requires consciousness and clarity so that we stay in the therapeutic zone and do not abuse the trust and become too distant or unaware or too overly involved. We are at risk of violating boundaries when our own needs or issues become more significant than the patient's. The Nurses Association of New Brunswick (2000) and the College of Nurses of Ontario (2004) published comprehensive standards for the therapeutic nurse-client relationship with an in-depth discussion of boundaries. I recommend both of these documents as valuable resources for deeper exploration of the therapeutic relationship. I have adapted their steps for managing the boundaries of the relationship along with some discussion points below:

1. The nurse establishes and follows a plan of care.

The plan is developed with the patient/family and provides guidance and direction for the approaches best suited to meet the patient's need. Once the plan is agreed upon, the nurse and patient/family have also mutually established the boundaries for care.

2. The nurse understands the nature and limits of the therapeutic relationship and meets his or her own personal needs outside the relationship.

This is a sensitive and complex boundary to manage. The nurse must maintain an ongoing awareness of the distinction between social and therapeutic relationships. The health and well-being of the patient and family remain the constant focus of the therapeutic relationship. Over-involvement occurs if a nurse becomes overly personal or familiar with the patient or a family member because of his or her own needs rather than the therapeutic goal.

Another example of over-involvement which is fairly common is sharing a work frustration with the patient/family such as being "short staffed." There is clearly nothing the patient/family can do about the situation, and therefore, this information is burdening to them. Examples of under-involvement include those actions or behaviors that keep the nurse at a distance rather than engaging the patient and family as individuals. Under-involvement denies the therapeutic relationship and is generally about self-protection. At a minimum it limits the patient's access to a caring and healing presence; at its maximum it is abandonment.

3. The nurse is aware of the context in which care is provided.

The context of care creates the parameters within which care is provided. The degree of involvement and the nature of the interventions are obviously affected by the needs and context of the situation. A short-term therapeutic relationship may be intense and highly involved when the patient and family are facing an emergency. A short-term therapeutic relationship may be one of teaching and guiding in the context of a clinic visit. A longer-term Primary Nurse-patient therapeutic relationship may exist in a rehabilitation center or intensive care unit or behavioral health setting. The nurse needs to be clear about his or her role and services and communicate those clearly so that the patient and family know what to expect and what the parameters of their relationship will be.

4. The therapeutic relationship is intentionally terminated.

At the beginning of each therapeutic relationship, the nurse has a responsibility to estimate and communicate the length of time he or she will be in the relationship. For example, in the case of an emergency department visit, the nurse may communicate, "I am the one who will care for you while you are in the emergency room. When you are admitted to the unit, one of the nurses on that unit will take over your care. When that happens, I will give him or her all of the information from your emergency visit and what I have learned about you so that he or she will be able to take over from where we left off."

On an inpatient unit, the nurse may say, "I am the one who coordinates all of your care while you are on our unit. I am your Primary Nurse. Other nurses and assistants will also care for you, but I am the one who will make sure everything is going according to our plan." In preparing for discharge, the nurse may say, "I will be teaching your family how to support you when you are discharged home, and if we determine you need more help we'll have a home care nurse see you after discharge."

Your Professional Nursing Practice

The therapeutic nurse-patient relationship is a sacred trust demonstrated in each act of respectful personal interaction care givers must:

- *know themselves,*
- *be aware of the inherent imbalance of power in the nurse-patient relationship,*
- *work to provide emotional safety for each patient and family served, and*
- *maintain professional boundaries.*

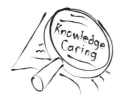

Nursing is a profession of giving, which is conscious, and knowledge-based. It is not a selfless giving, as some would have us believe—but a giving full of self. In every interaction, care givers make a choice about how they will *show up* in their own personal practice. The more aware we are of the dynamics of the therapeutic nurse-patient relationship, the better equipped we are to find meaning and fulfillment in our own practice, while making a significant positive difference for patients and their families.

References: American Nurses Association. (2001). *Code of ethics for nurses with interpretive statements.* Silver Springs, MD: Author.

College and Association of Registered Nurses of Alberta. (2005). *Professional boundaries: A discussion guide and teaching tool.* Edmonton, AB: Author.

College of Nurses of Ontario. (2004). *Practice standards: Therapeutic nurse-client relationship.* Toronto, ON: Author.

Felgen, J. (2004). A caring and healing environment. In *Relationship-based care: A model for transforming practice.* Minneapolis, MN: Creative Health Care Management.

Goleman, D. (1995). *Emotional intelligence: Why it can matter more than IQ.* New York: Bantam.

Johnson, M., Bulechek, G., McCloskey Dochterman, J., Maas, M., Moorhead, S., Swanson, E. et al. (2001). *Nursing diagnoses, outcomes, and interventions: NANDA, NOC and NIC linkages.* St. Louis, MO: Mosby.

National Council of State Boards of Nursing. (2004). *A nurse's guide to the importance of professional boundaries.* Chicago, IL: Author.

Nurses Association of New Brunswick. (2000). *Standard for the therapeutic nurse-client relationship.* Fredericton, NB: Author.

Seagal, S., & Horne, D. (1997). *Human dynamics: A new framework for understanding people and realizing the potential in our organizations.* Waltham, MA: Pegasus Communications.

Swanson, K. (1993). Nursing as informed caring for the well-being of others. *IMAGE: Journal of Nursing Scholarship, 25,* 352-357.

Watson, Jean. (2006). *Transpersonal caring and the caring moment defined.* Retrieved December 12, 2006 from http://www2.uchsc.edu/son/caring/content/transpersonal.asp

Williams, C., & Davis C. (2005). *Therapeutic interaction in nursing.* Sudbury, MA: Jones and Bartlett.

The Therapeutic Nurse-Patient Relationship, Part II: Theory Applied to Practice

—Mary Koloroutis

Nurse theorists and clinicians view the therapeutic nurse-patient relationship as the foundation of nursing practice and patient care. This relationship is anchored in the simple truth that care happens between people. In the most fundamental terms, it breaks down this way:

- *The primary* **tool** *at the disposal of nurses is the self.*

- *There is a specialized body of nursing* **knowledge**.

- *The* **tasks** *of nursing practice are procedures, treatments and other interventions.*

- *The* **true work** *of nursing is the creation of a relationship through which quality care can be effectively offered and received.*

It is in these relationships that patients and families receive the support and guidance necessary for them to recover and heal. It is in these relationships that trust and safety are communicated so that the conditions for healing are optimal.

Reviewing the Roots of Modern Nursing Theory

Nurse theorists have long cited the nurse-patient relationship as the most crucial dimension to nursing practice. A brief summary of their work will serve as a foundation for reflecting on the evolution of the therapeutic nurse-patient relationship from its earliest formalized incarnations until those of the present day.

Hildegard Peplau

Peplau was known as the mother of psychiatric nursing and is credited with first describing the explicit dynamics of the nurse-patient relationship. She identified nursing as a therapeutic, healing art and an interpersonal process. The interpersonal process is an interaction between two or more individuals with a common goal. The interaction is built on mutual respect and mutual learning (Peplau, 1952).

Peplau's concept of the therapeutic relationship included a deepening and building of the relationship over time. She described four phases of this relationship:

- *orientation—in which the patient and the nurse mutually identify the problem;*

- *identification—in which the patient identifies with the helping environment and thereby regains enough awareness of the situation to be able to accept help;*

- *exploitation—in which the patient makes use of the nurse's help and health care services; and*

- *resolution—in which the patient accepts new goals and frees himself or herself from the relationship (Belcher and Fish, 1995).*

Peplau's great contribution to nursing theory is her acknowledgment that the therapeutic nurse-patient relationship begins, progresses, deepens and recedes through a series of identifiable phases. While her theory was developed at a time when patient stays were much longer than they are today, we are better off adapting her theory to briefer interactions rather than discarding it. It can be very helpful to see each nurse-patient relationship—whether it be months, days or hours long—as occurring in stages much like those Peplau describes.

Joyce Travelbee

Travelbee, the author of *Interpersonal Aspects of Nursing* (1971), is recognized for describing the *significance* of the nurse-patient relationship. In her classic book she explores the nature of nursing in relation to concepts such as rapport, sympathy, hope and suffering. Travelbee defined a human being as a "unique and irreplaceable individual—a one time being in this world ... unlike any person who has lived or will live." This explicit focus on the uniqueness of each human provides the basis for the significant human connection that happens within the nurse-patient relationship.

> Peplau's great contribution to nursing theory is her acknowledgment that the therapeutic nurse-patient relationship begins, progresses, deepens and recedes through a series of identifiable phases.

Paterson and Zderad focus on the lived experience of the patient, including specific life circumstances, family relationships, experience with illness, cultural differences and any other factors that come into play.

The great value of Travelbee's contribution to the literature is the degree to which she humanized the patient. When we see patients as people it feels natural for us to establish relationships with them. Further, Travelbee offers a view of the nurse-patient relationship as one that allows for a personal connection within a professional setting.

Josephine G. Paterson and Loretta T. Zderad

Paterson and Zderad (1988) developed a theory of "humanistic" nursing practice. In a humanistic orientation there is a belief in the potential of human beings and that people can only be known or understood within the context of their own unique lived experience. The humanistic theory is built on the underlying belief that "nursing helps others develop well-being and more-being" through increasing the possibility of their making responsible choices." Paterson and Zderad's theory includes the following key concepts:

- *dialogue—in which there is genuine sharing;*

- *meeting—a coming together of human beings with the expectation that there will be a nurse and a "nursed";*

- *presence—the quality of being open, receptive, ready and available to another person in a reciprocal manner; and*

- *community—defined as two or more persons striving together. Nursing creates community and exists in community; people find meaning in their existence by sharing and relating to others (Paterson and Zderad, 1988).*

Paterson and Zderad gave nursing theory its first insight into the significance of knowing the patient's personal context. They focus on the lived experience of the patient, including specific life circumstances, family relationships, experience with illness, cultural differences and any other factors that come into play.

Watson's most significant contributions are her acknowledgment that a therapeutic relationship that reaches all the way into the transpersonal realm can be accomplished in an extremely short amount of time.

Jean Watson

Watson's theory of human caring, which describes the transpersonal relationship between the nurse and the other, has evolved from work that she began publishing in the 1980s. Watson emphasizes that the transpersonal relationship can happen in a "moment," while most of the earlier theorists emphasized the significance of how the relationship is built over time. Watson says that "Transpersonal caring calls for an authenticity of being and becoming, an ability to be present to self and other in a reflective frame; the transpersonal nurse has the ability to center consciousness and intentionality on caring, healing, and wholeness, rather than on disease, illness and pathology." The interpersonal relationship happens in what Watson calls "caring moments" (Watson, 2006).

Watson states, "A caring moment involves an action and choice by both the nurse and the other. The moment of coming together presents them with the opportunity to decide how to be in the moment and in the relationship as well as what to do with and during the moment. If the caring moment is transpersonal, each feels a connection with the other at the spirit level, thus [the moment] transcends time and space, opening up new possibilities for healing and human connection at a deeper level than physical interaction."

Watson's contribution is one that reflects not only the evolution of nursing, but the evolution of business as well. There is greater recognition now than ever before that all business is essentially about people, and that building a culture in which relationships are deeply valued and carefully tended to helps us to attract and retain business. One of Watson's most significant contributions is her acknowledgment that a therapeutic relationship that reaches all the way into the transpersonal realm can be accomplished in an extremely short amount of time.

Kristen Swanson

Swanson's Five Caring Processes provide care givers with a basis for caring and interacting consciously and therapeutically. Her processes provide an accessible and practical framework for relating, while helping us to see more clearly the roles, actions and behaviors inherent in the therapeutic nurse-patient relationship (Swanson, 1993).

Swanson defines nursing as "informed caring for the well-being of others." And in her framework, caring is put into action through five caring processes:

We don't simply "hand off" patients; we prepare them to be received—welcomed once again—into whatever comes next for them.

Maintaining Belief	*Maintaining Belief* in the capacity of the other to make it through an event or transition and to find his or her own meaning provides the context for the nurse-patient relationship. It is a fundamental belief that the other's experience and worldview are naturally distinct from those of the nurse and are to be respected and honored, etc.
Knowing	*Knowing* means seeking to understand the other and the meaning of an event in his or her life. This knowing provides the way to interact, and it happens through inquiry, listening, seeking cues and dialogue.
Being with	*Being with* means being present and emotionally accessible to patients and their families. It means establishing a relationship built on authenticity, compassion and empathy.
Doing for	*Doing for* others what they would otherwise do for themselves if it were possible is achieved through establishing rapport, creating conditions for safety, protecting dignity and privacy, and comforting.
Enabling	*Enabling* involves guiding and informing the patient and family through a life transition and unfamiliar events. The nurse serves as an advocate and guide informing, generating options, supporting, anticipating and preparing for future transitions.

Refining the Therapeutic Nurse-Patient Relationship for Today's Health Care Environment

Admittedly, there are significant challenges in relating to patients and families in the context of today's fast-moving and sometimes confounding health care environment. Because of the reality of these challenges, it has become more important than ever to build on and adapt the wisdom of our early theorists. Our aim is to strengthen our ability to hold the therapeutic nurse-patient relationship as the core nursing practice. We are called to be proactive and unwavering in developing the clarity, competence and confidence to establish therapeutic relationships in the moment and/or over time—whichever correlates to the patient's length of stay.

The model for therapeutic relationships that we endorse is one that brings the best of what's come before into the reality of today's care environments. The ideal health care environment would incorporate:

- *Peplau's recognition that the therapeutic relationship is accomplished in distinct phases,*

- *Travelbee's focus on the patient as a person,*

- *Paterson and Zderad's commitment to discovering the patient's lived experience and adapting practice to it,*

- *Watson's belief that significant acts of caring can happen in a single moment with intention and presence, and*

- *the consistent use of Swanson's Caring Processes to increase the "in the moment" presence of care givers as they tend to what may otherwise be seen as the routine tasks of caring for patients and their families.*

Three Phases of the Therapeutic Nurse-Patient Relationship

There are those who feel establishing a therapeutic relationship in phases is no longer relevant, given today's time of shorter patient interactions, more specialization of services and extreme acuity requiring technology and intermittent interactions. However, as Watson points out, a meaningful relationship between patients and their care givers can be experienced in a single moment. Even if a care giver's interaction with a patient is brief, both parties benefit from practice that is directly fostered by an awareness of three distinct phases of the therapeutic relationship and the purpose of each. I have adapted the concept of phases as defined in Peplau's work, and have identified the following three phases:

- *Receiving*

- *Engaging*

- *Transitioning*

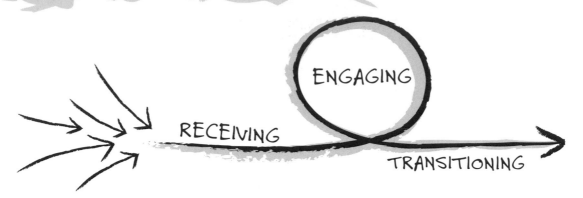

Phase One: Receiving

This phase could logically have been called initiation, or as Peplau called it, orientation, but the term *receiving* conveys one of the most important aspects of the phase. It is not simply that a nurse guides or informs patients in this phase (though that is part of what happens). In Relationship-Based Care, we receive patients into a relationship that continues for the duration of the patient's stay in a particular unit or area, even when that stay lasts no more than a few moments or hours.

In the receiving phase, patients and their loved ones are welcomed to their surroundings. The fundamental act of *receiving and welcoming* helps people cope with whatever they may be facing and conveys that they are seen and understood by somebody who knows them by name and anticipated their arrival. In this phase, we have the opportunity to set the tone for the patient's entire stay and to help them to understand the role the Primary Nurse will play in providing the best conditions for healing and recovery.

> The fundamental act of receiving and welcoming helps people cope with whatever they may be facing and conveys that they are seen and understood by somebody who knows them by name and anticipated their arrival.

This is the first opportunity we have to communicate to the patient that we see him or her as a person. (See "See Me as a Person," page 46.) We all know what it feels like to be seen as a number (or condition), and we know what it feels like to be seen as a person. When a Primary Nurse receives a patient and establishes a human connection, the therapeutic relationship is initiated.

It is also in this phase that the nurse puts Paterson and Zderad's theory to work as he or she seeks to understand the context through which the patient and family are experiencing the current episode of care. Although understanding begins in the receiving phase, like much of what else begins there, it is carried through all the other phases as well. In seeking to understand the context–this patient's individual story–the nurse may seek to understand the following:

- *Who is this patient as a person?*
- *Who are the people with the patient?*
- *What is the reason for the admission?*
- *What is the meaning of this illness (procedure, birth, surgery or trauma) for the patient and family?*
- *What aspects of this patient/family's life circumstances do I need to know about in order to deliver care?*
- *What is the patient/family's greatest concern or fear?*
- *What is this patient's number one priority for this care experience or for this shift?*

What is the meaning of this illness (procedure, birth, surgery or trauma) for the patient and family?

Phase Two: Engaging

This phase represents the core of the interaction–again, whether the patient's length of stay is months, weeks, days or hours long. This is when the plan of care is executed.

The LEARN Model, designed by E. A. Berlin and W. C. Fowkes (1983) to address cross-cultural communication issues in health care settings, is a great framework for engaging patients whether obvious cultural issues are in play or not. We know that each patient has unique life experiences and history; therefore "diversity" is inherent in every interaction. The LEARN model, adapted below, asks care givers to do the following:

- *Listen with compassion and understanding to the patient/family's perception of the problem or situation,*
- *Explain your perception of the situation,*
- *Affirm and discuss the differences and similarities,*
- *Recommend a plan of care, and*
- *Negotiate a mutual agreement for the plan including goals and priorities.*

The LEARN acronym is a way to guide a nurse's thinking so that the patient's experience is directed more by what the patient needs and wants and less by what the nurse intends to do. It's a subtle but important difference, and one that helps patients feel more in control of their experience despite being in a place and condition that could otherwise lead them to feel lost or helpless.

Swanson's Five Caring Processes are another great guide for all care givers to use in this phase. While the LEARN model provides direction for verbal communication and care planning, Swanson's processes deal with the broader and deeper spectrum of knowledge-based caring. Deep knowledge and conscious practice of the Five Caring Processes promote the therapeutic use of self on the part of the nurse and facilitates the patient's care and healing (see page 301).

Swanson's Five Caring Processes provide care givers with a basis for caring and interacting consciously and therapeutically.

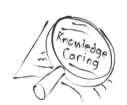

Phase Three: Transitioning

In this phase, we transition patients into their next setting, whether that setting is another medical setting, hospice care, a rehabilitation facility or home. In this phase we anticipate what patients and their families may need to know based on what we've learned about them and what we know about their condition.

The term *transitioning* implies that when patients leave us, it is in no way the end of their journey. We don't simply "hand off" patients; we prepare them to be received—welcomed once again—into whatever comes next for them. Transitioning, as is true of the two previous phases, may take place over moments or days.

Throughout each of the phases of the therapeutic relationship, nurses function in a number of practice roles (Koloroutis, 2004). In any given moment, a nurse may be called upon to act as:

- *Sentry*
- *Healer*
- *Guide*
- *Teacher*
- *Collaborator*
- *Leader*

The Six Practice Roles as Expressed in the Therapeutic Relationship: Practical Language for Caring Connections

While it is true that in any interaction, a nurse can be called upon to play more than one of these roles simultaneously, discussing them individually will help demonstrate how various situations can call care givers to play one role more prominently than another. Thinking in terms of "roles" also helps nurses put voice to what they are doing on behalf of the patient—and why. When a patient enters a facility, for example, an extremely important role the nurse fulfills is that of guide (one who informs and translates). When a patient comes out of surgery, he or she most needs for the nurse to be a sentry (one who watches over and protects), and the nurse accomplishes this by assessing, monitoring and preventing complications. Understanding the roles themselves and how they can be expressed within the nurse-patient relationship is useful in assisting nurses to more consciously engage in therapeutic relationships with patients and their families.

The six practice roles may be expressed differently throughout each phase of the therapeutic relationship.

SENTRY—One Who Watches Over and Protects

The nurse as sentry continually assesses, monitors and intervenes for the patient to prevent complications, promote healing and optimize safe outcomes.

Receiving: "I am the one who will watch over you during the next 12 hours to make sure that you are recovering as expected from your surgery. I will check on you frequently and here is the way you can reach me if I am not in your room."

Engaging: "I want to ensure that you are as comfortable as possible tonight. I will explain some of the options for managing your pain, and then we will decide what will work best for you."

Transitioning: "As we move to the unit where you will recover, I will tell your new nurse exactly what happened in the initial part of your recovery so that you and your Primary Nurse can make sure you continue to progress."

HEALER—One Who Cares for Another's Body, Mind and Spirit

The healer helps others improve their level of health and well-being.

Receiving: "I am your Primary Nurse and will be caring for you this evening. I will do everything I can to help you stay comfortable and continue your recovery."

Engaging: "What is your number one priority for today?"

Transitioning: "I will not be here tomorrow, and while I'm away, your nurse will be Sharon Jackson. Sharon will be joining us in just a moment so you can meet her, and we will talk with her about your care and what is most important to you."

GUIDE—One Who Possesses Intimate Knowledge of the Way

The nurse translates information and processes it into lay language, by clarifying and explaining procedures, and by making certain that the patient and family understand what to expect and can make informed decisions about their care.

Receiving: "We have been expecting you. Before I explain what will happen next, I want to let you know that there is no question you cannot ask me and there should be no language that is mysterious to you. I am here to make sure you know what is going on and what to expect."

Engaging: "My goal is to keep you informed and answer your questions."

Transitioning: "Before you leave for surgery, I will clarify anything you may still be wondering about."

TEACHER—One Who Imparts Knowledge

The care giver helps another gain knowledge and learn a skill. The nurse teaches the patient and family how to safely care for themselves in the health care setting and upon discharge.

Receiving (to a family member): "I am Mary Koloroutis; I'm the Primary Nurse who's been caring for your mother. Over the next few days I will help you learn how to care for your mother after she returns home."

Engaging: "How are you feeling about caring for your mother at home? What support do you have? What do you feel most comfortable with and what do you feel most concerned about?"

Transitioning: "I want to review the three most important aspects of caring for your mother as you prepare to take her home."

COLLABORATOR—One Who Works Cooperatively With Others to Achieve a Common Purpose

The nurse works with each member of the health care team to coordinate care. The nurse makes sure that the team receives and provides pertinent information regarding the patient and family.

Receiving: "Welcome, Mr. and Mrs. Franklin. I am John Caufield, your Primary Nurse. I am the one who will be caring for you tonight and coordinating your care during your stay. Your physician, Dr. Kaur, called and let me know that you would be coming. Mr. Franklin, the first thing I want to do is to help you settle into your room and give you the medication Dr. Kaur asked me to give you to relieve your pain. After you are more comfortable, I will complete your admission and discuss what is planned for tomorrow."

Engaging: "I will let your social worker and physician know about our conversation and your concerns about the discharge. The three of us will meet with you and your family tomorrow to make sure that all of your concerns are addressed."

Transitioning: "You are stable and we are ready to transfer you to the medical unit for your continued recovery. This is a milestone that shows that you are making good progress. Your Primary Nurse on the medical unit is Janet Lear. When we get on the unit, she and I will review your care with you and I will make sure that she has all the information she needs to care for you in the next phase."

LEADER—One Who Advocates on Behalf of the Patient and Family

The nurse as leader uses his or her authority to act on behalf of others; he or she possesses the capacity to affect change and influence direction. The nurse supervises, advocates for the individual patient and family, and delegates care to other members of the health care team.

Receiving: "We've been expecting you; welcome to our unit. I am Susan Wright, your Primary Nurse, and I'll be coordinating the care you will receive on this unit."

Engaging: "I learned from the nursing assistant that you are very concerned about this procedure. Will you talk with me about what is concerning you? I think it's important for your physician to know that you still have questions about this procedure. I will call her and share your concerns and make sure that all of your questions are addressed before we move forward."

Transitioning: "On this unit, I've been your Primary Nurse, and you will have a new Primary Nurse on the next unit. I have called her and let her know specifically about your questions regarding the plan for discharge. She will continue to work with your social worker to make sure the plan is right for you. I will accompany you to the unit and introduce you."

Looking at the therapeutic relationship through the lenses of the six practice roles is another way to see more deeply into "who we are" in the work we do. In every patient interaction, no matter what role you play, you have a valuable opportunity to choose language that promotes a meaningful therapeutic relationship.

Your Professional Nursing Practice

As we continue the evolution of the nurse-patient relationship, we must never lose sight of the power of the nurse's therapeutic use of self. Each nurse theorist who has come before has helped us to see something different about our role as healers, but in essence, they all point back to the importance of meaningful human connection itself. Each theorist helps us to understand a different way in which we may offer ourselves more fully to the service of healing our patients, helping them learn to heal themselves, and enabling their families to participate in their healing as well.

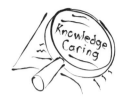

While the work of nurse theorists is important, it is best used as a jumping-off point for the personalization of every nurse's practice. While it is beneficial for us to review all of the theory available to us, the therapeutic use of self is inherently personal. It truly does exist, as Watson suggests, in each "moment." Each episode of care is a series of these moments—at best, a series of moments intentionally chosen and deliberately formed.

References: Belcher, P. & Fish, L. (1995). Hildegard E. Peplau. In George J. *Nursing Theories: The base for Professional Practice.* London: Prentice Wall

Berlin, E., & Fowkes, W. (1983). A teaching framework for cross-cultural health care: Application in family practice, In Cross-cultural Medicine. *Western Journal of Medicine*, 12:139, 93-98.

Koloroutis, M. (2004). *Relationship-based care: A model for transforming practice.* Minneapolis, MN: Creative Health Care Management.

Paterson, J., & Zderad, L. (1988). *Humanistic nursing.* New York: National League for Nursing.

Peplau, H. E. (1952). *Interpersonal relations in nursing.* New York: G. P. Putnam's Sons.

Swanson, K. (1993). Nursing as informed caring for the well-being of others. *IMAGE: Journal of Nursing Scholarship*, 25, 352-367.

Travelbee, J. (1971). *Interpersonal aspects of nursing.* Philadelphia: F. A. Davis.

Watson, J. (2006). *Transpersonal caring relationships.* Retrieved July 20, 2006, from http://www2.uchsc.edu/son/caring/content/transpersonal.asp.

Exemplar: Six Practice Roles and Therapeutic Communication

Background: *Putting words to each of the practice roles in a group process is an effective way to concretely apply principles of therapeutic communication and to benefit from each other's experience. The following examples are the result of group work at a Leadership at the Point of Care workshop. The group consisted of 22 nurses from UC Davis Medical Center who are continuing to evolve their Primary Nursing Practice.*

The six practice roles provide us with a way to put voice to the work of nursing.

Sentry Role (one who watches over, protects, keeps safe)	Pediatric Intensive Care Unit example "I'm your nurse and will be caring for your child today. You are in a children's hospital. What that means is that everyone here is committed to your child's recovery. We recognize how important it is for you to be here with your child. While I understand how scary this is for you, I promise you will not go through this alone. No matter what happens today I will be here for you and your child keeping you informed and involved."
Healer Role (one who cares for another's body, mind and spirit)	"Hello, my name is…. Welcome to UC Davis Medical Center. Are there any special needs I can meet for you or your family? Your doctor will be here shortly to assess your needs and write orders. In the interim we can discuss your concerns and start to develop our plan of care. What works best for you? I have found it helps if we work as a team."

Guide Role (someone who leads or directs another's way through unfamiliar circumstances; one who possesses intimate knowledge of the way)	"As your Primary Nurse, I will help you navigate the hospital and each department so that you may have a rewarding and positive hospital stay. I will explain all procedures and tests in a way that you and your family will understand. I will assist you in making informed decisions. I will help you to understand the role of each health care provider and how their jobs relate to your well-being. I will tell you specifics in words you can understand and in ways that will allow you to make your own decisions about your care."
Teacher Role (one who imparts knowledge; someone who helps another learn a skill)	"Tell me what you normally do at home." (Assessing knowledge base) "Do you know what to expect after taking this medication?" "Who is involved in your care?" "I am here to answer your questions." Return demonstration of care ... "Is anything making you feel anxious?" "Write down any questions that you have." "It is my role as a nurse to help you feel comfortable and confident and able to care for yourself when you are discharged."
Collaborator Role (one who works cooperatively with others to achieve a common purpose)	"As a nurse, I will work with the other disciplines to facilitate your plan of care." • Participate in MD rounds: "I will be at the bedside to help you talk to the doctors." • Care conferences: All disciplines will be pulled together to develop a plan of care. • Assertive patient advocate • Communication board • "I am your Primary Nurse." • "Before you go home, do you have any concerns for discharge arrangements?" • Patient involved in plan of care: "What will work for you?"

Leader Role (one who has the authority to act on behalf of others; someone who possesses the capacity to effect change and influence direction)

"As a leader of your care I will accept responsibility to ..."

- Ensure that your needs and expectations are addressed.

- Advocate for you and your family.

- Attend to any concerns/issues in your care and facilitate necessary changes with the health care team.

- Create with you an environment that promotes open communication in facilitating your care.

Therapeutic Relationships: Three Leaders' Reflections

—Mary Koloroutis

In preparation for writing about the therapeutic nurse-patient relationship, I sent e-mails out to colleagues in the field who had been identified by other colleagues as exemplars in establishing a therapeutic relationship with patients and families. I asked them to reflect on the nature of the therapeutic relationship as a privileged bond and sacred trust, and to reflect on how their practice relates to the following quote:

> *When a care provider crosses the threshold*
> *of a patient and family's door, he or she crosses a border—*
> *moving from the world of practical preparation*
> *into that of a personal healing relationship in which*
> *everything he or she does is in service to the patient....*

> *—Jayne A. Felgen*

I received responses from three exemplary healers who are clear about the power of the therapeutic use of self and the importance of the therapeutic relationship. I am pleased to share their words and stories here. They are instructional, inspirational and hope-filled.

Clifford Bond

Background: *Clifford is a chaplin who has worked in hospital and hospire settings in the Topeka, Kansas area since 1984. He also has extensive experience in the addiction and recovery field.*

What does the quote by Jayne Felgen mean to you in practice?

Theory is great preparation for what is real, but when we fall back into our training or theory we begin to speak in footnotes, which are safe but not very helpful. The helpful relationship involves risk of ourselves, which in a therapeutic setting will build trust. Without risk of self, trust lies dormant. I see five behaviors, actually, which build relationship and they are honesty, trust, risk, gratitude and humility. Felgen's quote says the same to me in different words.

> The helpful relationship involves risk of ourselves, which in a therapeutic setting will build trust. Without risk of self, trust lies dormant.

Describe a therapeutic relationship that you found meaningful.

My visit started as a "drive-by," meaning an exploration visit of very brief duration just to get a feel for dynamics without making the cancer patient and her spouse feel caught. My second visit included sharing my concept of spirituality with the young woman and her TV personality husband, who did not enter into any overtly religious dialogue. Over the months we have developed a trust that is honest at a professional level. Now the patient and I e-mail back and forth as she goes in and out of remission and goes to Mayo Clinic for a second opinion. The patient, her husband and I have a "close" therapeutic tie that does not violate boundaries. Cool.

What are some ways you create emotional safety for the patients and families you care for?

Trust means that they can process their situation without pressure from me, from the "shoulds" of society or religion or the medical profession or any other source, even from within themselves. Any feeling or thought is validated and encouraged. When we look at options it is at behaviors, not feelings. Some options may have better outcomes than others but feelings are not value rated. They know that I will enter into their situation with them as far as they have need, but they will also sense that I will not substitute my own experience for theirs or allow them to be care givers for me. That balance is probably the most difficult to maintain: to be helpful without taking over. The goal is to empower, not to create dependency, which is always easy to do even without realizing it.

Please respond to the following beginning sentences:

My relationship with the patient and family is ... one that allows distance without separation so that they can feel free to ask for help but not feel obligated or in need to do so.

The greatest challenge for me is ... to remember that I cannot "fix" things like I think they "should" be fixed but to remember that where trust exists healing can occur and I can be part of that healing.

I believe that ... all of us are afraid of the unknown and it is only in a healthy "we" that strength most fully comes so that we can accept without resignation and believe without unrealistic expectations, allowing hope to develop and flourish.

The interpersonal connection is what powers the work and transforms it into nursing care.

When people laugh, they sometimes put their guard down and we can get to authentic communication a little faster.

Sharon Melburg

Background: *Sharon Melburg recently retired from her position as a nursing director at UC Davis Medical Center. She is a facilitator of the* Reigniting the Spirit of Caring *workshop.*

What does the quote by Jayne Felgen mean to you in practice?

All the preparation that nurses (physicians and other healers as well) undergo prepares them for service to another. There is no compelling reason (other than curiosity, of course) to learn about human physiology and behavior except to apply that knowledge to improve the life of another—directly or indirectly. Because of what the nurse has come to understand, the nurse can enter into a unique relationship of trust and intimate service.

For me, this has meant being able to approach a patient with pneumocystis pneumonia (PCP), manipulate his chest tube, restart his IV, talk about his plans for the weekend, describe PCP as an AIDS-defining diagnosis, replace his condom catheter and talk about end-of-life care all in the same brief visit.

Often what nurses do is not at all glamorous. Providing personal care, manipulating invasive devices, remembering to deliver medications, fluids and nutrition accurately and on time, and teaching the same material to the 200th patient and

Once a fear is framed in words, it can be dealt with. As long as it has no name, it is infinite in size and ferocity.

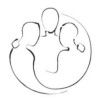

family may be exciting and challenging at first, but after years of practice, become mundane. What never gets routine is the response each individual patient and family has to the work the nurse does. The interpersonal connection is what powers the work and transforms it into nursing care. The nurse has been down the road before, with others—not the same road, maybe, but a similar one—and the nurse is not afraid. The nurse's willingness to be present to pain has healing potential.

Describe a therapeutic relationship of which you are particularly proud.

A friend's mother had been diagnosed with throat cancer. She was terrified, and unwilling to undergo what she described as "horrific" surgery when her physicians did not hold out significant promise of cure. Radical neck surgery with follow-up radiation would likely extend her life and might remove all of the cancer, but her ability to speak would be gone, her ability to eat would be gone, and the chances that she already had metastatic disease were high.

My friend's relationship with his mother had been rocky, but he wanted to be present to her and provide physical care and emotional support to her. He asked me if I would see her. We had not met before, but as we established our relationship, she shared her fear of pain with me and we talked about pain management options. We set up a kind of algorithm for decision making; if metastatic—what? If resectable—what? If laryngectomy required—what? If unable to swallow—what? We talked about her role as mother to my friend and about the things she wanted him to remember. We talked about the central crisis of her life—her divorce—and what it would take for her to be peaceful about that. She asked me at one point if I thought she was dying. Looking at the size of her tumor, how emaciated she was quickly becoming, and listening to the increased difficulty she was having speaking and managing her secretions, I answered—yes, I thought she probably was. She cried for a few minutes, and then seemed to brighten. She asked what her death might be like. She asked if I had ever been with someone as they died from her kind of cancer. She wanted to know if she could stay at home and what that would be like for her son and his wife. She asked some questions about my understanding of God and told me hers. We found things to laugh about and found some areas of common ground such that I believe she trusted me.

As she became more debilitated, I showed her son how to reposition her and how to give a back rub. She relaxed when we did this. She liked having a scented candle in her room. We put lots of pillows around to cushion all her bony parts. When tests showed lung metastasis, her decision to refuse surgery was affirmed in her mind and this brought some peace. She continued a gradual downhill slide and began to require pain medication in higher and higher doses. She lost her ability to swallow. Speaking became increasingly difficult. By this time she was enrolled in hospice. Her physician recommended radiation to shrink the tumor and relieve some of the pressure that was contributing to her pain. This would mean coming out of hospice. I helped her son understand how they could continue to do those things the hospice nurses had taught them while she was getting radiation. I tried to be a sounding board for his frustration with "the health care system." An appeal got her reinstated into hospice as soon as the radiation treatments were completed. As it became more difficult for her to manage her secretions and swallow, I intervened to get IV access with IV pain medication. Getting up to the bathroom became a problem, so we obtained an order for a catheter. This helped us keep the promise we had made to her that we would not let her die in pain.

My last visit to her was a few days before she died. In the night, her son snapped awake and went in to be with her. She died cradled in his arms. When he called, I felt good for her and for him and for me—gratified because I believe I was a catalyst for healing their frayed connections and I was able to use my nursing knowledge to make things easier for her and for my friend.

> I believe I was a catalyst for healing their frayed connections and I was able to use my nursing knowledge to make things easier for her and for my friend.

What are some ways you create emotional safety for the patients and families you care for?

I introduce myself. I try not to ask any yes-no types of questions, but say things like "Please tell me about ..." or "What has been your experience with...." I try not to come up with "solutions" too quickly. I use selective self-disclosure to find common ground. I try to find something really funny that we can share. When people laugh, they sometimes put their guard down and we can get to authentic communication a little faster. I try to grasp what they are most afraid of and put it into words—usually in a question. Once a fear is framed in words, it can be dealt with. As long as it has no name, it is infinite in size and ferocity.

Please complete these sentences:

My relationship with the patient and family is ... respectful and welcoming.

The greatest challenge for me is ... to not to take over and reduce their problems to fit my solutions.

I believe that ... there will be wonderful surprises.

Teresa Kellerman

Background: *Teresa Kellerman is a Clinical Nurse Specialist and facilitator for Reigniting the Spirit of Caring at St Francis Hospital in Topeka, KS.*

Describe a therapeutic relationship of which you are particularly proud. Consider how you established it, managed it and ended it. What can be learned from your experience that would guide others?

Many years ago, as I was beginning my Wound and Ostomy Care practice, I encountered an elderly gentleman who was newly diagnosed with bladder cancer and who would require a urinary diversion. He was hungry for information and was understandably concerned about the life changes that awaited him. I wanted desperately to prove my worth in this new role and to provide the patient and his wife with support and assistance to help them cope with their difficult news. As I educated this man and his spouse, our relationship quickly took shape; we learned about each other and forged a strong rapport and trust, making ourselves vulnerable to each other. He assertively recovered from his surgery, taking command of his situation. I offered encouragement and helped him to chart his own course. We worked as a team.

The following years provided opportunities for follow-up and counsel. He became one of my core Ostomy Support members and ostomy visitors, cheerleading and role modeling for other patients. He knew that he could call on me at any time for help, just as I could count on him. Leonard was an avid fisherman and fishing nearly every day of the year was his lifeline. On occasion, I would receive a voice message from him while he was in his boat letting me know that the fish were biting especially well that day.

Shortly after his metastatic lung cancer diagnosis was made, we had lengthy conversations about his treatment, his prognosis and his wife's well-being after he died. He was admitted a few times during his treatment period, but he remained an active member of the support group and continued to fish as often as he could. I was awed by his strength and determination, but we both knew the reality of his situation. He became a patient guest at our *Reigniting the Spirit of Caring* workshops and welcomed the opportunity to share his story and to impassion care givers. During this time, the mutual respect, appreciation and trust between us intensified. He knew that I would do anything within my power for him.

> Part of the lesson in this for me was the transition from a simple nurse-patient relationship to human-to-human relationship.

The day that I received the call that he had died was incredibly challenging. I did not anticipate the huge void that was left by his passing or the ache within my heart. I had lost a true friend. As I attended his visitation, I cried with his wife and daughters and held his hand for the last time, knowing that this man had left an indelible imprint upon my being and owning the impact that I had made in his life.

Part of the lesson in this for me was the transition from a simple nurse-patient relationship to human-to-human relationship. Neither of us felt threatened within our roles. We taught each other as our connection grew. I helped Leonard determine his own illness-wellness course by providing him with support and information and facilitating his making his own decisions. This provided him with control and autonomy, and he knew that I would provide support and not waver in our relationship regardless of his choices. He was confident that I would not abandon him. I believe that within our relationships with our patients, we are obligated to communicate this steadfast sense of compassionate duty and deliver it, not as a burden, but as a true privilege.

What are some ways you create emotional safety for the patients and families you care for?

There are a number of everyday interventions that nurses employ to create an emotionally safe milieu for patients and family. We begin by meeting people where they are as individuals with unique life circumstances.

By sharing appropriately with them the passion I feel for my work and demonstrating empathy for their situation, I hope to communicate that they are important to me. I consciously utilize appropriate touch, maintain a respectful, subdued tone and demeanor, actively listen, ask follow-up questions and allow time for responses. This interaction sets the stage for genuine sharing and storytelling. I present myself as "nonhurried"—and convey that these individuals are the most important people I will encounter. I believe this adds to the potential for a safe and honest exchange. I believe we each have the ability to create a safe harbor for those within our care.

The greatest challenge for me is ...to remember that I cannot "fix" things like I think they "should" be fixed but to remember that where trust exists healing can occur and I can be part of that healing.

Please complete these sentences:

My relationship with the patient and family is ... intentional, but not scripted; it must remain fluid given the circumstances and relationship.

The greatest challenge for me is ... time. My patients always come first. Projects, meetings and other such demands are secondary, but sometimes I feel as though administrative staff will see that priority as inappropriate. I am a nurse first and foremost. The other responsibilities are important and I take them seriously; however, they cannot supersede the clinical, emotional, spiritual needs of a patient and family.

I believe that ... being a care giver is a privilege and an honor not to be taken for granted or treated casually. We each have a gift for caring and an obligation to give the best that we have to offer. These gifts present themselves differently within individual care givers, yet the purpose remains the same—to serve others and to recognize our own needs in order to maintain a healthy balance of service. We are the essence of caring by virtue of what we do.

Caring Made Visible

—Kristen M. Swanson

Birth of the Five Caring Processes

My development of what came to be the Five Caring Processes started with a deep interest in understanding what it was like for women to miscarry. I was a doctoral student, and when I approached my chairperson, Dr. Jean Watson, who founded the Center for Human Caring in Colorado, she told me that she would work with me if I would explore what caring meant from the perception of women who miscarried.

At the end of that study, I suggested there were five basic caring processes:

- *Knowing*
- *Being with*
- *Doing for*
- *Enabling*
- *Maintaining belief*

During my postdoctoral studies with Dr. Kathryn Barnard at the University of Washington I further refined the processes through interviewing and observing care givers in a neonatal intensive care unit and by interviewing high-risk mothers who had received a long-term public health nursing intervention. Each of the Five Caring Processes is expressed through a number of specific acts. Each process and its common expressions are described in the following pages.

Editors' note: *In this adaptation of a 1998 interview with* Creative Nursing's *Pat Jakobsen, Swanson talks about the development of the Five Caring Processes.*

Knowing

In the context of care, **knowing** means "striving to understand an event as it has meaning in the life of the other."

The process of knowing involves trying to avoid assumptions about patients. That doesn't mean we let go of everything we know about the disease condition they may be experiencing or even the typical responses people might have to a diagnosis. But it means that we check out what we know and find out if it happens to be true for this individual. For example, many women feel angry when they're first diagnosed with breast cancer. So we might ask this woman to tell us how she's feeling or say, "This is hard, isn't it? What is this like for you?" You leave a space for her to fill in.

Knowing can be expressed as:

- *making the patient fully aware that he or she is the center of a conversation,*

- *assessing thoroughly—seeking what is said and not said on the patient's part, and*

- *understanding the other patient's situation to the extent that you become personally engaged with the patient as a person.*

When we are being emotionally present for our patients, they sense that no matter how bad the circumstances might be, we won't abandon them.

Being With

Once you have established the engagement of two selves, you can't help moving on to the next level, which is **being with**. I define this as being emotionally present with another. When we are being emotionally present for our patients, they get the sense that they really matter. They sense that no matter how bad the circumstances might be, we won't abandon them. Sometimes giving patients an extra minute and a half in an emergency says, "I'm here to listen." Sometimes it's when you're working in the middle of the night and you choose to have your cup of coffee alongside the patient's bed instead of at the station. It's that sense that you're willing to give them time and give of yourself.

Maybe what brings us to nursing is our belief in people, our ability to hold them in esteem and to see them as persons of dignity and worth.

> **Being with means:**
>
> - *you convey your availability to patients—even when you aren't free to spend as much time with patients as you desire to, you convey that desire,*
>
> - *you share your feelings—expressing a willingness to smile at a birth and get frustrated with someone when they just can't take that step, and*
>
> - *you safeguard that you are not burdening clients with your experience of their experience.*

Doing For

The next process is **doing for**. After you know the patient and are able to be with him or her, then the actions that you do feel so much more relevant to the patient. "Doing for" is doing for the patient what they would do for themselves if it were possible—but doing no more than that. You don't want to make your patients dependent on you. The goal is to let them be in charge and take care of their own life, whatever their life might happen to be at the moment.

Still, there are times when you realize patients are capable of, for example, brushing their hair. But you say, "Do you mind if I brush your hair?" and have a conversation with them as you brush. They're perfectly capable of brushing their hair, but for you it is an act of affection or a chance to comfort and massage; it is an act of "doing for," but it comes more from a "being with" stance.

> ### Doing for involves:
>
> - *comforting patients,*
>
> - *anticipating what the other will need in order to experience success,*
>
> - *performing competently and skillfully, and*
>
> - *protecting our patients by safeguarding both their physical well-being and their dignity.*

Enabling

Enabling is next. It means facilitating the other's passage through difficult events and life transitions. This is the teaching and learning component, done in such a way that we ultimately put the patient back on center stage and stop coaching so overtly. It's about empowering people, families and communities to know how to care for themselves.

> ### Enabling involves:
>
> - *keeping patients informed—explaining what is going on,*
>
> - *supporting patients both personally and professionally, and*
>
> - *allowing people to be "right where they are," focusing on the issue in front of them.*

The last caring process is **maintaining belief.** Maintaining belief means sustaining faith in the capacity of patients to get through an event or transition and face the future with meaning. Those events and transitions include episodes of wellness and illness, births, deaths and many of the other conditions under which we as nurses encounter people. When we believe in people, we are willing to maintain a hope-filled attitude when we work with people. As best we can, we offer optimism. And if nothing else, we go the whole distance; we don't abandon people no matter how bad the situation may get.

> ### *Maintaining belief includes:*
>
> * *helping patients find meaning for themselves— helping patients to make what they're going through sacred or special, and*
>
> * *working with people around their religious and spiritual needs.*

After having gone through the processes—knowing, being with, doing for, enabling and maintaining belief—you might think that I see maintaining belief as the end of it. But in fact, I believe it's the beginning of caring.

Maybe what brings us to nursing is our belief in people, our ability to hold them in esteem and to see them as persons of dignity and worth. When we stand by a parent whose child has been diagnosed with an end-stage disease, we stay and start talking about the child's play needs or teaching needs. We do this because we see a tomorrow, even if it feels like the end of the world for the family whose child is about to die. We might not explicitly say to the family, "Here is what your tomorrow looks like," but we talk about maintaining the child and his or her human growth and development needs. The family gets the message that there is a tomorrow and that tomorrow will still have meaning.

I believe that's what motivates nurses to act in a caring fashion: We believe in people and their right to get through events and transitions and find meaning. That's what gets us started, and if we keep feeling that way, we're going to try to understand what it's like for patients, make ourselves as available to them as possible, do for them all that they would do for themselves, keep them informed enough to make good decisions for themselves, and believe always in the possibility for meaning in each moment—no matter what the future will bring.

Reference: Swanson, K. (1998). Caring made visible, interview by Pat Jakobsen. *Creative Nursing*, 4(4), 8-11, 16.

The Role of the LPN or ... the Problem of Two Levels

—A Marie Manthey classic

The problem of defining two levels in nursing is still a painful impediment to sane, high-quality, cost-effective care. As Leah Curtin suggests in her May 1987 editorial we seem to have lost sight of the purpose of licensure; i.e., to protect society. Instead, the two levels in nursing are viewed as a step ladder to professionalization. If there are two levels, the ones carrying the title "professional" are on the top rung, and therefore identifiable and visible almost as if one becomes professional by standing on the shoulders of "technical" nurses.

Differentiation of practice has been problematic for at least the past four decades. Ever since the Second World War when the numbers of LPNs increased astronomically (from eight schools before the war to over a thousand after), explanations of the difference between RNs and LPNs have hovered from the ridiculous to the sublime.

Consider that in the early 1960s, LPNs were not allowed to administer medications to patients in acute care hospitals. Later they could pass orals, but not IMs. Then they could do IMs but not regulate the flow of IVs. Then they could regulate the flow of IVs, but not add medicated solutions. This is where the situation rests today, except in those jurisdictions where the law states or is interpreted to mean that they cannot even regulate IV flow. (In these jurisdictions, the RN role gets clarified quickly; she functions primarily as a plumber!)

Attempts to differentiate roles according to tasks performed perpetuate the notion that nursing can be defined as a task-based occupation. This nonsense continues to be articulated in the face of current discharge planning activities that have family members learning how to do almost everything nurses do in the hospital, including administering medicated IV solutions! Task-based differentiation attempts are so silly

Editors' note: *This classic piece was written in 1989, yet the issue is timeless. Are we differentiating nursing responsibility, authority and accountability by knowledge and complexity of clinical judgment or by tasks? Originally published in* Nursing Management, *20(2). Used with permission.*

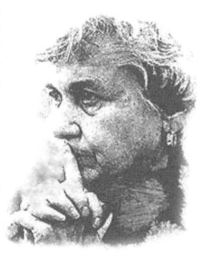

that the profession itself suffers from an enormous loss of self-respect every time the issue is discussed and reinforced.

The only rationale for differentiation that doesn't offend common sense is one based on the complexity of clinical judgment required to make clinically competent, knowledge-based practice decisions in the management of a patient's care. Very little work has been done to date on a logical definition of criteria for this differentiation, probably for the reasons mentioned in Leah Curtin's editorial. The absence of a consensus on the identifiable body of knowledge (core curriculum) required to practice any level of professional nursing hampers the development of complexity-based practice differentiation.

Several years ago (1965 to be exact), the University of California at San Francisco hosted a week-long exploration of the differentiation between practice and education. It was attended and conducted by leaders in both areas, and the results were available in the form of a manual for participants. A simple logic for differentiation has been in my mind ever since then. The rationale offered was intended to be used to differentiate between Associate and Baccalaureate degree educational preparation, but I have found it useful whenever differentiation criteria are needed. These criteria are especially helpful in deciding which patients are to be cared for by nurses prepared to function at a professional level and which are to be cared for by nurses prepared to function at a technical level. They are:

1. Patients whose care requirements are routine and standardized.

2. Patients whose outcomes are predictable.

3. Patients whose reaction to illness and hospitalization is not threatening to their sense of self and does not upset their emotional equilibrium.

These criteria provide a framework for decision-making that supports differentiation based on clinical judgment, rather than on task performance.

There are many reasons for shifting from task-based to judgment-based methods for differentiating practice. The strongest reason is that task-based methods support the notion that nurses' work is primarily a series of tasks. Moreover, we

> Task-based differentiation attempts are so silly that the profession itself suffers from an enormous loss of self-respect every time the issue is discussed and reinforced.

put ourselves in the awkward position of seeming to say that LPNs are not permitted to think. For example, assessment is essentially a cognitive attribute that all humans possess. Therefore, saying LPNs cannot "do assessments" is tantamount to telling them to stop thinking at the patient's bedside. It is akin to the game-playing between physicians and RNs: the RNs pretend they don't think diagnostically in order not to threaten their control over medical practice. Responsibility for a function such as decision-making doesn't mean others should not think about the decision—or even contribute to it. It simply means one person is responsible for doing it. Eliminating all assessment functions from the LPNs' role implies either that we would be just as well off using lobotomized LPNs or mechanical robots to do their jobs.

We get caught in these unholy positions because of our relentless use of task-based differentiation of function. In this case thinking (assessment) is the task not permitted, in order to differentiate level of education. And when the principals involved are an experienced, mature LPN and a new graduate RN, the situation can become downright Kafkaesque.

Another reason for moving away from this restricted thinking is the devastating effect it has on morale, as both LPNs and RNs are demeaned when so narrow, illogical and artificial a differentiation strategy is adopted. Registered nurses need to view practice as knowledge-based, and decision-making is the backbone of knowledge-based practice. Responsibility for decision-making about a patient's overall care activities should always be the RN's, regardless of the level of complexity of that care or the length of stay of the patient. Within the framework of those care decisions, LPNs, following the care plan designed by the RN, can be assigned to perform total care during a tour of duty.

The LPN should be expected to perform all the care activities required by that patient, and document and report on the patients cared for during that tour of duty. Requiring that certain tasks (assessment, documentation, IV management, etc.) be performed by RNs is demeaning and illogical and it supports a task-oriented definition of professional practice.

A careful analysis of the fundamental nature of past utilization problems points to poor management techniques

Responsibility for a function such as decision-making doesn't mean others should not think about the decision. It simply means one person is responsible for doing it.

in handling people with different role expectations. Modern managers must be skillful team-builders. Different levels of practice must be skillfully blended into a cohesive, unified and healthy work group. Failure to learn this management skill will ensure future problems.

The Dilemma of RN / LPN Role Confusion

—Susan Wessel

In many hospitals we find the unfortunate dilemma that registered nurses and licensed practical nurses are working in virtually the same roles. Often, RN and LPN roles are differentiated by task, such as IV push medication, rather than by judgment, licensure or education. Underlying this task-based differentiation is confusion about the scope of practice for both registered nurses and licensed practical nurses.

Some hospitals have stopped hiring LPNs to avoid this confusion. This unfortunately removes highly skilled nurses from the workforce. Eliminating LPNs for this reason would be analogous to eliminating the Nurse Practitioner role in physician offices and using only Medical Technicians to avoid confusion. A better option is to bring role clarity and the effective, intentional use of LPNs to the delivery system.

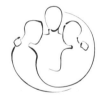

Leah Kinnaird developed the following model for use when performing *Work Complexity Assessments* (*see page 263*). Originally developed to explain the professional practice of nursing, it has proven effective in helping RNs and LPNs understand the important distinctions between their roles without causing defensiveness among the LPNs. When we spend time with RNs and LPNs analyzing how they work, we often learn that the true professional role of the RN—assessing, diagnosing and treating the human response to health problems—is not being visibly done at all. Instead, we find that RNs and LPNs are functioning in a task-based system that does not fulfill the responsibility, authority and accountability of the registered nurse.

When we ask about the differences between roles and responsibilities, the staff participants frequently have difficulty in differentiating the roles/responsibilities. The most common difference voiced is that RNs have a greater role for

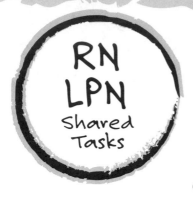

admission assessments. When the meaning of this is explored further, however, we often learn that the RN merely co-signs the LPN's admission assessment. What we find far too often in our *Work Complexity Assessments* is that RN and LPN roles are, in practice, almost identical.

In the graphic above, the inner circle represents the work that is to be done for a set of patients. Typically, patient assignments are divided between RNs and LPNs, so that the RN has his/her patients and the LPN has his/her patients. When the LPN cannot by law or policy do a task, the LPN finds an RN who can.

In these situations, the uniquely RN responsibilities are neglected or minimized. These responsibilities include:

- *Perform comprehensive assessment*

- *Recognize changes in condition and act to prevent complications*

- *Establish a plan of care using nursing diagnosis*

- *Evaluate responses to and effectiveness of plan of care*

- *Serve as Primary Nurse and coordinate care*

- *Manage and evaluate the practice of nursing*

When the RN role is not being fulfilled in a way that meets the true definition of professional practice, it's often that the systems are not designed to support the professional role.

These RN responsibilities go beyond the tasks that need to be done.

This graphic helps nurses (both RNs and LPNs) to see that most often it is not LPNs who are doing more than they have the authority to do. Rather, it is RNs who are not able to attend to their unique responsibilities. Patient care is compromised. When RNs and LPNs are clear about the uniqueness of their roles, they are able to partner to provide more comprehensive care. As a result, patients receive the best care.

It is essential that nurses realize that every patient needs to have an RN who has the responsibility for directing nursing care and tending to the decisions, advocacy and coordination of care that is needed. Working our way out of task-based care is not easy.

We have found that when the RN role is not being fulfilled in a way that meets the true definition of professional practice, it's often that the systems are not designed to support the professional role. These systems include things such as a clear nursing delivery system with all patients assigned to RNs, nursing documentation systems that facilitate all steps of the nursing process, and assignments, evaluations and report systems that promote continuity and give time and emphasis to the professional aspects of the RN role. The chaos and confusion on our patient care units have made it difficult (if not impossible) for RNs to fully carry out the responsibilities that define their professional role and differentiate and support their essential contribution to high-quality patient care.

It is helpful to begin with the American Nurses Association 1980 definition of nursing to describe the role of the professional RN in a concise and compelling way. This definition states that nursing is:

The diagnosis and treatment of human responses to actual or potential health problems (American Nurses Association [ANA], 2003).

This opens the way to a discussion of the independent role of registered nurses. For example, because we are often imprecise in our language, misunderstanding is prevalent about who may do the nursing assessment. The word "assessment" often includes two distinct steps: 1) data collection and 2) synthesis or interpretation of the data to form a nursing diagnosis. LPNs may perform data collection to contribute to the assessment according to their education and competence in doing so. The aspect of assessment that must be done by the RN is the synthesis and nursing diagnosis component. The experienced LPN may, of course, have a solid idea of the appropriate nursing diagnosis, but licensure requires it be discussed and confirmed by the RN.

Defining the Professional RN Role

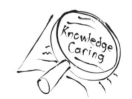

Patients desperately need RNs to fulfill their complete professional role as defined by law and by nursing's social contract with society

Each organization is guided by its own state practice act for nursing. An additional document that is instructive was developed by the National Council of State Boards of Nursing (NCSBN). This is a model nurse practice act, and it contains detailed descriptions of the scopes of nursing practice and standards of practice for both RNs and LPNs (National Council of State Boards of Nursing, 2004). The NCSBN reiterates the key distinction that the licensed practical/vocational nurse functions in a directed scope of nursing practice under the direction of an RN, licensed physician or other providers outlined by the state practice act. Registered nurses by license are independent in practicing the full scope of nursing.

Relationship-Based Care as a Pathway to Role Clarity

These principles, originally developed by Marie Manthey, recognize that the RN has the authority by law and by license to decide the amount, degree and kind of nursing care a patient will receive.

Patients desperately need RNs to fulfill their complete professional role as defined by law and by nursing's social contract with society (ANA, 2003). Relationship-Based Care (RBC) establishes an infrastructure to partner RNs and LPNs with a clear relationship based on specific responsibility, authority and accountability for each role. The principles of RBC require RNs to fulfill the full scope of their practice. These principles, originally developed by Marie Manthey, recognize that the RN has the authority by law and by license to decide the amount, degree and kind of nursing care a patient will receive. Patients and families are best served within systems designed so that registered nurses function within their full scope of professional practice which includes bringing their leadership and full expertise to the care of patients and families, and licensed practical nurses are affirmed for their valuable contribution to patient care.

References: American Nurses Association. (2003). *Nursing's social policy statement.* (2nd ed.). Washington, DC: Author.

National Council of State Boards of Nursing. (2004). *Model nursing act and rules.* Retrieved May 3, 2006, from http://www.ncsbn.org

I Am Your Nurse

—Vicki Bailey and Sharon E. Melberg

I am your patient.
I am afraid of the sounds and smells and machines.
I am cold.
I am alone.
Are you my nurse?

I am your nurse.
I am here and you are not alone.
I will answer your questions and bring you warm blankets.

I am your patient.
I don't know why I am here.
I don't know when I can leave.
Are you my nurse?

I am your nurse.
I will watch over you.
I will care for you.
I will treat you as the gift you are.

I am your patient.
I may get mad—I may say mean things—I may not listen.
Are you my nurse?

I am your nurse.
I will listen to your spirit; I will listen with my heart. Your
words will fall away.
I believe you are precious to God …
and I know you are precious to me.

I am your patient.
What if I don't make it? What if I can't see?
What if I can't walk? What if I have to die?

I am your nurse.
I will hold you, wash you, cherish you.
I will speak to you, and, if necessary for you.
And if it is your time to die,
I will miss you, I will grieve your passing.
If I never have another patient,
You are the reason I am a nurse.

Editors' note: *Vicki Bailey is a chaplain and Sharon Melberg is an RN at the University of California Davis Health System. They wrote the following poem in 2004 as part of a visioning exercise during a Reigniting the Spirit of Caring workshop sponsored by UCDHS.*

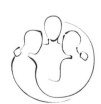

CHAPTER NINE

The Primary Nursing Role: The Foundation of Relationship-Based Care

Primary Nursing:
A Responsibility Relationship

—Colleen Person

The Primary Nursing Role

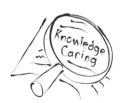

The Primary Nursing role is the responsibility relationship of a registered nurse for a therapeutic relationship and a plan of care for an individual patient. Typically the relationship is initiated by the nurse and is in effect for the length of the patient's stay in a service or unit. One of the hallmarks of the role is the clarity of the RN's acceptance of responsibility for decision making regarding the care of the patient. Another hallmark is that the relationship is known to the patient, family, other care givers and members of the interdisciplinary team. The Primary Nurse does not necessarily provide all of the activities of care. Typically the Primary Nurse transfers the relationship and plan of care to care providers in the next setting of care.

Primary Nurses experience the fullness of the professional role of nursing by accepting the responsibility for the individualized relationship and plan of care. The only factor that determines the presence or absence of professional nursing is the existence of a clearly established relationship between a member of society and an individual licensed by that society to administer professional nursing. The presence of that relationship is the essence of professional practice.

Other dimensions of nursing that impact the role are a defined care delivery model and a nursing theory. But the term "Primary Nurse" refers to the nurse who establishes and maintains the responsibility relationship with the patient.

The Primary Nurse uses the nursing process to determine the needs of the patient and to establish an individualized plan of care that is communicated to other members of the nursing team and the interdisciplinary team. The activities of care may be accomplished by Associate Nurses, Licensed Practical Nurses and Nursing Assistants within the context of the skill mix, care delivery model, practice acts and effective delegation.

The Primary Nurse is not responsible for providing all of the activities of care (as in Total Patient Care) but for the relationship and the plan of care. The activities of nursing—independent, dependent and interdependent—are the same regardless of the roles and the care delivery model. A defined Primary Nursing role and care delivery model provide the framework within which the activities of care are accomplished in an organized efficient and effective manner. The Primary Nurse determines what work requires his or her own time and attention and which work can be delegated to other care givers. Patient assignments are based on continuity of relationships, complexity of care and the skills and knowledge of the care giver.

The number of patients for whom a Primary Nurse is responsible depends upon the acuity of the patient population and the number of registered nurses in the skill mix. The skill mix should be based on patient acuity and work volume.

The term *Associate Nurse* is often used for the nurse who is assigned to care for the patient in the absence of the Primary Nurse and is responsible for following and/or revising the plan of care based on the patient's response to care and changing needs.

> The Primary Nurse is not responsible for providing all of the activities of care (as in Total Patient Care) but for the relationship and the plan of care.

> Primary Nursing has proven its worth in achieving the essence of professional nursing practice: healing within the context of caring relationships.

Within the context of the care delivery model specific Associate Nurses may be identified to be assigned to specific patients or the assignment may be more general.

The Patient Care Delivery Model

The patient care delivery model is an organized framework for accomplishing the responsibilities of basic nursing practice. There are four elements: relationship and decision making, work allocation, communication and management.

The first element references the role of the registered nurse and encompasses the definition of the fullness and extent of his/her responsibilities and the length of time of the responsibility relationship. The Primary Nurse role as defined typifies the fullness of a responsibility relationship.

The second element of a care delivery model is work allocation. The staffing schedule and assignments are the elements of a care delivery model that can be designed to support the Primary Nurse role and continuity of care givers with patients and with one another. Patient-centered staffing and scheduling principles can provide guidance in addressing the practical complexities.

The third element is that of communication between members of the health care team. In a Primary Nursing Model the Primary Nurse proactively provides information to others involved in the care of patients and seeks information from those who have it. Coordination of care is one of the essential aspects of the role.

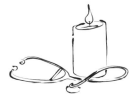

The fourth element of a patient care delivery model is that of management. The skills, attitude and behaviors of the unit managers are key to the success of the care delivery model. Managers need to be skilled in supporting registered nurses as autonomous decision makers and creative problem solvers regarding patient care.

Since its development almost 40 years ago the concept of the role and responsibilities of the Primary Nurse has proven its worth in achieving the essence of professional nursing practice: healing within the context of caring relationships. Because of misinterpretations over the years the time has come to clarify the Primary Nurse role so that both nurses and patients and their families can experience the benefits of relationships of caring and continuity.

Primary Nursing After Ten Years

—Ellen Kissinger (Interviewed by Mary Koloroutis)

Background: *Ellen Kissinger has been practicing on a 36-bed pediatrics unit at UC Davis Medical Center for the past 24 years. She is recognized as a clinical leader in making Primary Nursing come alive on her unit and sustaining it over the past ten years. The success of Primary Nursing on the pediatrics unit led to the implementation of Primary Nursing in all units at UC Davis. Ellen was interviewed by Mary Koloroutis*

Ellen, I appreciate your talking with me so that we can learn more about the background of Primary Nursing on your unit and what it has taken to structure and sustain it over the years. I'd like to hear about how it began.

I have been working on the same pediatric unit for the past 24 years. We actually believed that we were practicing Primary Nursing all along. The truth is, we were practicing bits and pieces of Primary Nursing. We were practicing only the concepts we wanted to and our practice was focused on meeting the needs of the nurse, not the patient. We had patients and families who loved us, who were very happy with the consistent coordinated care they were receiving; however, in the bed right next to them we could have a patient and family that were very frustrated and unhappy with the care they were receiving. No one wanted to take care of them. They did not have the consistent care the other patient/family was receiving and no one was advocating for them.

Were the "happy" families receiving Primary Nursing care?

Yes. For some reason we had patients that groups of nurses always wanted to take care of. Nurses coordinated care for them; they collaborated with the physicians and interdisciplinary team members to expedite discharge. I observed wonderful care for these patients. I called them our "See's Candies" patients. The patient was happy, families were happy, there weren't any complaints. They brought in See's Candies for the nurses and the hospitalization was wonderful for them. So these patients were well taken care of, their care was planned and coordinated and discharge teaching was anticipated and completed.

What about the families that you describe as being "not happy?"

We had patients and families that we as nurses labeled "difficult." These patients did *not* receive consistent care. In fact nurses advocated to not take care of them. These patients received a different nurse each shift. There wasn't communication between staff members about these patients—other than stories about them being difficult. Some of these patients required the most complex care and had poor resources and coping skills. There were times I would be assigned such a patient on the day of discharge, and absolutely nothing was done in preperation for discharge, even though they had been in the hospital for an extended time. The complex teaching wasn't started and there had been no advocacy to meet their discharge needs. There were times I had to go to the physician and tell him that we were not able to discharge a patient because we (nursing) had not prepared the patient and family for discharge. Some of these patients had been with us a few days or weeks. Nurses didn't accept responsibility for these patients and no one was held accountable.

What do you think could explain such a difference in care?

We didn't have a framework or structure for our practice. Patients were assigned geographically. The nurse was the center of focus, not the patient. We didn't have any system or structure in place for assignment making or tracking of patients. We were practicing in chaos; nurses on every shift were just trying to get by. We had unhealthy relationships between staff members. We didn't collaborate with the physicians, and, in fact, some physicians had requested not to have certain nurses take care of their patients.

We didn't develop nurses' competence. We were territorial. Certain nurses took care of certain types of patients and

> We were practicing in chaos; nurses on every shift were just trying to get by. We had unhealthy relationships between staff members. We didn't collaborate with the physicians, and, in fact, some physicians had requested not to have certain nurses take care of their patients.

things were done because they "were always done that way." Some nurses wanted to practice the bits and pieces of Primary Nursing while others came to work just to fulfill their hours. We lacked teamwork. In fact it reminded me of being in high school. We had cliques and some staff made it very clear who they would help and eat lunch with. It was difficult to take care of the patients because we were not taking care of ourselves or each other. It was not a healthy work environment.

And, you said earlier there was not a good mechanism in this system to hold nurses accountable for care?

That's right. Nurses were not accountable to themselves, their colleagues or their patients. It wasn't our culture back then to be able to have a professional conversation about a patient's care. Instead, the conversation was confrontational and not effective. So it was very difficult to collaborate and improve patient care, improve our own practice, or learn from each other.

What inspired you as a group to implement Primary Nursing?

As a group, we knew we had to do something. Our unit was very unhealthy. We would often go home feeling "beat up" from our colleagues, physicians and patients. We knew we had to turn the chaos off. We wanted to increase our professionalism. Our patients deserved more. The bottom line is we did it for the patients and their families.

How did a more systematic approach for Primary Nursing come to pass?

There were several of us who complained to our manager constantly about our toxic environment. We had a nurse that was going back to school and asked at a staff meeting what type of delivery care model we practiced. We all agreed it was the chaos model. The timing was right because there was a group of us who wanted to increase our professional practice. Lynne Boehret, our nurse manager, was visionary. She and Angie Marin, our assistant nurse manager, heard Marie Manthey speak back in the '80s. She told us how Marie Manthey inspired her and how she believed we could increase our professional practice. She recommended we read Marie Manthey's book, *The Practice of Primary Nursing.*

We wanted to increase our professionalism. Our patients deserved more. The bottom line is we did it for the patients and their families.

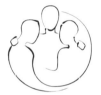

We no longer had "difficult patients" because nurses started to care and advocate for them.

What was most inspirational for you as you began the change to a Primary Nursing model for your entire unit?

The families and the patients. It was inspirational when everyone was receiving the same care. We no longer had "difficult patients" because nurses started to care and advocate for them. Nurses stepped up their professional practice. The nurses seemed happier; they were collaborating with colleagues, physicians and the interdisciplinary team. They truly felt valued and that they were making a difference.

We can never fully understand what the families are going through. What we can do is listen to what is important to them at that moment. This is the relationship that is developed with Primary Nursing. Sometimes their needs are not even related to the disease.

I have established some wonderful relationships with my patients and families. They always motivated me. I have always been amazed at the way families confide and open up to me during a crisis. Nurses are neutral to them and safe. I can see how accepting and nonjudgmental we have become.

Communication with the patient and the family starts right at admission when our key message is: "We are here for you." We partner with them immediately. We say, "You tell me your preferences and how you think this will work best."

What are some of the key factors that define your system of care delivery—that make it work well?

Communication is probably the most important factor. Communication with the patient and the family starts right at admission when our key message is: "We are here for you." We partner with them immediately. We say, "You tell me your preferences and how you think this will work best." I think it's important to give the family as much control as possible; it helps them cope. We developed tools to help staff communicate with each other and we saw a tremendous change in teamwork and respect for one another.

How are patient assignments made?

Assignments now are much more equitable than they were in our previous system. We have increased accountability and the competency of every single nurse on our floor so that we all are competent to care for the patients admitted to our general pediatric unit. In 10 years we have gone through several tracking systems from a file box with a colored dot to several different spreadsheets and now our electronic medical record. Patient assignments are patient focused, not nurse focused. When the Primary Nurse is on she always gets her primary patient back. If another nurse had the patient for two days and they were going home today, the Primary Nurse will have the authority to make the decision to keep the patient or let the associate nurse care for that patient. When we make out the assignments we assign patients to their Primary or associate nurses.

Has Primary Nursing affected scheduling?

We have always been very flexible with scheduling. We did not change this when we implemented our model. Obviously, working on a pediatrics unit means we love kids. And, we all have our own children. Many of us work set days because of child care issues. With our model of Primary Nursing, we divided the nurses into three teams. When we make out the assignment we start by assigning patients to their Primary Nurse, then associate nurse. If neither Primary nor associate nurses are working, we will assign the patient to a nurse that is on that color team. This has given us structure with assignment making.

How does the Primary Nurse take responsibility and accountability for the patient's plan of care?

The Primary Nurse starts to develop the plan of care with the family. Ideally this begins on admission by assessing home routines and preferences. This written plan of care is communicated to other members of the team. The plan of care is updated by team members as needed. We have given a lot of responsibility to the Primary Nurse and, as a result, we have seen the mutual respect among staff members flourish. I am a nurse with 24 years of experience; I may get report from a new colleague who has started a plan of care for her primary patient. I have to trust and respect her plan and carry it out. She is the expert in that relationship. I think this is where people may have difficulty with the model—extending respect and trust to less experienced colleagues.

We developed a communication sheet when we started Primary Nursing. It was a tool that helped staff communicate the plan of care to each other. It cut down on the frustration families were having with the lack of communication

We have given a lot of responsibility to the Primary Nurse and, as a result, we have seen the mutual respect among staff members flourish.

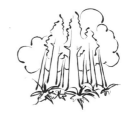

between staff. If the family requested or preferred something, the Primary Nurse communicated that on the communication sheet. For example, with children, it may take a nurse a half-hour to help a child take oral prednisone because it is difficult to swallow and it tastes terrible. She may try several different strategies before she is successful: strawberry jelly, chocolate syrup, grape jelly. Once the nurse determines what works, that becomes the plan with the family. Imagine if you will, the next nurse starting from the beginning (going through the same trial and error) 12 hours later. The family is going to lose their trust in everyone! So it's very important to write the plan of care you have established, what has worked out with the family and date it. If something changes, the plan needs updating and that should be done by the Primary Nurse or an associate nurse.

We have raised the bar on our practice. We care about each other, we trust each other, and we give all that we can for the patients and family.

What does the communication sheet look like?

There are five sections to it: medication and treatment, home routines, plan of care, discharge needs and psychosocial. It is a highly individualized communication sheet and all free text. Each plan is different because each nurse-patient relationship is different.

What would you say works really well with your Primary Nursing system?

The relationship with families, the relationship between the nurses, and the relationships with the physicians. All are healthy. We have raised the bar on our practice. We care about each other, we trust each other, and we give all that we can for the patients and family. When we see a patient and their family preparing to leave and yet wait for half an hour to say goodbye to "their nurse," give her a hug and thank her for their care, we know the nurse has touched them—has made an important difference in their child's care.

As we advocated more for our patients we started to realize areas that were lacking. We were consistently doing more teaching so we needed to improve our educational tools. Nurses developed educational handouts and videos. We learned how to write grants for resources to develop educational tools. I had a primary patient with diabetes and the mom said to me,

"I wish you could come to school with us on Monday and help us explain all this." That inspired my colleague Becca Billing and me to write a grant through Children's Miracle Network so that the Primary Nurse could go with the patient to the school, develop an individualized program, speak to classmates about the illness and help that patient transition into the school. We call the program *Tell My Classmates I'm Still Me.*

That is extremely inspiring, Ellen. What obstacles have you needed to overcome in designing and implementing Primary Nursing?

There were some members of our unit who didn't want to participate, but we set the date we were going to start and we just kept chipping away at it every day. We just kept focusing on the advantages and did not give energy to the negative people. When it became very strong, people bought into it, liked it, and it was successful. We started to be recognized for it within the hospital and beyond.

We have learned that we have to stay focused on Primary Nursing. It's not a model that happens by itself. We have to lead and cheerlead for it everyday. It is part of our language. We discuss it every day and work at maintaining it. When we moved into our new unit, there was so much that needed to be done and Primary Nursing was so strong that we neglected it. We thought it would flourish on its own; our nurse practice council stopped meeting routinely because our delivery care model practice was "strong." Because it was successful we figured we didn't have to nurture it; the work was done and it would sustain itself. However, everyone started going back to their old behaviors. So we learned that even though we believe in Primary Nursing and want it, in order for it to live every day, we must constantly tend to it, talk about it and refine it. It is part of my language every day. Even though we know the outcomes and the rewards and we have pride in the success of our care, unless we work at it, it will not happen. It is like a marriage.

> We just kept focusing on the advantages and did not give energy to the negative people. When it became very strong, people bought into it, liked it, and it was successful.

As we consider evidence of the success of Primary Nursing, patient satisfaction is a key indicator. When you began many years ago, patient satisfaction was not good. Where is patient satisfaction today?

We have seen incredible results with our patient satisfaction. Our discharge planning improved tremendously. We start at admission, we make everyone feel welcome, we have a sleep chair at every bedside which is comforting for the family and says that they are welcome and considered an important part of the care. I would love to see the same thing on adult units.

What is your vision for Primary Nursing on your unit from here?

I am going to take it further. In the last few years I have been talking with staff from other units and hospitals about Primary Nursing. I try to remember where we were 10 years ago and I encourage them to focus on moving forward with small steps and see that care is improving and build on those successes.

For our unit, we are focusing on strengthening our partnerships with other disciplines and are seeing incredible results. For example, we have been intentional about involving our housekeeping staff in celebrations and recognition as they are part of us, and they certainly contribute to the experience of patients and families. Their work is very structured and they have a routine that needs to be followed. But when they understand the need to be flexible to provide personalized care, they respond gladly. For example, we may say, "Cliff, this patient is in surgery; please do this room first." Cliff gladly does it because he is part of our team and understands that the patient/family is center. Our new manager, Angie Marin, was part of the original nurse practice council; she is just as visionary as Lynne Boehret was. It is crucial to have manager support for success. She believes in Primary Nursing and holds us accountable to that practice. Our next goal is to work with radiology to personalize schedules to patient needs.

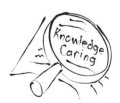

Thank you, Ellen. We celebrate with you and your colleagues who make extraordinary care happen every day. We look forward to hearing about your work with other disciplines.

An Expert Answers Common Questions about Primary Nursing

—A Marie Manthey classic

Primary Nursing is still a "hot topic" in nursing service departments throughout the United States and Canada. As reduced lengths of stay shrink hospitals, fewer patient days are used by people in the convalescent stage of their illnesses. This has created a dramatic rise in the acuity of patients, which coupled with the need to reduce expenditures, has resulted, in some cases, in changes in the use of ancillary personnel. Changing acuity ratios have necessitated changing staffing ratios in a way that definitely favors Primary Nursing.

This article was originally published in Nursing Management, *20(3), March 1989. Adapted with permission.*

The following questions and answers are those that have most frequently been asked in hospitals implementing Primary Nursing.

Does Primary Nursing require an all-RN staff?

No. An all-RN staff is not required for Primary Nursing. There is a great deal of care to be given to patients by other staff members, and there is no reason why this work can't be done by an LPN, nursing assistant, student nurse, or even, if need be, by an agency nurse.

Is there a role for nursing assistants in Primary Nursing?

Yes, there has always has been a role for nursing assistants in Primary Nursing. The most economical implementations of Primary Nursing have retained some nursing assistant coverage to perform unit-wide care activities (both direct and indirect) that don't require technical training. Some hospitals that practice Primary Nursing have even incorporated nursing assistants into daily care activities, and assign them to function as aides to the nursing staff. The important principle to keep in mind is that total patient care is the most economical way to assign

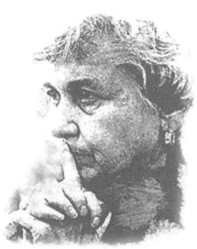

daily care and that Primary Nurses must do enough hands-on care to be able to make appropriate decisions about how that care should be given. Parts of the care may be delegated by the Primary Nurse without jeopardizing Primary Nursing.

Can part-time nurses fit into Primary Nursing?

Assignments are made on the basis of matching up need and ability first, and then taking a look at the location of the patient's room.

It depends on how time-off is scheduled on the unit. The following answer applies equally to the 11- or 12-hour shift-nurse. If the nurse works enough shifts during a span of days to manage a caseload, she can function as a Primary Nurse. Thus, if a part-time nurse works three shifts one week, has two days off and works two shifts for the next week's hours, during those seven days she easily can be a Primary Nurse, especially for a patient whose length of stay is less than seven days. If not, she can fit in very well as an associate—one who cares for a patient whose Primary Nurse is off duty.

Does Primary Nursing cost more to staff?

No, because staffing should be based on patient care needs, not the requirements of any given delivery system. As patient acuity has risen in the past decade, so have nursing care costs. The rising acuity has dictated an increase in ratio of licensed to non-licensed staff, simply because there is a definite limit to how much care a nurse's aide can give an acutely ill patient. If a hospital opts for an all-RN staff, salary costs will indeed rise. However, this decision is not necessary for the successful implementation of Primary Nursing.

Do all patients need a Primary Nurse?

If some patients do have Primary Nurses, while others do not, both patients and all those who visit patients become aware of a two-class system.

Yes, Primary Nursing is a delivery system (and a responsibility relationship). As such, all of its patients have a right to receive all of the elements in that system. If some patients do have Primary Nurses, while others do not, both patients and all those who visit patients become aware of a two-class system.

Do short-term patients get Primary Nurses too?

Short-term patients have the same right to know who is coordinating their care as do long-term patients.

How can care plans be done on short-term patients?

They usually cannot be, but then Primary Nursing is not synonymous with care plans. Primary Nursing requires that each patient know the name of his or her Primary Nurse. Primary Nursing also requires that each Primary Nurse be responsible for administering and coordinating whatever care the patient receives during the hospital stay.

Our staff likes the fact that we self-select patients, but what about the patients who are not selected? Does this show a lack of commitment on our part?

Although self-selection has advantages, it should not be relied upon as the sole means of matching patients with nurses. Nurses do not select patients for a number of reasons, and most of those reasons have little to do with a nurse's lack of commitment. Without enumerating all of the reasons, suffice it to say that a back-up system of patient-nurse assignment is the most effective way of dealing with a situation in which self-selection fails to match a patient with a Primary Nurse within the 24-hour period following admission.

Why must a Primary Nurse introduce herself to her patient by her name and title?

A Primary Nurse's relationship with a client is based on the nurse's role as a professional. When the nurse explains her role as a Primary Nurse, with particular emphasis on the meaning of her title, she establishes herself as a professional and creates the bond that is necessary for a "contractual" professional client relationship.

How does Primary Nursing work for the chronically ill patient who is hospitalized for an extended period of time?

This question usually leads to a broader issue: What do you do when a nurse becomes tired of a patient or who is not, for one reason or another, getting along with the patient? Since the essence of Primary Nursing is the establishment of a therapeutic relationship, the failure to achieve or to maintain such a relationship is adequate justification for a reassignment. This is a completely normal situation, which should be handled without chastising either the patient or the nurse.

> Since the essence of Primary Nursing is the establishment of a therapeutic relationship, the failure to achieve or to maintain such a relationship is adequate justification for a reassignment.

Does the patient have anything to say about who his or her Primary Nurse is?

Yes. An important factor in the Primary Nursing assignment is the patient's right to participate in the decision-making process. Since most nurses are not usually known to newly admitted patients, participation at the point of admission is limited to patients who have been previously hospitalized on the unit. If, at any time during a patient's hospitalization, he or she expresses the desire to change Primary Nurses or expresses an inability to relate well with his Primary Nurse, reassignment should be made quickly and with impunity. Nurses frequently ask how to handle a situation in which they do not get along with patients. My answer is always that you should be able to request reassignment without it becoming an issue. The same is true when a patient does not get along with a nurse.

Physicians appreciate having a nurse become really knowledgeable about their patients' care.

How does Primary Nursing work when you are short staffed?

Short staffing is handled in Primary Nursing just like it is in any other delivery system; the staff will choose which activities are the most important and do those, while maintaining the therapeutic relationship with their patients at all times. Other activities will be left undone, which is a reality that must always be accepted whenever the amount of work exceeds the amount of staff available.

Can Primary Nursing work in an emergency room?

Yes, Primary Nursing can work in an emergency room when the same guidelines noted above are followed. Again, patients need to know the name of the person who is responsible for administering and coordinating their nursing care.

How do physicians react to the concept of Primary Nursing?

Most are positive when the concept is implemented in a common-sense way. Physicians appreciate having a nurse become really knowledgeable about their patients' care. They come to rely on the nurse's input around overall decision making. It is important, however, that in the absence of the Primary

Nurse others are able to answer day-to-day questions. In faulty implementation, the communication flow about patient care can become so narrow that no one but the Primary Nurse can answer a question. This situation will eventually have a negative effect on the overall quality of a patient's care.

How can you do Primary Nursing when you are so short staffed that there isn't enough time to do care plans?

Primary Nursing is not about care plans. Primary Nursing is a relationship; care plans are conceptual exercises designed to facilitate an analytical process. Care plans have become the "tail wagging the dog" of Primary Nursing practice. I have seen excellent care given in the absence of what is called a nursing diagnosis-based, process-oriented comprehensive care plan, but I have not seen it given in the absence of common-sense communication. The current attitudes about care plans, however, are causing so much trouble in daily practice that good communication is practically impossible. In nursing practice, the energy must be devoted to simple, straight-forward communication of decisions about the patient's care—not about many columned splendors of a care plan.

Primary Nursing is not about care plans. Primary Nursing is a relationship

What do you think about starting Primary Nursing modules as a first step?

I think it is a disastrous mistake since this approach focuses attention on structural changes which actually result in the formation of mini-teams. While there may be some improvements in care in the short range, the lasting changes in attitudes and interpersonal relationships required for the effective practice of Primary Nursing may never take place.

How do Traveler Nurses and Agency Nurses fit into Primary Nursing?

At least one large medical university has developed a practice whereby Traveler Nurses, not Agency nurses, who will be on the unit for an extended period of time, may function as Primary Nurses.

CHAPTER TEN
Professional Colleagueship

Editors' note:
Relationship-Based Care emphasizes the importance of leadership at all levels of an organization. Personal leadership begins with owning one's work and experiences. Cohen's suggestions for self-management are a recipe for self-awareness and personal leadership.

Self-Management: Taking Responsibility for Our Own Experience in the Workplace

—Michael Henry Cohen

Why Self-Management?

Self-management is a strategy for successfully dealing with on-the-job stress, change and interpersonal conflict. Self-management calls for you to look more objectively at the common frustrations that are an inevitable part of your job. When you practice self-management, you learn to accept the actions of the people around you, and you learn how to get understanding and cooperation from them so that your work is more effective as well as pleasant.

When you practice self-management you demonstrate:

1. Flexibility and Adaptability

You are not paralyzed by change. You are able to adjust to an increasingly fast-paced, highly competitive and constantly changing work environment.

2. Versatility

You make yourself more valuable when you are willing to learn new skills and apply them to organizational needs. You demonstrate versatility when you accept input from others without getting defensive and when you experiment with new behaviors that lead to personal growth.

3. High Tolerance for Ambiguity

In the midst of change and uncertainty, you don't just wait for your marching orders. You take the initiative and act affirmatively within your scope of responsibility. You focus on those things that are within your control and do the very best you can, thereby creating your own structure and positive spheres of influence.

True motivation has to come from within as it is a product of your own work ethic.

4. Respect for Differences of Opinion

You effectively manage conflicts, always maintaining integrity and respect for yourself and others. You do this by addressing issues in a collaborative and constructive manner rather than personally attacking a co-worker with whom you are in disagreement.

5. Excitement about New Possibilities

You view change as a challenge and a new opportunity for growth and contribution to the organization. You don't look back to the "good old days," because things will never be the same. As Thomas Wolfe said, "You can't go home again."

Self-management is a strategy for successfully dealing with on-the-job stress, change, and interpersonal conflict.

6. Responsibility

You understand that you are ultimately responsible for your own success and happiness on the job. To succeed, you must take personal responsibility and hold yourself accountable for effective work performance.

7. Pursuit of Excellence

You acknowledge that your number one objective on the job is to make a meaningful contribution. Pursuing excellence means taking pride in your work. It means being part of a successful team in which communication is respectful and efficient. Regardless of work constraints and limitations, your primary focus is always on the contribution that you are making on behalf of the patient.

8. Realistic Expectations

You understand that there exists no perfect working environment free of frustrations or irritations. You take full advantage of the positive aspects of the job, try to improve those things that are within your control to change, and adjust to those things you can't change. You remain flexible in your dealings with patients, managers and co-workers.

When you practice self-management, you learn to accept the actions of the people around you.

9. Effective Manager Relationships

You accept the fact that you don't have to like your manager on a personal level in order to have an effective professional relationship. Of course, it's nicer and easier to work with a manager you like, but it's not a precondition for a successful working relationship. The best manager in the world cannot make you successful, and the worst manager cannot make you fail. You always have choices to make regarding where and for whom you are going to work. But if you choose to stay, you owe it to your patients to secure a harmonious working relationship with your manager. Successful staff members, in fact, "manage the manager" as effectively as the manager manages them. And if you want to be managed less by your manager, you have to manage yourself more.

10. Self-Motivation

You realize that even the most talented manager cannot motivate you to do an outstanding job. Managers can, on occasion, de-motivate you through a litany of management missteps, but true motivation has to come from within as it is a product of your own work ethic. As a self-managed staff member, you approach the job with a strong sense of commitment that demonstrates:

- *"I'm able to work as the schedule requires on a consistent basis. You can count on me to be here. I am reliable."*

- *"I will take the initiative and follow through on tasks to successful completion. I am independent and self-directed."*

- *"I feel good when I do something nice for someone. I enjoy serving others, and I will go the extra mile to ensure that I fully meet (or exceed) their expectations."*

You acknowledge that your number one objective on the job is to make a meaningful contribution.

Your manager's job is to effectively select personnel who possess these work values from the start, lead by example, provide recognition and reward for achievement, and create a positive work environment that facilitates your success. If you possess the technical skills, creativity and desire to succeed, your manager can channel this energy toward constructive ends consistent with a common vision. But it's your responsibility to make yourself successful. No matter how inspiring or charismatic managers may be, they cannot light a fire beneath you unless you provide the initial spark or will to achieve. Self-managed people are self-motivated members of the organization.

Intrinsic motivation encourages the employee to enjoy work because the activity is enjoyable and meaningful as well as a source of income. When the motivation is essentially extrinsic, the terms of achievement are imposed from outside oneself and are, therefore, outer-directed rather than self-directed (Katz & Liu, 1991).

Self-Management is Motivated Primarily by Intrinsic Rewards

When Motivation is Extrinsic or Outer-Directed	When Motivation is Intrinsic or Self-Directed
The person's desire is fueled by the pursuit of material rewards, praise or recognition.	*The person's desire is fueled by passion, pride and a responsible work ethic.*
The person is preoccupied with the performance of manager, co-workers and organizational politics.	*The person's primary concern is being the best he or she can be and making a significant contribution regardless of how others act.*
Hard work or challenging situations are resented by the person for the amount of extra energy and time required to complete the task.	*Hard work or challenging situations are not regarded as a personal sacrifice, because the employee "owns her job" and wants to follow through to achieve positive results.*
The person's focus is on competition, getting credit, and on "looking good" in comparison with others.	*The person's focus is on personal and professional fulfillment. The job itself is highly valued and has meaning in the individual's life.*
External success (raises, promotions, job security, prestige, adulation) is largely determined or provided by others.	*A sense of intrinsic success is determined by the person.*
The pursuit of external success can easily lead to "workaholism" and burn-out at the expense of personal fulfillment. Work can be all-consuming and exhausting.	*The pursuit of intrinsic success usually leads to a healthy balance between personal and work life because the individual is in touch with his or her own feelings and values.*
The person's focus is on competition, getting credit, and on "looking good" in comparison with others.	*The person's focus is on personal and professional fulfillment. The job itself is highly valued and has meaning in the individual's life.*
External success (raises, promotions, job security, prestige, adulation) is largely determined or provided by others.	*A sense of intrinsic success is determined by the person.*

Reference: Katz, S., & Liu, A. (1991). *Success trap: Rethink your ambitions to achieve greater personal and professional fulfillment.* New York: Dell.

Interdisciplinary Teamwork: Bringing Expertise to the Table

—Susan Lampe

Today quality patient care demands the expertise of a variety of providers. Teams collaborating to assess, plan, implement and evaluate patient care are the norm and are necessary in the face of complex patient needs and shorter lengths of stay. The question for many of us is now "How do I as an individual participate and contribute to the team?" I discovered a satisfying answer to this question in Stephen Covey's book *The Seven Habits of Highly Effective People*–specifically in his "Maturity Continuum," which he defines with three levels:

- *Dependence (you need others to get what you want);*

- *Independence (you can get what you want on your own); and*

- *Interdependence (you get what you want by working in cooperation with others).*

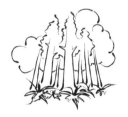

The "aha" for me is that this is a continuum, which means that it is progressive–one moves from one step to the next as one matures. Therefore, according to Covey, one needs to be independent before one can be successfully interdependent. He says: "As an interdependent person, I have the opportunity to share myself deeply, meaningfully, with others, and I have access to the vast resources and potential of other human beings. Interdependence is a choice only independent people can make" (Covey, 1989, p. 51). When I apply Covey's idea to my professional work it means that when I attend an interdisciplinary team conference, I need to be securely grounded as an *independent professional* in my discipline before I can enter into a successful effort to establish an interdependent relationship with others on the team.

We are all equal, but we are not all the same.

Being securely grounded in my discipline means that I have a set of values and beliefs about my skill and my role and the value that these bring to patient care, no matter what profession I represent at the interdisciplinary conference. I am clear and confident in the value of my participation in assessing, planning, implementing and evaluating patient care. I believe that others will respect my judgment and my contributions. Not only is it okay for me to come to the conference thinking and saying, "I am here as the patient's nurse," it is in fact imperative that everyone understand that the reason I am here is that I bring nursing expertise to the table. The same is true for each discipline.

Collaboration means that each member is valued for his or her expertise—that each is brought to the conference specifically to achieve our goal of providing quality patient care. Each team member is equally important to the process of helping the patient and family meet their goals. Each team member has an important role in assessment, planning, intervention and evaluation. We are all equal, but we are not all the same. What makes me a valuable team member is that I have a special expertise that others do not have—and that my strength complements the strength of others.

It is important that I be skilled and confident in my independent area of expertise and that I respect the expertise of every other team member. When we come together as an interdisciplinary team, we put forward the goals of the patient and family and then work collaboratively to determine who has the resources and expertise to contribute to the accomplishment of each goal. Successful professional interdependence is made possible by professional independence.

Reference: Covey, S. (1989). *The seven habits of highly effective people.* New York: Simon & Schuster.

It is important that I be skilled and confident in my independent area of expertise and that I respect the expertise of every other team member.

Honest Reflections about "Difficult Patients"

—Laurence A. Savett

One of the largest groups of patients whose needs are not being met are the so-called difficult patients. Sometimes, despite our best efforts, the patient distrusts the physician or nurse, and it becomes challenging to establish a relationship and rapport. The "difficult patient" is often one who is dealing with important psychological or social issues. Identifying these issues can be transformative in providing integrated and thoughtful continuity of care (Savett, 2002).

But one cannot take these steps in their care without this insight: Just as the problem, congestive heart failure has a list of symptoms that, taken alone or together, suggest a differential diagnosis, so does the problem, difficult patient.

Editors' Note: *Portions of this article have been adapted from* The Human Side of Medicine: Learning What It's Like to be a Patient and What It's Like to be a Physician *written by Savett and published by Greenwood Publishing Group and from "Spirituality and Practice: Stories, Barriers and Opportunities" an interview by Savett published in* Creative Nursing, *3(4):7-11, 16. Used with permission.*

Congestive heart failure: symptoms and differential diagnosis

Symptoms: shortness of breath, poor exercise tolerance, rapid heartbeat, ankle swelling

Differential diagnosis: coronary heart disease, valvular heart disease, primary disease of the heart muscle (cardiomyopathy)

Difficult patient; symptoms and differential diagnosis

Symptoms: anger, distrust, absence of rapport

Differential diagnosis: psychosocial problems, "difficult doctor," "difficult nurse," "difficult system"

Just as one may name the problem "congestive heart failure" on the basis of one or more symptoms—and then look further to see what specific problem is causing the altered physiologic state—so one should consider the problem statement "difficult patient" on the basis of one or more specific criteria and then investigate the cause of the problem. Approaching the problem "difficult patient" in this precise way can defuse the tension and lead to a precise, clear plan of action.

Two Stories From My Practice

ONE

On a weekend I received a call from a nurse who told me that an 80-year-old patient had fallen at the nursing home, was eating poorly, was hypoxic, and was clearly failing. My partner, her primary physician, was away. A chest x-ray done a few days earlier showed no evidence of pneumonia or congestive heart failure, two conditions high on the list of causes of hypoxia. The patient, who also had Parkinson's disease, was a "full code." The nurse reported that the patient's son was "very difficult and unrealistic." When I spoke by phone with the son, whom I had never met, he became increasingly agitated as I suggested continuing to care for his mother at the nursing home. I hospitalized her and arranged to meet with him.

In a long conversation, her son told me his mother's story—and his own. His widowed mother had been the family's breadwinner. His father had been abusive to her. During the previous two years, the son remained at home with his mother, unable to leave her alone. She had once said to him, "Promise me you'll never put me in the nursing home," and so it was a major step for him to do so. He spoke with passion and feeling. It was a better conversation than we had had on the phone; I understood him better and he was able to perceive my commitment to his mother's care. (Savett, Hatgidakis, Timko, Plotnikoff & Gale, 1997)

TWO

Though I generally see my patients at their scheduled time, I was five minutes late for a first meeting with a 75-year-old man who greeted me with, "You're late! Who the hell do you think you are?" This guy is really difficult, I thought. Angry and defensive myself, I was inclined to respond, "I sense that we're not going to get along. I think you should find another doctor." Instead I asked myself, "What's his anger all about? What's my anger all about?" I recognized that he reminded me of a relative who had been depressed for many years; his anger was an expression of his depression. Instead of dismissing the patient, I relaxed, continued the interview, and used that insight in his care. He was indeed depressed.

These stories offer many lessons:

- It is always a disservice to the patient, the professional and the care process to label someone as "difficult." It limits inquiry and compromises effective, appropriate care.

- Patients who are angry or distrustful offer us a cue to dig deeper in order to figure out the full scope of issues they may be bringing to the care experience.

- Listening to the patient's (and often the family's) story and reflecting on it are important steps in integrating the insights in planning care.

- Though all of this takes time, time spent early on saves time later on. It is time well spent.

- A confrontation signals a need for a longer conversation (see page 532).

- A face-to-face conversation is better than a phone conversation.

As part of the differential diagnosis of "difficult patient," I included on page 364, "difficult doctor," "difficult nurse," and "difficult system." If we consistently deal with each patient with equanimity, then how the patient behaves can be seen as significant data. If, on the other hand, we are inconsistent and uneven, if the patient cannot trust that we will be the same on each encounter, if our demeanor is provocative, then how the patient behaves cannot be seen as data, and we will always have to ask ourselves, "Was it the patient who provoked this response or was it me?" Or additionally, "Did the system contribute to making him a difficult patient by not meeting his needs?"

It is always a disservice to the patient, the professional and the care process to label someone as "difficult." It limits inquiry and compromises effective, appropriate care.

What Leads Us to Label Patients as "Difficult?"

We don't inquire.	When a middle-aged woman made many phone calls to her physician in preparation for a breast biopsy, he labeled her "manipulative and demanding," instead of recognizing that there were good reasons for her concern and cascade of questions. She had a chronic disease and she was concerned about how long she would have to be off medication. In addition, she had a number of prearranged speaking engagements and needed to know which to reschedule. And she was frightened. Her concerns and questions were valid; calling her "manipulative and demanding" was unfair and squandered the opportunity to build a relationship
We stifle our patients' expressions of feelings.	We interrupt a weeping patient, instead of remaining silent and allowing the emotion to express itself. We don't allow the patient to express anger, fear, anxiety, doubt, and so we squander the opportunity to explore these issues to expand our awareness of the patient's story.
We may not recognize where the patient is in the story.	When the patient has been dealing with another illness, physician, hospital and set of assumptions for a long time, it's no wonder that a new physician and his opinions might initially be rejected.
We expect patients to make decisions too quickly.	Difficult decisions take time.
Patients and families may misinterpret our motives.	When a nursing home resident's son called to request psychiatric consultation for his mother, who had become confused, I suggested an alternative: "I'll see her first to look for nonpsychiatric causes of her confusion." He rejected the proposal, accusing me of "trying to save the state some money by being 'the gatekeeper.'" A relationship would have helped.

A colleague of mine suggested that "any difficult patient started out as a complex patient." Patients whose illnesses are complex or who have complex dramas going on in their lives may have difficulty in finding someone with enough patience to address all the issues. Incomplete attention may leave the patient dissatisfied and frustrated. When that happens, we also become frustrated, label the patient "difficult," exacerbate that difficulty in our self-fulfilling prophecy, and no one feels satisfied.

But not all complex patients become difficult and those we may be tempted to label "difficult patients" aren't all that complex in the right hands. Just as we see serious illnesses as challenges and opportunities, many of us see "difficult patients" as challenges and opportunities too. The search for the solutions to these challenges can be fascinating and their resolution elevates everyone. Anyone can deal with easy problems or patients. The test of a real professional is how he or she deals with the "difficult" ones.

References: Savett, L. (2002). *The human side of medicine: Learning what it's like to be a patient and what it's like to be a physician.* Westport, CT: Greenwood Publishing Group.

Savett, L., Hatgidakis, J., Timko, E., Plotnikoff, G., & Gale, C. (1997). Spirituality and practice: Stories, barriers and opportunities. *Creative Nursing,* 3(4), 7-11, 16.

Genuine Collaboration in Physician-Nurse Relationships

—Laurence A. Savett

Editors' note: *Some of this material was origi-nally published in L. A. Savett and S. G. Savett, "Genuine Collaboration: Our Obligation to Our Patients and to Each Other,"* Creative Nursing, *13(5): 11-13. Used with permission.*

Good relationships are built on reciprocal honesty, trust, respect, consistency—and continuity. A guiding principle in providing care is "The patient is the center of the drama." Really good health care often involves a complex collaboration among many professionals, each bringing his or her own fund of knowledge and professional paradigm, which often overlap. At best, we complement each others' skills, enhance patient care, and enrich the joy in our careers (Savett, 2004).

But sometimes there are problems, because physicians and nurses have separate rather than joint training, because each can lack information about what the other does, and, sadly, because we don't always treat each other respectfully. However, when we work together, share information, and draw on each other's special skills, training, insights and experiences, we quickly discover how much our roles overlap. This kind of highly interactive, mutually respectful collaboration is better for patients. And it's better for nurses and physicians—in terms of job satisfaction, joy in our work, retention, and protection against early disenchantment and premature retirement. All of us connect with very interesting people as we work with each other. How we relate to one another is critical. We should do nothing that undermines that relationship; we shouldn't squander that opportunity.

Establishing a Collaborative Relationship

The key to genuine collaboration between nurse and physician is easy access to each other and exchange of information about the following questions:[1]

1 Originally described in a more extensive article, L. A. Savett and V. Good, "Continuing education for nurses: A problem oriented system," in Minnesota Medicine, Supplement No. 2, vol. 56, pp. 19-23, October 1973. Used with permission.

- *Nurses must ask physicians, "What sort of information do you need from me to help care for our patient?"*

- *Physicians must ask nurses, "What sort of information do you need from me in caring for our patient?" and "What sort of recurring observations do you make in the course of managing a patient with diabetes (or chest pain or hypertension) that require decisions?"*

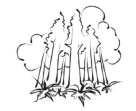

For example, for a patient hospitalized for diabetes as a primary or secondary diagnosis, the physician and the nurse share information about these potentially co-occurring conditions for which the patient is at greater risk: hypoglycemia (the prime, urgently treatable condition) and its various ways of presentation (including agitation, confusion, erratic behavior, diaphoresis, and seizures), ketoacidosis, cystitis, dehydration, myocardial infarct, peripheral and visceral neuropathy, stroke, and arterial insufficiency. For each of these conditions, there are observations that provide clues to early recognition. Joint preparation by nurse and physician of a protocol for care, stimulated by the above questions, helps each to genuinely collaborate.

Together they construct a protocol for care, which includes:

- *initial questions of patient*

- *initial observations*

- *ongoing observations*

- *what clinical conditions often co-occur in the context of the illness and how one recognizes them*

- *the side effects of drugs commonly used to treat the illness*

- *the meaning of certain regularly seen observations in the illness*

- *what should be reported to the physician*

- *other general comments*

Once the habit of collaboration is established, the patient is better served. Absence of collaboration can adversely influence patient outcomes or delay recovery as much as incorrect diagnosis or inappropriate treatment can.

Characteristics of Genuine Collaboration

When we collaborate—genuinely collaborate—we enhance our ability to serve our patients, streamline care and generate ongoing opportunities to learn and enhance trust, not only between our patients and ourselves, but also with each other—nurses and physicians.

In genuine collaboration, all those who need to be involved—nurse, physician, other health care professionals, patient and family—are consulted. *The goals are negotiable; where conflict exists between professionals or a professional and the patient, those conflicts are recognized and clarified, as they often represent disparate or incomplete versions of the same story.*

In genuine collaboration, there is ongoing critical review and oversight. *In any complex system of care, the process may falter, but each participant knows that it can be fixed by talking it over.*

In genuine collaboration, no artificial boundaries exist between the professions; each has equal worth.

Genuine collaboration is liberating. *From time to time, both nurses and physicians are faced with tasks that exceed their skills. Tackling them alone is inefficient and unsatisfying. Calling upon others speeds up the process and allows each to concentrate on what he or she does best.*

Genuine collaboration takes time. *Attending to the whole story of the patient's illness and the psychological and social context in which it occurs; reflecting on the meaning of the information; identifying, clarifying and validating the issues among all the participants; evolving a strategy for care and altering it when appropriate all take time. But in the end, it's far more efficient than not collaborating, because each of the collaborating partners does his or her job with special skill.*

> In any complex system of care, the process may falter, but each participant knows that it can be fixed by talking it over.

Genuine collaboration allows the patient to develop trust in the system. *Trust is reciprocal. When we trust and respect patients for their observations and personal values, they can trust those upon whose expertise they rely.*

Genuine collaboration gives everyone an ongoing opportunity to learn. *From other professionals, we learn better ways to explore the patient's story, to identify the issues, and to enlarge our knowledge of resources. We learn what works and what doesn't. By sharing our observations and inferences with others, we correct each other's misperceptions.*

Collaboration in Action

In the course of genuine collaboration, interactions like those that follow take place routinely. All of them enhance the relationship between physician and nurse, benefiting patients and their families in numerous ways.

I

Nurse: Doctor, it's 4 p.m. and your 16-year-old patient, who has diabetes, insists on signing out AMA ("against medical advice").

Doctor: I wonder if she's having an insulin reaction.

This leads to a broader discussion for the staff about subtle manifestations of hypoglycemia.

II

Nurse: Mrs. S., who is recovering from a heart attack, is confused. I wonder if she's hypoxemic from congestive heart failure or pneumonia.

Doctor: Great call! I'll be right over.

This leads to a broader discussion for nurses and physicians on the meaning of change in mental status.

III

Doctor: Nurse, I'm having trouble really connecting with my patient and his family. What's your sense of what's going on?

This provides an opportunity for the nurse and physician to exchange observations and insights.

In genuine collaboration, no artificial boundaries exist between the professions; each has equal worth.

In our daily practices, we must know that when the needs exceed our own skills and resources, collaboration is necessary. We must know not only what institutional resources are available to us, but also the people within them and how they work. Can we trust their perceptions and assessments? Are they thoughtful or do they jump to conclusions? Are they consistent in their approach? Do they ask, "What can I learn from this patient and from others with whom I work?" Do they genuinely collaborate? We must know what questions to ask and be able to formulate the questions clearly. And each person in the collaboration must know when and how to expand the inquiry. Such collaborative relationships are essential to the delivery of Relationship-Based Care.

> When the needs exceed our own skills and resources, collaboration is necessary

Reference: Savett, L. A. (2004). "On the nurse-physician relationship." Creative Nursing, 10:4, 3.

Savett, L. A. and Good, V. (1973) , "Continuing education for nurses: A problem oriented system." *Minnesota medicine,* Supplement No. 2, 56, 19-23.

Savett, L. A. and Savett, S. G. (1994). "Genuine collaboration: Our obligation to our patients and to each other." Creative Nursing, 1:1, 11-13.

Calling the Physician:
A Tool to Facilitate Communication

—John W. Nelson

Communication between nurses and physicians has been shown to have a significant measurable effect on patient outcomes (Baggs, Schmitt, Mushlin, Mitchell, Eldredge, Oakes & Hutson, 1999; Mahlmeister, 2005), patient mortality (Estabrooks, Midodzi, Cummings, Ricker, Giovannetti, P, 2005; Knaus & Draper, 1986), ability to rescue hospitalized patients from severe physical decline (Estabrooks, 2005; Knaus & Draper, 1986; Simpson, 2005), and nurse job satisfaction (Manojlovich, 2005; Rosenstein & O'Daniel, 2005).

What follows is a tool to facilitate effective phone communication between the nurse and physician for changes in patient condition. Readers are encouraged to use this tool to improve nurse-physician communication and collaboration, and to measure the impact on any of the factors noted above that relate with communication.

Baggs (1999) reported that as communication between the nurse and physician improved, negative patient outcomes declined. These findings were consistent with the case study presented by Mahlmeister (2005), where the negative outcomes in an obstetrics case presented were largely due to poor communication. No study to date could be found that has documented the importance of communication better than the 1986 study conducted by Knaus and Draper, which revealed a 41% decline in mortality in the hospital with good nurse-physician communication and collaboration when contrasted to other hospitals in the study. Estabrooks et al. (2005) have also documented a decline in mortality rates when good nurse-physician communication and collaboration was present.

If negative patient outcomes and mortality are to be curtailed, it is vital that nurses identify and communicate changes in patient status to the physician. Simpson (2005)

If negative patient outcomes and mortality are to be curtailed, it is vital that nurses identify and communicate changes in patient status to the physician.

Calling the Physician Guide (CPG)

Below is a guide for gathering pertinent information when calling the physician.

If you are a nurse who has less than one year of experience or if you are working temporarily on this unit for the day or for a period of less than one year, please inform the charge nurse of your intent to call the physician. The charge nurse will then work with you in gathering any additional information that the physician from that specialty or group may request of you. This is meant to be a tool to facilitate communication between you and the physician and to ultimately help the patient.

Please gather the information below before calling the physician.

Patient's name:

Date of admission:

Primary physician:

Primary Nurse:

Patient's admitting diagnosis:

Reason for call:

Baseline information:	New since admission information:
Chronic illnesses:	Acute illness:
Baseline vital signs:	Changes/trends in vital signs (if applicable):
Baseline lab work: (CBC, electrolytes, BUN and Creatinine most frequently requested by most physicians)	Changes/trends in lab work:
Home medications:	New medications since admission:
Living situation and power of attorney:	Currently involved/updated family:
Dynamics unique to patient situation:	New dynamics in patient situation:

asserts that clear articulation of the changes in patient status to the physician is essential if the appropriate response is to be prompted by the physician. Even subtle changes may need to be reported to avert any chance of miscommunication between nurse and physician (Burke, Boal, & Mitchell, 2004). Nurses must be able to competently communicate the changes of patient status from the baseline to the physician so that trust is established, and a collaborative plan of care can be co-created. A tool to guide the nurse in this conversation has been shown to help (Nelson & Venhaus, 2005). Such a tool may be especially helpful for nurses who are new to a unit, or must float to a unit in which they are unfamiliar with unit routine and physician preferences.

References: Baggs, J., Schmitt, M., Mushlin, A., Mitchell, P., Eldredge, D., Oakes, D., & Hutson, A. (1999). Association between nurse-physician collaboration and patient outcomes in three intensive care units. *Critical Care Medicine*, 27(9), 1991-1998.

Burke, M., Boal, J., & Mitchell, R. (2004). Communicating for better care: improving nurse-physician communication. *American Journal of Nursing* 104(12), 40-47.

Estabrooks, C., Midodzi, W., Cummings, G., Ricker, K., & Giovannetti P. (2005). The impact of hospital nursing characteristics on 30-day mortality. *Nursing Research*, 54(2), 74-84.

Knaus, W., & Draper, E. (1986). An evaluation of outcome from intensive care in major medical centers. *Annals of Internal Medicine*, 104(3), 410-418.

Mahlmeister, L. (2005). Preventing adverse perinatal outcomes through effective communication. *Journal of Perinatal Neonatal Nursing*, 19(4), 295-297.

Manojlovich, M. (2005). Linking the practice environment to nurses' job satisfaction through nurse-physician communication. *Journal of Nursing Scholarship*, 37(4), 367-373.

Nelson, J., & Venhaus, R. (2005). Improving retention through nurse/physician communication. *Nurse Leader*, 3(1), 54-56.

Rosenstein, A., & O'Daniel, M. (2005). Disruptive behavior and clinical outcomes: Perceptions of nurses and physicians: Nurses, physicians, and administrators say that clinicians' disruptive behavior has negative effects on clinical outcomes. *American Journal of Nursing*, 105(1), 54-64.

Simpson, K. (2005). Failure to rescue: Implications for evaluating quality of care during labor and birth. *Journal of Perinatal Neonatal Nursing*, 19(1), 24-34.

Exemplar: Listening to Colleagues in New Ways through Human Dynamics at Centegra Health System

—Frances Glosson

> *Most of us listen through a screen of resistance.*
> *We are screened with prejudices, whether religious or spiritual,*
> *psychological or scientific, or with daily worries, desires and fears.*
> *And with these fears for a screen, we listen. Therefore we listen really to our*
> *own noise, our own sound, not to what is being said.*
>
> *—J. Krishnamurti*

Listening in New Ways

Ten years of offering Human Dynamics (see page 396) at Centegra Health System has resulted in enhanced listening skills, serving to remove the screen of resistance Krishnamurti describes in the quote above. At Centegra, improved listening has contributed to this organization being recognized nationally as a best-practice institution which has received numerous prestigious awards (see table page 375).

The quality of an individual's listening is a sign of respect for other people. Mutual respect and trust among colleagues are critical for excellent outcomes in Relationship-Based Care, and both can be conveyed, at least in part, by active listening skills. Our study of Human Dynamics led us to discover that good listening actually begins with listening to one's own voice and becoming aware of our own natural processing during communications and while learning new skills. Self-knowledge has been enhanced as direct-care providers have become aware of their unique ways of thinking, observing and interacting.

Because we have integrated Human Dynamics so thoroughly into our culture, it has become second nature for most of us to recognize the "dynamic" of the person or persons with

374 •

whom we are speaking. We are able to tailor our communication to best fit the person with whom we are communicating—and specifically, we can tailor how we listen. We know that individuals of different dynamics will offer different perspectives, all of which are inherently valuable, but only really useful to us if we know how to listen for them. For example:

mental-physical	While communicating with mental-physical colleagues, we know to listen intently for the essential points, the structure, and the values. We listen for the logic and the vision and the precision required for implementation.
emotional-mental	While communicating with emotional-mental colleagues, we listen intently for new forms or new ways of accomplishing a goal. We listen for any critical action steps and future direction in a project.
emotional-physical	While communicating with emotional-physical colleagues, we listen intently for connections amidst diversity, feelings and personal interpretations. We know to listen for vital relationships and essential links—especially any interpretations connecting the present experience with a past experience.
physical-emotional	While communicating with physical-emotional colleagues, we listen intently for missing pieces to complex systems and for practical applications to problems. We listen for the facts, the continuity, the context of the speaker, and potential practical applications.
physical-mental	While communicating with physical-mental colleagues we listen intently for the purpose and the structure or roadmap that might assist in attaining goals in the most efficient manner. We listen for the pertinent background and the strategy to achieve the purpose.

At Centegra, we listen to both the patient and the co-worker in new, more respectful ways, resulting in improved relationships and outcomes. Our goal is to have each individual understand the other person's worldview and to accurately identify the gaps in expectations. The other individual involved listens reflectively and demonstrates an active understanding of what the speaker is saying.

Powerful listening is an essential competency for direct-care providers to create a genuine connection and serve patients and co-workers in a respectful manner. By incorporating Human Dynamics knowledge into their day-to-day interactions, individuals at Centegra are listening in new ways and genuinely seeking mutual purpose and mutual respect.

Summary

Listening is an essential building block in positive Relationship-Based Care. There clearly has been a significant positive impact at both the individual and the team level as it relates to listening to each other after 10 years of Human Dynamics at Centegra. An awareness of these positive effects is invaluable for better health care team relationships and the leveraging of a learning culture. Human Dynamics is a body of knowledge that has served to engage individuals in a transformational journey toward self-knowledge and ongoing development. This strategy has also resulted in team transformations which are directly linked to organizational excellence.

Centegra Health System has been recognized by the following organizations:

- HealthGrades Distinguished Hospital Award for Clinical Excellence, 2006

- U.S. *News and World Report Top 100 Hospitals in Respiratory Care, July 2005*

- Solucient 100 Top Hospitals in "Performance Improvement Leaders Award," 2005

- National Fire Starter of the Month, Studer Group, March 2005

- American Association of Retired Persons (AARP) for the second consecutive year as one of the "Best Employers for Workers Over 50," 2004 and 2005

- Press Ganey "Success Story," 2003

- Aon Loyalty Institute "Number One in Associate Opinion Survey," 2003 and 2004

PART

IV

Education

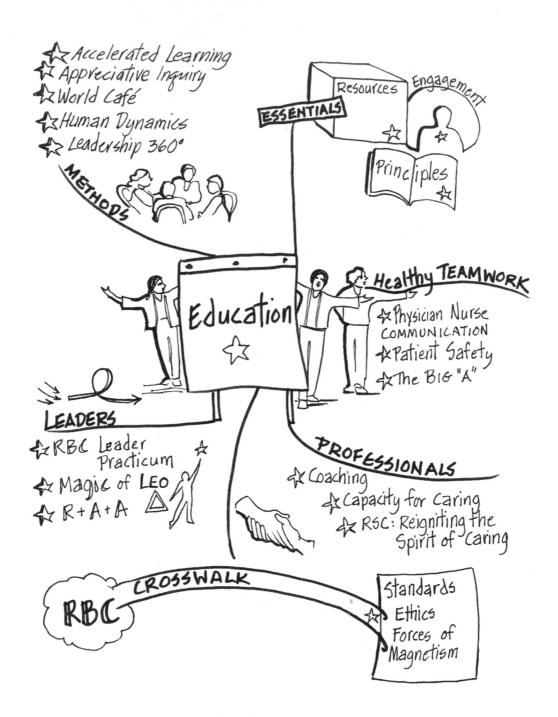

☆ Accelerated Learning
☆ Appreciative Inquiry
☆ World Café
☆ Human Dynamics
☆ Leadership 360°

METHODS

ESSENTIALS

Resources   Engagement
☆
Principles ☆

Education ☆

Healthy TEAMWORK
☆ Physician Nurse COMMUNICATION
☆ Patient Safety
☆ The BIG "A"

LEADERS
☆ RBC Leader Practicum
☆ Magic of LEO
☆ R + A + A △

PROFESSIONALS
☆ Coaching
☆ Capacity for Caring
☆ RSC: Reigniting the Spirit of Caring

CROSSWALK

RBC

Standards
☆ Ethics
Forces of Magnetism

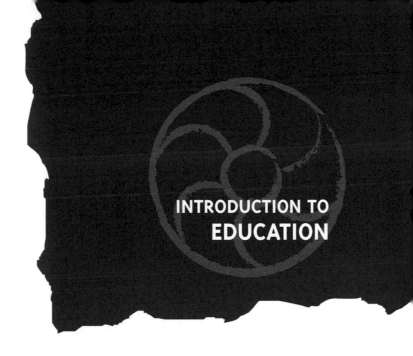

INTRODUCTION TO EDUCATION

Relationship-Based Care (RBC) seeks to optimize the capacity and direct the focus of all members of an organization toward the enhancement and continuity of patient/care giver relationships. With a shift of focus of this magnitude, not only will practices change, requiring some degree of "un learning," but the culture of the organization will also change, requiring that knowledge and skill development be offered pertaining specifically to the "new way of being." For this reason, education plays a significant role in the transformation to Relationship-Based Care.

In an environment undergoing substantive cultural change, it is inevitable that individuals will have much to learn, but the timing of that learning is also important. It is important to provide education early enough in the change process so people are confident in their new skills and feel prepared to take an active part in the change. One of the marks of a good learning experience is that participants walk out of it more enthusiastic about the changes than when they walked in. Adequate education makes us feel competent and well-prepared; excellent education makes us feel eager to use the new skills and practices we've learned.

Clarity & Competency   Confidence   Collaboration

COMMITMENT

Ability to ENGAGE in Change

There are five conditions (see page 480) required for people to engage in change. First, people need to have **clarity** about the purpose of the change, why their individual contribution matters, how their role and that of others "fits," and which systems of daily practice enhance their personal and professional efforts. Second, they need to learn the new knowledge, skills and attitudes (**competency**) required to work effectively with the change. These competencies need to cover all four domains (clinical/technical, interpersonal, critical/creative thinking, and leadership) so that they can meet the new expectations and standards. When people have clarity about both their role and direction and have the competence to meet the requirements, they are **confident** and therefore more likely to own their part in the change. Additionally, with clarity, competence and confidence people begin to **collaborate** with others to co-create the desired transformation. The **commitment** to do what is right for patients, families and colleagues is held dear by most people who have chosen the field of health care. When this commitment is combined with the first four Cs, individuals feel they are a vital part of the change and their insight is valuable. As a result, they have the courage to challenge the status quo.

Adequate education makes us feel competent and well-prepared; excellent education makes us feel eager to use the new skills and practices we've learned.

We believe that it is essential for those transforming to RBC to feel like experts in what RBC means in their areas of practice and leadership. This is achieved through educational initiatives designed especially for leaders of change at all levels. Part IV spells out what it takes to prepare leaders of change from the boardroom to the point of care to bring their organizations into the full realization of the RBC vision. It provides information on how creating effective teams, rethinking work practices, enhancing healthy communications practices and tending to our own self-development are all essential to the successful implementation and sustainability of Relationship-Based Care.

CHAPTER ELEVEN

Learning Methodologies and Resources

Accelerated Learning: Achieving Personal and Organizational Results

—Mary Koloroutis

Education is essential in the transformation to Relationship-Based Care (RBC). But it is important to remember that education can only take hold when it is grounded in reality and facilitated so that its meaning is apparent.

The following four fundamental conditions must exist within organizations in order for substantive transformation to occur:

- *Leaders are visible, engaged and consistently focused on reaching the desired vision.*

- *Education is designed to support insight-based learning and individual ownership for ongoing learning and growth.*

- *People are open to learning and committed to putting their new insights into action.*

- *Individuals and groups "own their part" and do what it takes to change old mindsets, routines and habits.*

As education is only one part of the larger wave of transformation, it would be illogical to design an education program that feels to its participants like it stands apart from the greater transformational design. Traditional education has long been information driven with lecture and presentation as the most common delivery method. But in order for education to really help individuals be an integral part of a transformation, it must inspire personal ownership for what is being learned along with a meaningful connection to the whole picture and what it means to the individual's work specifically. Accelerated Learning does just that.

Accelerated Learning, as described by Dave Meier (2000), is based on current research on the brain and learning. Meier defines Accelerated Learning as "an integrated philosophy of life and learning" (p. xxii). As such, it's a whole new view of things that de-mechanizes and rehumanizes learning and puts the learner (not the presenter or materials) squarely in the center of things. Its roots are ancient—it has been practiced by every child ever born—but in our Western culture, it is revolutionary.

The key to Accelerated Learning is engaging learners in their own learning. It leaves behind any semblance of the old instructor-in-front-of-the classroom model. Accelerated Learning means that the majority of the knowledge used in the course surfaces as a direct result of engaging the participants in what is most relevant to their own work or practice. They actually create new knowledge while discovering innovative applications for both new and existing knowledge.

In the insight-based coursework we offer, facilitators act as guides for the participants. We know where we're starting, we know where we'll end, and we know what stops we'll make along the way. But the real substance of the course is co-created with the participants in answer to what each participant needs in order to grow and develop in his or her own professional practice.

For example, in the *Reigniting the Spirit of Caring* workshop (see page 524) we present and discuss the Five Caring Processes (a midrange theory of caring) from Dr. Kristen Swanson's research regarding what constitutes caring behaviors. Patients and families are invited into the workshop to describe what caring means to them. Everyone present

> Accelerated Learning means that the majority of the knowledge used in the course surfaces as a direct result of engaging the participants in what is most relevant to their own work or practice.

connects the patients' experiences to Swanson's framework, bringing the theory alive. Through dialogue and storytelling, participants gain insight far beyond what they would have gained if the theory had been presented through a didactic methodology. Through this insight-based learning, we support each individual's understanding by validating and cultivating his or her own wisdom and applying the learning to their lived reality.

If our goal is for all team members to interact effectively with their colleagues and to be effective, critical and creative thinkers on the job, we need to give them opportunities to experience and validate their own competence through learning initiatives that draw on their own hard-won wisdom. Accelerated Learning helps individuals realize that they really are co-creating RBC in their organizations as it is largely the knowledge and skill they offer that shapes their organization's emerging practice of Relationship-Based Care.

Because we use participants' own knowledge to augment their understanding and facilitate the link between theory and application, they are clear about how to move what they have learned into action. The question that weaves through every topic is "What will it take to put this into practice?" While we provide some of the "hows" through time-tested experiences in implementing RBC, many of them come from the participants themselves, and that's when the light bulbs really come on. Insight-based learning helps us to move very quickly from "How has it been done before?" to the far more meaningful "How will *I* do it?"

In planning the educational initiatives for your transformation to RBC, consider integrating these elements of Accelerated Learning:

Accelerated Learning provides a whole new view of life and learning that de-mechanizes and re-humanizes learning and puts the learner squarely in the middle of things.

Create a Positive Learning Environment. People learn best in a positive physical, emotional and social environment—one that is both relaxed and stimulating. A sense of wholeness, safety, interest and enjoyment is essential for optimizing learning.	**Implications:** The physical space we choose for learning communicates our respect for the participants and the learning process. The physical space sets the stage. The space should have good lighting, comfortable and quiet surroundings, and room for participants to work in small groups and to convene in large groups for dialogues. Think of the learners as VIPs, and the learning experience as an investment in your most valuable asset—the people in your organization.
Create a structure that allows for total learner involvement. People learn best when they are totally and actively involved and take full responsibility for their own learning. Learning is not a spectator sport but a participatory one. Knowledge is not something a learner passively absorbs, but something a learner actively co-creates. Accelerated Learning is more activity based than materials or presenter based.	**Implications:** We design our programs to be 80-90% active participation and 10-20% presentation. The power of engagement and collective thinking is demonstrated repeatedly in the insights reported by our participants during the programs and in the endurance of personal and professional change following the programs. The goal is for the participant to "embody" the learning. Active engagement is an integral part of what makes embodiment possible.
Create a structure that allows for collaboration among learners. People generally learn best in an environment of collaboration. Whereas traditional learning emphasizes competition between isolated individuals, Accelerated Learning emphasizes collaboration between learners in a learning community.	**Implications:** If we wish to cultivate collaboration rather than competition on the job, it makes sense to provide opportunities to put collaboration into practice—particularly in educational offerings. A learning community is one in which all participants share responsibility for the learning that takes place. The facilitator serves as a guide and leads the way, but it is through individual ownership and interdependence that "the way" takes shape and deepens in meaning.
Integrate variety to appeal to all types of learners. People learn best when they have a rich variety of learning options that allow them to use all of their senses and to exercise their preferred learning style. Rather than treating a learning program as a one-dish meal, Accelerated Learning treats it as a results-driven, learner-centered smorgasbord.	**Implications:** We use the knowledge and work of Human Dynamics (see page 396) to inform our thinking about diverse learning styles. We integrate structure, logic, vision, interaction and technology with human diversity foremost in mind. We encourage participants to understand their own learning requirements and to ask for what they need.
Ensure that all learning is contextual. People learn best in context. Facts and skills learned in isolation are hard to absorb and quick to evaporate. The best learning comes from doing the work itself in a continual process of "real-work" immersion, feedback, reflection, evaluation and reimmersion.	**Implications:** One of the goals of education is to build confidence in individuals—confidence to make decisions and take action in their real-life work environments. Education preparing individuals for Relationship-Based Care takes place in a healing and caring environment. The participants are immersed in learning designed to build confidence and competence in creating and sustaining therapeutic, healthy relationships.

Adapted from D. Meier, *The Accelerated learning handbook*, McGraw-Hill, 2000.
Used with permission of the author.

Meier reminds us that effective learning is not merely "head learning" but involves the whole body/mind with all of its emotions, senses and receptors (p. 41). Remember to engage participants in creating (not just consuming) the course content in active collaboration with others. These experiences of whole body/mind creative collaboration provide real-life learning that guides and inspires individuals to own what they have learned and to put it into practice to achieve results.

Reference: Meier, D. (2000). *The accelerated learning handbook*. Columbus, OH: McGraw-Hill.

The Power of Appreciation, Affirmation and Celebration

—Colleen Person

Concepts about change are changing! For years the field of psychology has emphasized the power of positive thinking on behavior, which in turn has been validated through scientific research on psychoneuroimmunology. In motivation theory, attention is shifting from the use of external rewards to an appreciation for the intrinsic motivators that give us energy. The new quantum sciences teach us that energy flows in the direction in which we place our attention. And Appreciative Inquiry (AI) methodology has demonstrated the power of affirmative processes in organizational change.

Once we become aware of the power of the positive, we may wonder why we ever focused on the negative in any of our social and/or work interactions. Is it a habit culled from the way we were disciplined at home or educated at school? Is it a holdover from the old Newtonian approach to science that focuses on problems, deficits and gaps? Regardless of the cause, it's time for a shift to the positive in both our personal and organizational behaviors.

At Creative Health Care Management (CHCM), we have noticed for years the difference in the responses, energy and effect generated by complaining about what's going wrong versus appreciating what's going right. If we ask an organization, a group or an individual to describe the problems in their work setting we get a long list. During the recitation of problems, the energy of the group or individual spirals downward to frustration, anger, even hopelessness. Conversely, if we ask appreciative questions, there is pause for reflection followed by comments or stories that are positive, heartfelt, energetic, and not surprisingly, energetically positive.

This phenomenon first came to our attention years ago when Marie Manthey, in one of her former roles as a nurse executive, was making rounds with Esther Lucille Brown, a noted anthropologist. As Marie tells the story, she was "doing the typical nurse executive thing—asking how things were—if they had enough staff, if there were problems," and sure enough she got a list of problems. Then Ms. Brown intervened and suggested she ask the questions on the next unit. Her first question was, "what are you doing of interest to you professionally today?" The response she got every time was a thoughtful pause, followed by a touching story of patient care.

Appreciation is expressed most often through recognition, valuing and gratitude. *Appreciate* is a verb that carries a double meaning. It refers both to the act of recognition and to the act of enhancing value. A number of thought-provoking definitions of appreciation are offered in Diana Whitney, Amanda Trosten-Bloom, and David Cooperrider's *The Power of Appreciative Inquiry: A Practical Guide to Positive Change* (2003). They say that to appreciate is:

- *to recognize the best in people and the world around us,*

- *to perceive those things which give life, health, vitality and excellence to living human systems,*

- *to affirm past and present strengths, successes, assets, and potentials, and*

- *to increase in value (as in, the investment has appreciated in value).*

People long for recognition for their contributions in family, in society and in organizations. They long to have their work linked to their values, to experience meaning, even joy, in their work. During organizational assessment using the Reflective Practice Cycle and with the *Reigniting the Spirit of Caring* workshop (see page 524), participants find new joy, meaning and purpose (Leider, 2005) in their ever demanding work when that work is connected to their values. Participants tell us that when they experience their work as connected to their values, they reconnect with their purpose for going into health care in the first place—they want to make a difference in people's lives. That connection brings renewed energy and meaning into the workplace. It's the connection that allows us to join Katharine Graham, former editor of the *Washington*

It's time for a shift to the positive in both our personal and organizational behaviors.

Post, in saying "To love what you do and feel that it matters ... how could anything be more fun?"

Affirmation is the assertion that something exists or is true. In practice we note that when behavior, comments and contributions are affirmed, people smile, relax and continue the behavior that is affirmed. Affirming something amplifies it.

People long for recognition for their contributions in family, in society, and in organizations.

Affirmation and appreciation can both appear as statements or as questions. The most important insight we have learned with AI to date is that "human systems grow toward what they persistently ask questions about" (Cooperrider & Whitney, 2000). The act of asking questions (inquiry) affects individuals and organizations because it focuses attention and promotes reflection on the subject of the question; it increases awareness by providing for the pause necessary for reflection. Questions make us think. And when asked from the affirmative, appreciative mode, questions help individuals increase their awareness of what worked, what was learned, and what to do again. When the topic is related to core values and issues critical to the success of an organization, new energy—and new potential—is released.

As the new sciences are applied to organizational development, they help us to realize that we don't necessarily need to have the answers, but rather to ask a question from which new answers can emerge from others' perspectives. Questions evoke generative thought and invite others into change. Questions also shape our dialogues with others. Margaret Wheatley, in her book *Turning to One Another: Simple Conversations to Restore Hope to the Future* (2002, p. 3), says:

I believe we can change the world if we start listening to one another again. Simple, honest, human conversation. Not mediation, negotiation, problem-solving, debate or public meetings. Simple, truthful conversation where we each have a chance to speak, we each feel heard and we each listen well.

Inevitably these conversations in which we "each feel heard, and we each listen well" lead us back to what we truly care about: relationships—those within our own personal lives, with our patients and their families, and with our colleagues. In these conversations we reconnect with our values. We gain new ideas along with an appreciation for other perspectives, and we often even experience a renewed commitment to the things that we can do to make a difference.

Celebration, unlike affirmation and appreciation, is a more formal recognition of significant events. It's been a long tradition of CHCM's to encourage organizations embarking on new initiatives to mark events along the way with special celebrations—the "kick off" of a new care delivery model, the first day of the official implementation on a unit, special recognition of groups, individuals and events (such as Nurses' Week)—both spontaneously and routinely. Participants in *Leading an Empowered Organization* (see page 483) have been taking the notion of celebrating individual "Moments of Excellence" into their organizations. It's a practice whereby an individual announces—sometimes spontaneously—that he or she is having a "moment of excellence" for a significant idea, contribution or experience. This helps people to take notice of and celebrate daily successes.

The questions on the following page will help you begin a daily practice of appreciation, affirmation and celebration.

Affirming something amplifies it.

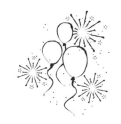

"What" and "How" Questions That Leaders Can Ask on a Daily Basis

Patient care:

What do you feel good about in your work with patients/families today? Tell me a story of patient care that made you proud to be a nurse, an aide, etc.

How did you make a meaningful difference for that person today?

What challenged you to new learning today?

Teamwork:

What do you want our work environment to be like?

What is important to you?

What did you do today to contribute to that environment?

What's an example of teamwork that made a difference for you today?

What's it going to take for us to come together to make the most of everyone's contributions to meet our challenges today?

What did we learn today that we will want to remember in the future?

Organization:

What are the three things that you value about this organization? About this unit?

What attracted you to this organization?

What keeps you here?

Appreciation, affirmation and celebration are practices which cost little or no money but achieve invaluable results in honoring individuals and groups for their contributions to the relationship-based culture of caring. Deliberately placing our attention on each—appreciation, affirmation and celebration— cannot help moving us toward what we desire to create in our experience, in our organization, on our unit, in our lives.

References: Cooperrider, D., & Whitney, D. (2000). *Appreciative inquiry: Collaborating for change.* San Francisco: Berrett-Koehler.

Leider, R. (2005). *The power of purpose: Creating meaning in your life and work.* San Francisco: Berrett-Koehler.

Wheatley, M. (2002). *Turning to one another: Simple conversations to restore hope to the future.* San Francisco: Berrett-Koehler.

Whitney, D., Trosten-Bloom, A., & Cooperrider, D. (2003). *The power of appreciative inquiry: A practical guide to positive change.* San Francisco: Berrett-Koehler.

World Café: Roundtable Conversations That Matter

—Jayne A. Felgen

The World Café facilitation process refers to both a philosophical vision of creating collective wisdom and another innovative, yet familiar method of dialogue. It evolved out of conversations and experimentation one evening at the home of colleagues Juanita Brown and David Isaacs of Whole System Associates.

World Café conversations are an intentional way to create a living network of conversations that matter. A Café Conversation is a creative process for leading collaborative dialogue, sharing knowledge and creating possibilities for action in groups of all sizes. These conversations are one method that communities, businesses, governments and people from all walks of life are using to create a common purpose, share knowledge, make intelligent decisions and create life-affirming presents/presence.

The method is simple: People sit four to a table and have a series of conversational rounds lasting 20 to 45 minutes about a selected question that is personally meaningful to them. At the end of one round, one person remains as the host and each of the other three travels to separate tables. The host of the table welcomes the travelers and shares the essence of the previous conversation. The travelers also relate any conversational threads which they are carrying, so the conversation deepens as the round progresses. The facilitator may continue with another round, or interject a new question, or suggest a deepening of the original question.

After two or more rounds, those at each table are asked to reflect upon essence of their themes and an individual is selected to report their insights to the whole group. These lessons are captured in creative ways on flipcharts to make them visible and allow further reflection. Creative ways include car-

Participants were able to recognize their own potential to contribute to the field as well.

tooning, mind mapping, graphics and even the use of mimes, musicians and artists.

Juanita, David and the World Café Community have generously shared this process and their learning. Their Web site, www.theworldcafe.com, and their book, *The World Café: Shaping Our Futures Through Conversations that Matter*, are treasure troves for leaders inspired to engage others in meaningful dialogue using this innovative method.

We have used the World Café in a variety of settings and circumstances in our health care consulting practice. In all cases we have integrated Appreciative Inquiry principles consistent with our leadership philosophy.

This highly interactive collegial experience showed them they were not alone.

Several years ago more than a hundred participants at the Creative Health Care Management client conference experienced World Café as the method to respond to a panel of speakers each reading their part, or representing their "voice," which is an adaptation of Dynamic Dialogue (see page 410). The stories of a patient, family member, nurse, nurse manager, and chief nurse were told individually, then "run" simultaneously as context for engaging the participants in a dialogue about this health care situation.

Questions deepened understanding as participants traveled among the tables for two rounds. Then, for the next two rounds they were asked to explore insights specifically about what's working in this system. The final two rounds focused on what was needed to achieve greater successes in compassionate health care outcomes.

At the end of the day the table hosts shared the essence of these conversations with the whole group, thus completing the first day's objective and setting the stage for determining what actions are required by participating leaders to make a difference in their organizations and beyond.

Similarly, World Café was employed at another gathering of more than 300 nurse leaders from around the world assembled at a preconference for the first Summit of Sages featuring six distinguished nurse leaders. Our objective was to communicate that we are all sages, and that the world of health care needs what each of us has to offer.

We integrated Appreciative Inquiry concepts (see page 96) and our rounds were centered on four key questions related to "discover, dream, dialogue and design." We asked participants:

1. To describe a time when they were part of an extraordinary innovation in nursing that had a significant impact on patients, families and/or care givers;

2. What their hopes and dreams for the future of nursing in the next decade were;

3. What, given the realities in health care today, it would take for them to accelerate the impact of their efforts on behalf of patients, families and care givers in order to achieve their future vision; and

4. What steps they could take now to make their desired future a reality.

This design and the full engagement of the participants proved to be highly effective in setting the stage for the following 2-day conference. Participants said the process was so affirming and inspirational and they were so "tuned into" listening to reflections from the celebrated sages that they were now more able to recognize their own potential to contribute to the field as well. One leader shared that this conference was the zenith of her professional career!

Another highly successful application of World Café involved 800 nurses who were returning to share their accomplishments in making changes on their units as a follow-up assignment to previous participation in a 3-day workshop, *Leadership at the Point of Care.* More than 26 sessions were offered so that groups of 30 to 35 could assemble and tell their success stories.

The initial rounds featured participant success stories about the changes they had made in their patient care practices or colleague relationships. In the next round, participants addressed what factors contributed to their success. In the final round, they discussed what was needed to enhance their successes. The energy was mesmerizing, and the participants left exhilarated by their individual accomplishments and reinspired to continue their quest for patient care innovations because this highly interactive collegial experience showed them they were not alone.

World Café is a remarkable dialogue method that builds on the assumption that we already have the answers; we simply need to ask the right questions, then listen and act.

In another workshop setting, a 3-hour presession was held the evening before the first in a series of three full-day workshops to take place over 8 months. Participants included teams from a variety of hospitals from a health care network. This series was designed to introduce Relationship-Based Care (RBC) concepts to nurse leaders who desired to make changes on their patient units and within the nursing or patient care services division.

Participants were asked to introduce themselves and state their hospital, position and years in health care. They were also asked to describe a time when a patient or family received exactly the care they needed.

Following a dinner and formal welcome, we reconvened the Café with teams of colleagues sitting together. Each table was asked to review the predinner stories and select which one they told or heard that best reflected their values about patient and family care as they would hope it to be.

Then each table was asked to record their responses to a series of questions from Dynamic Dialogue, which uses a 360° approach as follows (see page 410):

- *Perspective: What are the different beliefs and dynamics at work in the group? What cycles or patterns do you see?*

- *Purpose: What is this system designed to teach? What seems to be its purpose?*

- *Effect: How does it feel? What aspects deserve appreciation? What lessons are to be learned? What feelings were elicited? What core truths emerged?*

- *Boundaries: What is included or excluded in the system? What hard truths must be spoken? What actions are you inspired to take?*

The World Café process was explored and discussed before adjourning for the evening. The flipchart responses were organized into like categories and affixed to each of the four walls so participants could review all responses in the morning as a welcoming exercise before the next day's workshop began.

This immersion process into what really mattered most to them—providing the best compassionate care for patients and their families—was quite effective. The collective wisdom of the participants, which exceeded 1,000 years in nursing and was gathered in such a short period of time, touched them deeply, and set the stage perfectly for launching this workshop series designed to inspire leaders to action.

World Café is a remarkable dialogue method that builds on the assumption that we already have the answers; we simply need to ask the right questions, then listen and act.

Brown, J. (2005). *The world café: Shaping our futures through conversations that matter.* San Francisco: Berrett-Koehler.

Human Dynamics Overview

—Sandra Seagal and David Horne

Editors' Note:
Sandra Seagal and David
Horne are co-authors
of Human Dynamics:
A New Framework for
Understanding People *and*
Realizing the Potential in
Our Organizations (Pegasus
Communications, 1997) For
more information, go to
www.humandynamics.
com. Adapted with authors'
permission.

The outcome of an ongoing investigation begun over 25 years ago that has so far involved more than 80,000 people from more than 25 cultures, Human Dynamics is a body of work that identifies innate distinctions in people as whole systems of mental-emotional-physical functioning. Nine such different human systems (termed "personality dynamics") have been identified. These different "ways of being" appear to be so foundational in the human makeup that they can be seen the world over, identified at every age level (even in infancy), and observed in males and females equally. In other words, these distinctions are more fundamental to who we are and how we function than age, race, culture or gender.

Mental, Emotional and Physical Centering

While each individual comprises a continual interplay of mental, emotional and physical life, we have discovered that people seem to be "wired" in such a way that one of these three aspects of human functioning is central to each individual's total functioning. Some people are "centered" mentally (rationally), some emotionally (relationally), and some physically (pragmatically). Our innate centering determines how we naturally "experience experience" and take in and process information.

For example:

Mentally centered people process information in a linear, logical and sequential way. They are characterized also by an innate detachment. They experience life as if they were standing on a hilltop, with a bird's-eye view of events. It is therefore natural for them to maintain objectivity and a long-range perspective.

Emotionally centered people, on the other hand, process information in a nonlinear, associative, interactive way that incorporates feelings and intuition, rather than through a strictly rational process. This relatively spontaneous way of proceeding often results in the generation of new ideas and the exploration of new avenues of thought or action that might not have emerged through a more linear process. For emotionally centered people, engaging in dialogue with others is essential as a means of clarifying thoughts, feelings, and intuitions, as well as for establishing the sense of personal connection with others that makes life meaningful for them.

Finally, **physically centered** people process information in a systemic way. They gather and assimilate large amounts of factual data, and think in terms of the interconnections that make up whole systems of functioning. Because of their affinity for the systemic, they may be fascinated by the patterns they observe in the flow of events across time, from past to present and projected into the future, while on a more concrete level they often have a keen interest in the mechanical functioning of things. They seem to instinctively understand how parts interact for the successful functioning of the whole.

Five Predominant Personality Dynamics

We have found that there are three variations on each of these ways of being centered. Mentally centered people may be "mental-mental," "mental-emotional" or "mental-physical." Emotionally centered people may be "emotional-mental," "emotional-emotional" or "emotional-physical." And physically centered people may be "physical-mental," "physical-emotional" or "physical-physical," making the nine personality dynamics to which we have referred. Whereas the first principle indicates how one naturally processes information, the second indicates what one processes—the kind of material or events that are the natural focus of attention. However, of the nine personality dynamics we find that five are by far the most prevalent, and it is these five that will therefore be the focus of this article. The five consist of one variation on the mentally centered theme—mental-physical; two variations on the emotionally centered theme—emotional-mental and emotional-physical; and two variations on the physically centered theme—physical-mental and physical-emotional. Some combination of representatives of these five very different kinds of people will be present in any group anywhere—in any management or clinical team, for example, in any family, in any classroom, at any international conference or meeting of heads of state—each characterized by inherently different processes of taking in and processing information, of learning, communicating, relating, undertaking tasks and contributing to groups or teams. Each will tend to take leadership in different ways. Each also experiences stress differently and depends upon different conditions for optimum health and well-being. Most importantly, the path of development toward greater integration and wholeness is different for each. While the members of each personality dynamic group share basic common characteristics, each individual is unique and each is at a different place along the group's developmental path.

Each dynamic tends to take leadership in different ways. Each also experiences stress differently and depends upon different conditions for optimum health and well-being.

Following are thumbnail sketches of each of the five predominant personality dynamics, to provide a sense of their similarities and distinctions, and also of the most commonly arising misinterpretations of each. No value judgments are to be attached to the different personality dynamics. One is not inherently "better" than another. Anyone of any personality dynamic may be more or less intelligent, caring, contributive or gifted. They simply comprise the particular mental-emotional-physical structures through which we operate. Our responsibility is to understand how our "instrument" works and to continually expand our capacities to use it well.

Mental-Physical:

The thinking process of mental-physical people is linear, logical and sequential.

Being mentally centered, the thinking process of mental-physical people is linear, logical and sequential. The secondary principle being physical, the mental-physical person's thinking is typically focused upon events in the external world (as opposed to emotional data). Because of their "hilltop" perspective, mental-physical people tend to focus on the long term and to think in terms of enduring principles and values. Because of their innate detachment (which does not imply disengagement), their emotional life is typically extremely even. Mental-physical people offer to others emotional stability, objectivity and their gift for perceiving and articulating what is essential—key points, principles, values, goals and information. They value clarity in thinking and communication. For this reason, they often have an affinity for the written rather than the spoken word. They are usually precise and meticulous in any task they undertake.

Mental-physical people often ask the questions "Why?" and "What do you mean by ... ?" However, they are frequently silent in groups, either because they feel no need to speak if others are saying what needs to be said or because they think carefully before speaking and cannot find the space to participate if a process is less than orderly. Because of their natural detachment and reticence, and because they do not readily express their feelings, others may interpret mental-physical people as being aloof, disengaged, uncaring or unwilling to be approached. None of these interpretations is necessarily true. If you want to know what a mental-physical person is really thinking or feeling, just ask. Such questions will help him or her to connect and communicate.

Mental-physical people often ask the questions "Why?" and "What do you mean by ... ?"

Emotional-Mental:

Being emotionally centered, emotional-mental people process in a nonlinear, associative way. Because their secondary principle is mental, their primary focus is the world of ideas.

Emotional-mental people deeply enjoy a highly interactive brainstorming kind of communication in which one idea triggers another, leading to the generation of new ways of thinking or acting. They have a deep affinity for movement and change. They are often innovators, drawn to the new and untried. They intuitively sense new possibilities in people, situations and events, and endeavor to promote their realization. They commonly do not enjoy communication that is highly detailed, preferring a flow of ideas that moves in big steps. In taking on new projects, emotional-mental people can move into action with a strong sense of the general direction to be taken, but with minimal data and little or no concrete planning. This experimental movement leads to new events, which in turn suggest next steps. The specific form of the outcome that emerges at the end of this repeated process may be entirely unanticipated.

Emotional-mental people deeply enjoy a highly interactive brainstorming kind of communication in which one idea triggers another, leading to the generation of new ways of thinking or acting.

Because emotional-mental people are focused on the future, they typically carry from the past only what they consider to be essential information or experience. However, their memory for the data required for, or related to, any undertaking on which they are currently focused is usually excellent.

The physical signals that emotional-mental people receive from their bodies tend to be subtle and not readily apparent. For this reason they are often able to work long hours without becoming aware that they may be hungry or tired. They also may not be fully aware of being hurt or becoming sick, and need to learn to take "minor" symptoms seriously.

Others may sometimes misinterpret emotional-mental people as being either "pushy" or, because they initiate movement with little or no prior planning, even irresponsible. Rather, they are following their natural instinct to move events forward and light the fires of new endeavors.

Emotional-Physical:

Emotional-physical people are sensitive to others' feelings and can often experience those feelings in their own bodies, even when others aren't outwardly expressing them.

Emotional-physical people also think in a nonlinear, associative way—preferably through dialogue with others. But since the secondary principle is physical, their focus is on the physical world of things, events and, especially, people. They experience constantly changing emotional responses to their environment, and all the objects, people and events in it. In relation to the concrete world, they typically have an intuitive sense for how materials (e.g., fabrics, colors, foods) will work well together aesthetically. With regard to people, they are sensitive to others' feelings and can often experience those feelings in their own bodies, even when others aren't outwardly expressing them. This ability can be a gift, providing helpful information and insights; it can also be a burden if those feelings are negative or painful. Emotional-physical people may sometimes be uncertain whether feelings they are experiencing are their own, or whether they are picking them up from someone else.

Emotional-physical people value personal connection and communication with others. They bring to groups and teams both a high degree of creative thinking and a concern for establishing harmony. The tone and quality of the group's interactions are as important to them as the outcomes they achieve. They themselves can only offer their full capacities if they feel comfortable and "safe." Feeling threatened or judged in any way may cause them to withdraw and stay silent.

Emotional-physical people typically relive emotion-laden events from the past as if they were occurring again in the present. Sometimes others judge them as "too sensitive," "using too many words," or as insufficiently logical. The truth is that their sensitivity is a gift to be valued—facilitating understanding of individuals and interpersonal situations. Their sometimes extensive communication results from their need to establish personal connections and to ensure that misunderstandings don't arise. Their nonlinear thinking has an emotional logic, frequently reflecting a "knowing" that they cannot rationally explain. This intuitive gift often goes unused and unappreciated in organizations.

Sometimes others judge them as "too sensitive," "using too many words," or as insufficiently logical.

Physical-Mental:

Being physically centered, physical-mental people think systemically. Their secondary principle being mental, they are consciously focused upon creating mental structures to organize the data they collect to achieve systemic goals. They have a capacity for discerning patterns in varied data or in the complex flow of events, from which they make projections into the future and devise action plans accordingly. They plan systematically as well as systemically. They want to know the purpose of any endeavor, and then create a logical step-by-step plan for achieving that purpose. They tend to have a conscious strategy for almost everything they do, whether professionally or in their personal lives. They like to create efficient systems of operation, then refine those systems to be even more efficient and, if possible, applicable to multiple situations. They typically use such visual aids as models, diagrams and charts to assist their thinking and communicate their ideas.

Physical-mental people have a detailed factual memory in areas of particular interest to them. In communication with others, they are usually listening for the action to be taken or problem to be solved. They like communication to be factual and initially concise. A common misunderstanding about physical-mental people is that they do not care about people or their feelings. This misperception can occur because they may

Physical-mental people want to know the purpose of any endeavor, and then create a logical step-by-step plan for achieving that purpose.

be so focused on creating the logical steps to achieve results that they may fail to take into account human factors and people's personal responses. Moreover, they do not usually find it easy to express personal feelings. They typically express their caring more readily through offering their gifts for practical problem solving, rather than through their words.

Physical-Emotional:

Physical-emotional people also process information in a systemic way; their secondary principle being emotional; however, their attention is on the highly detailed web of interconnections among data, events and people, and their natural process of thinking, planning and learning is not systematic but organic. When approaching any new endeavor, they immerse themselves in gathering and absorbing data without initially sorting or prioritizing it, because for them everything is connected to everything else, and they cannot know initially what might be relevant and what not. They then assimilate, sort and link all of this information in a process that may be as much unconscious as consciously directed. This process, like digestion, takes its own time, until at some point everything comes together in a highly detailed, systemic understanding of a situation, or plan of action or product. Because the entire process takes place internally, typically without the aid of notes or charts or diagrams, others may think that nothing is "going on," when in fact very much is "going on," though the individual may not be able to clearly articulate what it is until the process is complete.

Physical-emotional people are sometimes labeled "slow" in a negative sense. In classrooms they may be categorized as "slow learners," with the implication that they may not be as smart as other students who respond more quickly. A more accurate descriptor would be "thorough." Their organic process takes time, but they typically assimilate and synthesize more data, and are able to comprehend more complex situations, than people of any other personality dynamic.

Physical-emotional people typically have a prodigious capacity to remember data. They can recollect events from even the distant past in which they were fully engaged in extraordinary sensory detail. Because they naturally think

> Immerse themselves in gathering and absorbing data without initially sorting or prioritizing it, because for them everything is connected to everything else, and they cannot know initially what might be relevant and what not.

and experience in terms of detailed interconnections, they appreciate communication that provides "the whole story," that gives the full context for any event or issues. They themselves characteristically convey information through detailed stories, not by enumerating points.

Some Implications

We hope that through these sketches we have been able to convey some sense of the distinctiveness of these different human systems, with their very different, sometimes totally contrasting, natural processes of experiencing, thinking, communicating, relating, learning and undertaking tasks. Each has characteristic gifts; each has characteristic needs. Each potentially complements the others—"potentially" because the realization of this complementarity depends upon two important precursors: consciousness and intention.

When we do not recognize these differences, we can easily misunderstand others and misinterpret their behavior, fail to "connect" in communication, engage in less than optimum teamwork, and in classroom and training sessions at every age level offer teaching methodologies that do not match students' specific learning processes. Awareness and understanding of the differences, on the other hand, opens the way for us to appreciate both our own and others' natural way of functioning, to understand and accommodate each other's needs, and to relate, manage and teach in ways that enable each group member to perform at his or her best. A shared base of such understanding helps families to live together more harmoniously, colleagues to work together more effectively, and all of us to better meet the needs of our "clients," whether in the realm of business, education or health care.

Awareness and understanding the differences, opens the way for us to appreciate both our own and others' natural way of functioning, to understand and accommodate each other's needs, and to relate, manage and teach in ways that enable each group member to perform at his or her best.

Human Dynamics:
A Pathway to Enhancing Self-Awareness and Improving Interpersonal Effectiveness

—Sandra Seagal

Background: *This piece comes from Sandra Seagal's work with individuals on the impact of Human Dynamics (see page 396) on their self-awareness and leadership performance. The following is based on an interview with a health care leader who has extensive training in Human Dynamics and is emotional-physically centered.*

The person whose story follows is what is termed "emotionally centered," and her personality dynamic is one of the variations on this theme which is termed "emotional-physical" because of the strong and continuous connection between her emotional experience and her physical experience.

Increasing Self-Awareness Through the Study of Human Dynamics

Human Dynamics has created a pathway for self-awareness and self-acceptance for me which then naturally enhances my ability to understand and accept others. I remember the moment when I learned, understood, embraced and accepted that I am emotionally centered. It was a life-changing moment of insight and helped me to understand why I respond as I do, why I seem to carry others' feelings in my heart and soul at times, and why I just seem to "know" what is going on emotionally before I am able to put it into words.

The difficult part of being "so emotional" (as I described myself prior to understanding my dynamic) was that at times I felt controlled by my emotional responses. It felt like I carried the emotions of the group in my body to the extent that I sometimes found myself physically depleted and mentally fogged. Learning that my emotional way of being was natural—and a *gift*, not something to resist—allowed me to surrender to it and value it. I am now able to feel and recognize the emotional dynamics in another or a group and, through conscious intention, prevent myself from absorbing the emotion. I have learned to mentally detach without disengaging and to stay clear about where my own emotional field begins and ends. This has been a huge development for me and allows me to be much more effective in working with complex and emotionally laden situations (pretty much the norm in health care) without relinquishing my gift of intuitive knowing and perceptions.

I also learned through studying Human Dynamics that I am gifted as a connector—an integrator of both people and concepts. I possess a natural understanding of people and their emotional needs and responses. I value meaningful communication and often take the lead in bringing people together to discuss important and difficult issues. I love helping others gain insight into their own gifts, actions and contributions. It is a natural role for someone with my dynamic.

When there is a disconnect—say, for instance, a lack of integrity between what we say we will do and what we *do*—I experience distress. Because I cannot "not see" when there is a disconnect between espoused values, beliefs, and principles and the actions that come from them, I move into action to find a way to achieve integrity—to integrate what is disconnected. For example, when I'm involved in a change initiative I expect substantive change—meaning that what we say we will do actually happens in day-to-day practice. I am particularly driven to achieve the principles of compassionate care in each patient/family interaction. If there's a mismatch in what we've said we want to do and what we're actually doing, I see it and work harder to achieve congruence. This way of being earned me some very descriptive nicknames at a number of different organizations. I was called the "Conscience of the Organization," "the Torch Burner," and (my personal favorite) "the Velvet Steamroller." I doubt you'd find anyone who wasn't ultimately pleased with the changes I helped bring to these organizations, but as you can imagine, not everyone found me easy to be with when a vision didn't execute in daily actions as planned.

When there is a disconnect—say, for instance, a lack of integrity between what we say we will do and what we do— I experience distress.

I had a watershed experience a few years ago as a participant in a Human Dynamics seminar. I was working in a group and I started feeling a lot of the same feelings I'd felt in my family of origin growing up—I was actually starting to have a bit of a meltdown emotionally. It was all about wanting to control the situation so that things would go better for everybody. As the facilitator came back to our group after having been away for a few minutes, she could see the distress written all over my face; I was actually considering walking out of the training. As I said earlier, one of the things that happens to me under emotional stress (when I am not conscious of it) is that I physically absorb the emotions of others. My whole body feels very heavy and I feel tired. I also experience "mental fogging," which means I find it difficult to stay focused on content or remain clear and objective as I process the content or interact with others.

The facilitator asked me what I was having difficulty with and I told her I was tired of trying to make things work in the group. *She asked me if I thought I could just stop trying.* It was so simple, but it was one of the most liberating moments of my life. She suggested that I stay engaged mentally and physically as part of the group, but no longer experience being *responsible* for the group. I stayed involved mentally and physically, but unplugged myself emotionally. She coached me to become aware of what was happening for me both physically and emotionally. I had been feeling extremely vulnerable and was not distinguishing my own emotions from the emotions of the individuals within the group. Through some inquiry and guided reflection, the facilitator helped me identify what was going on, clarify boundaries and differentiate myself emotionally, physically and mentally. She then used imagery to guide me into achieving a position of mental detachment. She helped me do it and feel it.

Since that day, I have had the capacity to access mental detachment on my own, which is a tremendous gift, and have continued to work on my development relative to differentiating myself, creating appropriate boundaries, and gaining greater objectivity and detachment. I have accomplished this through a meditative practice using the music of Paganini, which is part of the Human Dynamics "tool box." It involves focusing one's attention at a point above the head, which has the effect of building a capacity for detachment to balance my natural gift for emotional connection. A particular piece of music by Paganini that has properties of structure and clarity is used to help support this "position" of mental detachment.

After working with Human Dynamics I have a broader and deeper awareness of the natural distinctions in people and their unique gifts and capacities. I no longer tend to personalize differences in people or become emotionally flooded in conflict situations. I'm certainly not 100 percent there, but awareness is a major developmental step! Since I have developed my ability to set personal boundaries and to detach mentally, I have greater courage and capacity to work with differing points of view and I now even actually seek them out.

When I am able to keep a detached perspective without compromising my emotional sensibilities, I can sense more clearly what people really mean to say, what problems can and cannot be solved. I am more objective and I have more tools at my disposal now. It's not that the emotional part of me is discarded or even minimized; it's more like I choose to use my emotional ability as the gift that it is, and to access my mental capacity to maintain greater integration and balance.

I found it significant, too, that relief from emotional upset doesn't ultimately come through countering or opposing the emotional principle in me. The experience of focusing at the level of the heart–just deliberately putting my attention there–connects me with the emotional principle comfortably, allowing me to peacefully feel my own feelings. There are a variety of simple and effective practices that I can use to realign myself as needed. The key is knowing what is needed and taking conscious action. It's really a gift to be able to consciously shift your position energetically and at will.

I am fascinated by the possibilities for applying what we know about Human Dynamics to patient care. Human Dynamics can be extremely helpful for us in our clinical interactions with patients and families. Because being in a hospital setting usually puts people under extreme stress and in a high

How Increased Self-Awareness Benefits One-on-One Interactions

When I am able to keep a detached perspective without compromising my emotional sensibilities, I can sense more clearly what people really mean to say, what problems can and cannot be solved.

The key is knowing what is needed and taking conscious action. It's really a gift to be able to consciously shift your position energetically and at will.

state of vulnerability, their ability to take in information is naturally compromised. If we understand a patient's personality dynamic we can interact with greater intention and consciousness. We will be more likely to provide information in a way that can be absorbed and meet the patient's needs more effectively.

How Increased Self-Awareness Benefits Group Effectiveness

Human Dynamics has helped me to identify and be more confident about my strengths. It taught me that I am a skilled communicator (which didn't come as a surprise), but it also taught me that for me, process and outcomes are inexorably linked. Individuals with the emotional-physical dynamic see how everything is interrelated, and we also always see how things that are not already overtly related can be integrated. In the ideal work group, you'd have individuals representing all five dynamics, but you might also find, if you don't understand Human Dynamics, that it's hard to appreciate people who see things differently from how you do.

We are born with our dynamic, but we have the infinite potential to develop.

As we learn about our different dynamics, we learn to rely on each other to create a whole systemic approach to making things happen as a group. It helps us to see and appreciate as simple differences the things we once saw as disagreements. When we learn to rely on each other, we actually tend to seek out others who approach things differently, rather than feeling sideswiped by them when their differing opinions are brought to the table. I've worked in group situations in which everyone was trained in Human Dynamics and they were some of the most effective groups I've ever been part of. Once we understood the different dynamics that could be represented in groups, we recognized the great value there is in having people with overarching visioning, those who linked outcomes to processes, the detail people, the conceptual thinkers, and those who thought about what the impact on people would be.

In one group I was part of we took this value for diverse thinking very seriously. When we found that our team was not diversely represented enough—that one of the dynamics was not represented at the table—we would place an empty chair and recognize that the absence of a person with that dynamic created a hole in our process. We would stop periodically and discuss what the person with that dynamic would add if he or she were present. It was extremely helpful to the creative process and it was a big "aha!" for all of us.

How Increased Self-Awareness Benefits Ongoing Self-Development

Because there are three possibilities for our centering—mental, physical and emotional—and our dynamic is based on the two centerings that are primary and secondary for us, each of us then has an area for development. In my case, since I'm *emotional-physical*, I can make some of the best developmental strides in my life by strengthening my *mental* capacity and awareness. We are born with our dynamic (it is the way we are hardwired), but we have the infinite potential to develop, so if I develop my third dimension it helps me to become more integrated and whole. In Human Dynamics terminology, I would say that "my developmental track is the mental principle." It's a transformational path. When I had the experience in which the facilitator guided me to engage mentally rather than emotionally, I experienced what that felt like as well as the impact it had on my stress level and mental clarity. It was an insight and experience that changed my consciousness and my life.

In Human Dynamics, I learned that momentary loss of detachment under stress for *emotional-physical* people is part of their journey, and it was liberating for me to have this information presented as a simple statement of "how it is." It validated who I am and short-circuited any thoughts I'd had about being deficient in my ability to handle stress. The greatest gifts of Human Dynamics for me are a deeper sense of self-awareness, self-acceptance and well-being. I am more intentional and understanding in my interactions with others and live a more centered and purposeful life—both professionally and personally.

Dynamic Dialogue: Inspiring Clarity and Action Through Active Learning

—Jayne A. Felgen

Dynamic Dialogue is a unique learning practice particularly suited for engaging participants in exploring any current situation for the purpose of uncovering deep levels of wisdom and clarity about what should be changed.

It is particularly effective in bringing together diverse perspectives and groups around common, core values such as those embedded in Relationship-Based Care. It is innovative, inspiring and applicable in a variety of learning circumstances. According to Mitch Saunders and Tom Daly:

In Dynamic Dialogue, participants don't just talk about the patterns and energies present in the organization. They enact and experiment with them, using a wide range of methods, activities and tools. In addition to addressing immediate challenges, Dynamic Dialogue offers an opportunity to:

- *explore the interaction of the parts of an existing system,*

- *examine the functioning and emergent nature of the system as a whole, and*

- *generate and experiment with something entirely new.*

(Saunders & Daly, 2000, 1)

In one instance, while I was facilitating the status reports of action planning from three Unit Practice Councils, Dynamic Dialogue successfully led to a major shift in the group energy overall, and in one group in particular. This unit had been mired in negativity and staff were resisting change on their unit because they "already enjoyed a reputation for excellent patient care" and did not believe that "raising the bar" was necessary. Their negative energy was adversely affecting their relationships with each other and their cohort groups. After one hour of Dynamic Dialogue, that changed, and the whole group embraced their roles as leaders of innovation on their respective units. The project was immediately back on track.

In another instance, Dynamic Dialogue was used by a group of health care consultants who were striving to learn what clients were really asking for or needing, what talent the individual members had to offer and what possibilities could be considered for strategic or perational relationships among themselves. Because they each shared a passion for service to health care leaders and providers, but were each practicing independently, there was a desire to determine an ideal forum for collaboration. Dynamic Dialogue was fully utilized throughout the full-day gathering and the outcomes were thrilling! A strategic vision was formed, an operational plan was conceived and individual tactical assignments were readily made to complete the desired business plan.

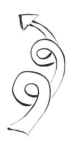

Dynamic Dialogue is available as a powerful tool to learn new insights and therefore to inspire oneself and others to consider changing the status quo.

Reference: Saunders, M., & Daly, T. (2000). Dynamic dialogue: Practice for learning from experience. *Leverage*, 43, 1

Mind Mapping:
The Harmonizing of Knowledge

—Phillip Schwartzkopf

Mind mapping, an organizational process that helps promote harmonizing, or the "inspired blending," of knowledge, is used regularly by Creative Health Care Management (CHCM) consultants in workshops, such as *Work Complexity Assessment,* and in Appreciative Inquiry.

Mind maps can be powerful tools, and even business moguls such as Bill Gates are seeing the potential of mind mapping, as he discussed in a recent article he wrote in *Newsweek.* On the evolution of mind mapping and its impact on how we gather, organize and make knowledge accessible, Gates (2006, paragraph 5) writes that "a new generation of 'mind mapping' software can be used as a digital 'blank slate' to help connect and synthesize ideas and data—and ultimately create new knowledge."

Mr. Gates, as you might expect, relates mind mapping to software, but its implications are much farther reaching. Consider how powerful it is to realize that merely by organizing known information effectively and making it visually logical and easily accessible, it can be transformed into new ideas and knowledge.

Software and other tools may make mind mapping easier and provide even greater access to information (stored documents, databases, and Internet links), but first we need to understand the basic concept of mind mapping. Mind mapping requires simply picking a central theme, branching out ideas from that theme into categories, and then expanding and supporting those categories with specific details.

Look at the following mind map examples and see how they start with the broad theme: *Nursing Interventions.*

> Consider how powerful it is to realize that merely by organizing known information effectively and making it visually logical and easily accessible, it can be transformed into new ideas and knowledge.

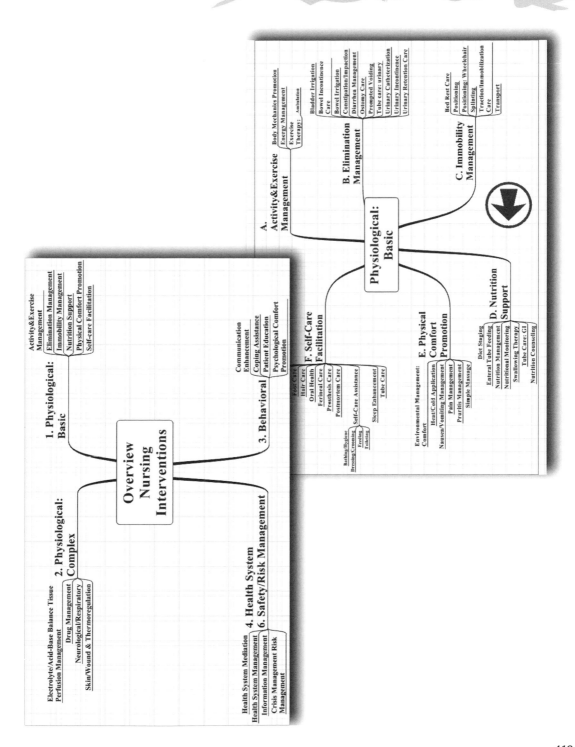

As you can see from an example used in *Work Complexity Assessment, Nursing Interventions* then branches out into the categories of *Physiological Basic, Physiological Complex, Behavioral, Health System* and *Safety/Risk Management.* Specific details are then broken down from there. In the example, you can see the progression into more specific detail as *Physiological Basic* becomes the central theme and its details become categories of their own, which then expand into even further explanation. Though a mind map initially looks nothing like an outline and is created using highly generative, nonlinear thinking, a mind map created using MindManager® software can be printed as an outline. Because different individuals understand and process information differently, having both a linear and a nonlinear way to present the same information is invaluable.

Creating a mind map stimulates both left-brain logic and right-brain creativity so that the creation of the map itself has a great impact on the memory and learning of those who generate it. We have also found that those who create mind maps in group learning settings tend to take tangible ownership of the information generated. The benefits of mind mapping can be measured in terms of productivity improvements and time savings in note taking, increased idea generation, simplified communication and group problem-solving processes. Individuals or groups can use mind mapping in a variety of settings, and we have seen it consistently lead to more meaningful, productive, satisfying meetings.

Reference: Gates, B. (2006). The road ahead: How 'intelligent agents' and mind-mappers are taking our information democracy to the next stage. *Newsweek–2006 Issues.* Retrieved January 31, 2006, from http://msnbc.msn.com/id/11020787/site/newsweek/

Using Leadership 360-Degree to Develop Leaders

—Susan Wessel

One of the greatest challenges in achieving truly excellent results is selecting and developing managers. Good managers have the capacity to develop the knowledge and skills necessary to achieve the organization's vision. In our experience, education, though necessary, is not enough to ensure a high-functioning leadership team. This article will highlight a powerful 360-degree evaluation and coaching tool with a particularly effective component that improves leadership behaviors.

The leadership style and competence of all leaders, but particularly first-line managers, either sets the stage or derails efforts for an empowered staff and excellent patient care. Unfortunately, most of us have a blind side as far as how we are perceived by our co-workers. An effective 360-degree feedback process should give us more than just feedback; it should include tools to modify our behavior. The best process avoids fear and defensiveness and places responsibility for development in our own hands and with the assistance of an objective coach.

The Leadership Effectiveness Analysis (LEA) 360, also known as Leadership 360, has proven particularly successful in achieving these goals. This tool was developed by psychologists at Management Research Group in Portland, ME. The LEA combines 360-degree feedback with personal coaching and a robust set of strategies for developing new leadership behaviors that match an organization's needs.

The LEA process differs from other "360" evaluation tools in some significant ways. This tool has been tested all over

Assuming Ownership for One's Own Development

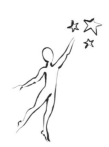

the world by Management Research Group for reliability and validity in all fields of business. The survey itself has a unique normative semi-ipsative design. Its strength is that the choices for each question are equal in their social desirability, that is, one choice doesn't seem any better than the others. This takes the subjectivity and rater biases out of the process. The survey is generally completed online, and feedback is obtained from subordinates, peers, immediate supervisors and the test taker. This test is particularly helpful in allowing participants to compare their own self-perceptions with those of others.

Combining The LEA With Identification of a Strategic Direction by the Executive Team

Leadership 360 can be used alone or combined with a broader initiative for the executive team to establish the strategic direction for the organization. Strategic Directions is a unique process in which the executive team identifies high-priority leadership skills and behaviors necessary for achieving the mission and strategic plan of the organization. These high-priority leadership skills and behaviors become the standard against which each manager's Leadership 360 profile is aligned. Individual leaders then choose behavioral modification strategies to move them in the direction that the organization has chosen. It allows them to develop the leadership style necessary for success as determined by the executive team.

The LEA can also be combined with an Individual Directions Inventory (IDI). This personal inventory deepens the insights gained by leaders into the emotional satisfaction derived from various situations. It provides them with a profile of their motivations and preferences in life. When combined with the LEA and coaching, the IDI helps leaders understand the types of settings and job roles that will provide them with the most satisfaction, interest and success.

Snapshot of Leadership Effectiveness Analysis

The best way to illustrate the output of Leadership 360 is to see an example. The LEA tool measures 22 distinct leadership behaviors and the degree to which an individual manager uses these behaviors in his or her role. The results include feedback from the self-appraisal and from one's boss, peers and subordinates. Results are given as percentiles, which show

how one's score compares with those in a large database of business executives.

Below are results for four of the 22 leadership behaviors.

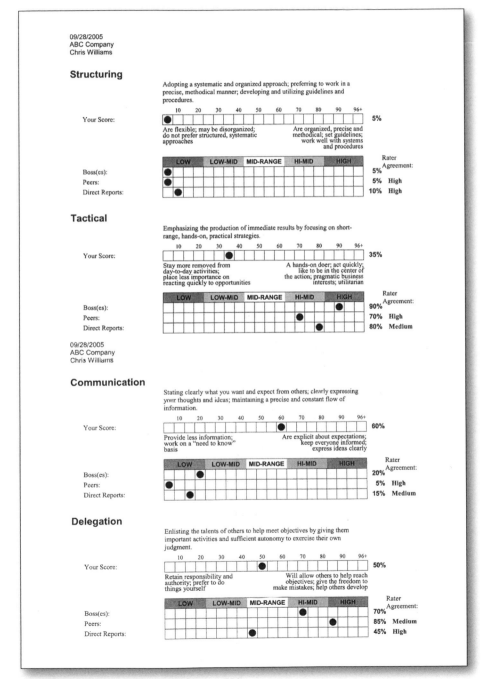

Notice that this fictitious manager, Chris Williams, scores very low in his use of communication. He scores lower than 80% of midlevel business executives in the database. During the LEA workshop and individual coaching, managers carefully examine scores that are extremely high or extremely low. They are given a Resource Guide that examines both the potential assets and the potential liabilities of these extreme scores. The resource guide also gives specific action steps for increasing various behaviors that would make managers more successful in their roles.

To continue with the Chris Williams example of very low communication scores, below is a partial list of the resources that would guide Chris in developing his own action plan with the help of a personal coach.

Communication

Low Communication Score—Potential Assets

    May be concise

    May be discreet and know when to keep quiet

    May let people do the job without interference

Low Communication Score—Potential Liabilities

    May confuse others by providing too little information

    May hold back needed information

    May have poor results because people don't know what is wanted

A menu of 15 potential action steps is provided in the resource guide to assist managers who want to increase their use of communication. Similarly, action steps are offered for each of the remaining 21 behaviors measured by the LEA. Some of these are general; others are targeted toward one's boss, peers and direct reports. A few of these action steps are highlighted below. During the coaching process, managers choose a few key action steps that best fit their situation.

Sample Action Steps for Strengthening Communication Skills

1. **Design your communication to meet the needs of your audience.** Determine the most effective ways to communicate with the people in your network. Some people want written reports, while others prefer informal meetings; some like all the details, while others want only the broad picture. Once you have determined an individual's preference, communicate in the appropriate manner.

2. **Analyze your own communication style.** Try to determine its specific strengths and weaknesses. Ask other people—most will be only too glad to tell you. Work to strengthen your communication approach and eliminate any gaps you discover.

3. **Keep your boss informed.** Try to meet with your boss on a regular basis to update him/her on how things are going. Unless your boss dislikes written reports, try to write memos or send e-mail on a regular basis to keep him/her informed. Keep these meetings and messages brief.

4. **Determine the critical communication needs of your boss.** Try to identify what information, thoughts or ideas you have that would be useful to your boss in carrying out his/her role.

5. **Know where the weak links are.** Identify the crucial points in implementing unit responsibilities where there are likely to be communication failures. Design your communication to avoid such failures at these critical junctures.

6. **Communicate freely.** Go beyond communicating expectations. Communicate your thoughts, ideas and opinions as well, and encourage your direct reports to do the same.

7. **Analyze the communication needs of your peers.** See if you can get them to work with you in determining what priorities they have for your unit (i.e., how your unit may be more helpful to them by providing information or ideas).

A Real-Life Example

It may be helpful to see a practical example of results from a nurse manager and actions she selected to increase her effectiveness. A nurse manager with more than 80 direct reports selected two priority areas to focus on in her action plan. Her boss's rating, her direct reports' assessment and her self-assessment were all in the 15th to 20th percentile range for "delegation," indicating that she demonstrated delegation behaviors less often than 80-85% of business people in the database. It was also significant that in the general area of achieving results, her boss and she herself rated her "production" in the 30th percentile. Production measures the extent to which a person demonstrates a strong orientation toward achievement, holding high expectations for oneself and others.

During her individual coaching we discussed the potential relationships between her low scores in producing results and the low delegation scores. She was asked to consider whether enhancing her strengths in delegation might also improve her ability to produce results. Although we discussed her scores in all 22 behavioral areas during the coaching session, during action planning she selected delegation and production as the two priority areas to work on. She identified three specific methods of increasing delegation and two methods of enhancing production using the LEA resource guide for ideas. She was encouraged to discuss her action plan with her immediate supervisor and ask for feedback on progress in 3 months, 6 months and a year.

These are just a few examples of how Leadership 360 can be used in the growth and development of managers at any level. The process is structured to ensure individual accountability for action plans and follow-up with the personal coach.

The LEA is effective in helping successful leaders to reach an even higher level of performance. For marginal performers, the LEA is a supportive strategy to help them develop in the direction that is required for success.

Leadership 360® is a registered trademark of Management Research Group.

Strategic Directions™ and Individual Directions Inventory™ are trademarks of Management Research Group.

CHAPTER TWELVE

Essential Education for Relationship-Based Care

Educational Resources For Relationship-Based Care

—Susan Wessel and Mary Koloroutis

Preparing an organization for Relationship-Based Care (RBC) involves educating nearly every group in the organization, including the board. The ideal education plan is tailored to the needs and frame of reference of each group. The curriculum overview presented here will serve as a starting point for the education subcommittee as they design the 12 to 18 month education plan. Table 1 (page 429) provides educational content by stakeholder group.

The actual education plan should take into consideration the strengths and developmental needs of your own staff. Some requests for education may come from Unit Practice Councils (UPCs) based on their understanding of the level of competence of their peers. The education department and others involved in educating should be prepared to repeat key messages often and in a variety of ways.

At Creative Health Care Management (CHCM) we use some of our classic workshops during implementation of RBC in order to:

- *provide inspiration,*

- *prepare leaders to lead in a culture of true empowerment, and*

- *prepare the staff for their role on Unit Practice Councils.*

The following summary of several of these workshops highlights educational content that has proven most effective over the years.

Leading an Empowered Organization

- *Leading an Empowered Organization (LEO) is a 3-day workshop intended to provide both novice and experienced leaders with a conceptual framework for leadership, practical skills and an opportunity to develop those skills in personal action planning. The LEO workshop includes concepts of:*

- *Decentralized leadership*

- *Articulating expectations*

- *Responsibility, authority and accountability*

- *Healthy interpersonal relationships*

- *Developing staff*

- *Creative problem solving*

Leading an Empowered Organization culminates with attendees developing a personal action plan for growth and development and an action plan to resolve a problem impacting patient care in their department.

Relationship-Based Care Leader Practicum

The *Relationship-Based Care Leader Practicum* is an intensive 5-day workshop which provides organizational leaders with the clarity and competence essential for leading transformational change for Relationship-Based Care. The program blends a variety of experiential methodologies to develop competencies, integrate learning relative to RBC and design customized strategies and outcomes for individual organizations. The curriculum includes:

- *I_2E_2 —Inspiration, Infrastructure, Education, Evidence—a time-tested formula for leading sustainable change.*

- *The 5 Cs for Actionable Change: Clarity, Competence, Confidence, Collaboration, Commitment*

- *Appreciative Inquiry*

- *Organizational leverage points*

- *Organizational challenges*

- *Engaging key stakeholders*

- *Council structure: Results Council; Unit Practice Council*

- *Six phases of implementation*

- *Project management*

- *Strengthening essential relationships*

- *Transformational leadership: An individual action plan for leading change day to day.*

Relationship-Based Care Overview Workshop

The *RBC Overview* workshop helps executives, managers and staff participants gain insight about the seven dimensions of Relationship-Based Care. Participants begin the process of assessing how many elements of RBC already exist in their organization's culture. The day culminates with individual and shared visions for how RBC can impact colleague relationships and patient/family care. Participants begin to develop ownership for this transformational change. The content is adapted to each organization and the needs of the audience. Some common elements include:

- *Relationship-Based Care—connections to the organization's existing mission and vision*

- *Feedback on your organization—Appreciative Inquiry findings*

- *Seven Dimensions of RBC; Organizational Self-Assessment Exercise*

- *Visioning—individual and collective exercise*
- *Roles and Responsibilities for Optimal Implementation*
- *I_2E_2: The Formula for Sustainable Change*
- *Commitment to Action: Next Steps*

Reigniting the Spirit of Caring

Reigniting the Spirit of Caring (*RSC*) is a 3-day workshop that grounds and renews care providers of all disciplines and their managers in the many dimensions of caring. The focus of the workshop is caring for self and others. Participants experience a renewed commitment to purpose and meaning in practice and a new perspective on collaboration with colleagues.

Diverse experiential learning techniques make this a unique, life-changing experience. Learning methods include dialogue circle, reflection, journaling, storytelling and visioning. Content includes:

- *Body, mind and spirit balance and self-assessment*
- *Strategies for maintaining energy and reducing stress*
- *Principles of healthy interpersonal relationships*
- *Techniques for strengthening collegiality and teamwork*
- *Patient and family interviews to understand perceptions of caring behaviors*
- *Shared vision and actions for transforming the work environment to optimize self-care, healthy teamwork and compassionate care for patients and families*

Leadership at the Point of Care

Leadership at the Point of Care (*LPC*) is a 3-day workshop for nursing staff that builds on the inspiration provided by *RSC*. It helps participants achieve clarity about their own professional role and the systems that support them. The participants are able to recognize and strengthen their innate leadership skills and accept ownership for professional practice. Content includes:

- *Self-care and stress management*
- *Thriving in the workplace*
- *Human Dynamics (working with different personality types)*
- *Healthy colleague relationships*
- *Conscious communication and listening*
- *Dealing with difficult interactions*
- *Nursing scope of practice (responsibility, authority and accountability)*
- *Six practice roles of professional nurses*
- *Relationship-Based Care and Unit Practice Councils*

Woven through the curriculum are reflective and application exercises and each day ends with a commitment to action in the form of individual action plans. A key outcome of this experience is that nurses declare ownership for their practice an d their relationships with patients, families and one another.

Relationships at the Point of Care

Relationships at the Point of Care (RPC) is a one-day companion workshop to *LPC* that helps ancillary and support staff, who "touch" patients and families, to develop caring and healing relationships with everyone with whom they come into contact. Like nurses, ancillary and support staffs have chosen to work with people who are at their most vulnerable, and they too want to make a difference in the lives of the patients and families they serve. The *RPC* workshop helps participants turn their desire into action by teaching them skills that will have a positive effect on patient healing and the environment of care. The seven major areas of the curriculum are:

- *Effective communication skills,*
- *Cultural and generational diversity,*
- *Emotional intelligence,*
- *Team building and working relationships,*
- *Stress management,*

- *Concepts from The Caring Model, and*
- *Conflict resolution.*

Participants are given practical applications for each major area.

The Caring Model Workshop

This is a customer service program perfectly suited to support professional practice. The Caring Model involves a six-step intervention used by all hospital employees. The intent of the program is to focus on improving patient loyalty and satisfaction. Content includes:

- *Environmental forces for a renewed emphasis on caring*
- *Connection of The Caring Model to the mission, vision, values and strategic plan*
- *Strategies for implementation and maintenance of The Caring Model*
- *Action planning to integrate the behaviors into interdisciplinary practice, customer service and performance improvement initiatives*
- *Identification of specific outcomes indicators derived from current satisfaction data*

Results Councils and Unit Practice Council Development Curriculum

This program may be used as results councils and unit practice councils begin their work. Selected topics should be reinforced during status check meetings as needed. Content may include:

- *Group process*
- *Meeting management: developing agendas, keeping minutes, evaluating meetings*
- *Conscious communication (i.e., nondefensive; listening skills; assertive and open)*
- *Council Responsibilities and Authority*
- *Principles of change management— I_2E_2; 5 Cs*
- *Creative problem solving*

- *Consensus decision making*
- *Using the communication network*
- *Healthy team relationships and conflict resolution*

The Human Dynamics Program for Individual and Team Development

Human Dynamics offers a unique approach to individual and group transformation based upon each individual's understanding and appreciation of himself/herself and others as a particular system of mental-emotional-physical-spiritual interplay, each characterized by distinctive processes of "experiencing experience," processing information, learning, communicating, relating, undertaking tasks and developing. This inspiring 4-day (or 2-day) program has been successfully conducted at every level of organizations, from executive management to direct care and service providers. Specific areas of focus include:

- *Building remarkable teams that recognize value and leverage each member's instinctive inherent gifts and processes*
- *Building community within work areas and organizations as a whole*
- *Recognizing and accommodating individuals' processes of learning and task accomplishment*
- *Personal and leadership development*
- *Appreciating and leveraging diversity*

Competency Assessment

These workshops and consultations help participants to discover a new way of thinking about competency assessment— a way that is focused on outcomes and based on accountability. This program will help participants accomplish the following:

- *Collaboratively identify competencies that are reflective of the dynamic nature of health care work and mutually identified by staff and leadership*
- *Create an employee-centered verification process*
- *Identify verification methods and appropriately match them to the competency categories*

- *Bring competency verification forward to the organization*
- *Help leaders create a culture of organizational success with a dual focus*
- *Focus on the organizational mission*
- *Focus on supporting positive employee behavior by helping managers follow through appropriately and consistently with employee problems and deficits*

This competency assessment process helps lighten the load for achieving competency assessment and meeting standards. It provides a great way to carry out competency assessment with only a few focused competencies that reflect the ever changing nature of health care. It creates an environment of accountability and ownership, and helps recognize excellence in practice every day.

Creative Health Care Management also offers other workshops designed to meet a variety of organizational needs, such as:

- *How to Delegate Without Losing Your Friends, Your Job or Your Nursing License*
- *Communication: Why Is It So Difficult?*
- *Keys to Successful Precepting*
- *Celebrating Moments of Excellence*
- I_2E_2: *Leading Lasting Change*

Education must be woven throughout the implementation and evolution of Relationship-Based Care. Though we have included a basic plan here, your own assessment during all stages of implementation will reveal the specific education needed for each of the groups based on your organization. You may find that with the introduction of Primary Nursing (an important component of RBC) some nurses may need strengthening of clinical skills, including critical thinking and delegation. As each organization is unique, it is important to remain aware of what educational offerings are available to address the various issues or areas for knowledge and skill enhancement that may surface throughout RBC implementation and beyond.

Selected Educational Content by Stakeholder Group						
TOPIC	TRUSTEES	EXEC TEAM	MEDICAL STAFF	LEADERSHIP	UPCS	STAFF
Achieving the Mission & Vision through RBC	XX	XX	XX			
Transformational Leadership		XX	XX	XX	XX	XX
Five Cs for Leading Change		XX		XX	XX	
Dimensions of RBC (varying length)	XX	XX	XX	XX	XX	XX
Roles and Responsibilities for Implementation	XX	XX		XX	XX	
I_2E_2 Change Methodology	XX	XX	XX	XX	XX	
Engaging Stakeholders: Practices of Circle and Dialogue		XX		XX	XX	XX
Appreciative Inquiry		XX	XX	XX	XX	
Empowerment and Decentralization		XX	XX	XX	XX	XX
Relationship Management		XX	XX	XX	XX	XX
Principles of Caring			XX	XX	XX	XX
Human Dynamics	XX	XX	XX	XX	XX	XX
Creative & Critical Thinking				XX	XX	XX
Outcomes Measurement	XX	XX	XX	XX	XX	XX
Conscious Communication & Conflict Resolution			XX	XX	XX	XX
Delegation				XX	XX	XX
Competencies		XX		XX	XX	XX

Principles of Education for Relationship-Based Care

—Colleen Person and Jayne A. Felgen

In a recent *Reigniting the Spirit of Caring* (*RSC*) workshop, one insightful patient participant devised the following formula:

> ### *Clinical Competency + Compassionate Caring = Healing*

This patient had reflected on the two times when she had been the recipient of inpatient care. In retrospect the more positive experience had involved a combination of both clinical competency and compassionate caring while the less-than-desirable experience had only the clinical competency dimension.

The formula is both simple and accurate; it highlights the two areas of focus for education in any organization transitioning to Relationship-Based Care (RBC). In the transition to RBC, organizations will continue to provide the ongoing clinical education needed for clinical competencies, but now they will also need to put greater emphasis on the skills that comprise "compassionate caring."

Because of the nursing shortage and new education programs, the mix of Registered Nurses has shifted from a greater number having baccalaureate degrees to a greater number having 2-year associate degrees. Those with 2-year degrees are coming into work environments with solid clinical skills, but fewer have been offered the opportunity to develop the skills and capacities necessary to establish knowledgeable, caring and therapeutic relationships with patients. Most have the skills to develop social relationships with patients and their families, but caring and healing relationships reach beyond the social and serve a distinctly different purpose.

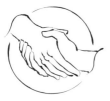

Establishment of the therapeutic nurse-patient relationship is central to the daily practice of Relationship-Based Care. Development of compassionate caring behaviors is the essential foundation in the educational plan devised for transition to Relationship-Based Care. A variety of insight-based work-shops and seminars can help practitioners discover their own unique expressions of therapeutic caring. The key concepts are as follows:

1. Compassionate Caring starts with the Self.

We know that compassionate caring requires care givers to be clear about their impact on patient healing and to be as authentic as possible with patients and families. When they are authentic they form unique human-to-human connection that Jean Watson addresses in her Caring Theory. For this reason, it would be of limited value for us to provide care givers with an "RBC script" from which to read. Instead, insight-based courses provide educational experiences that help increase participants' awareness of their own power to make choices at the point of care. This empowered awareness is central to each care giver's ability to be authentic and therapeutic with patients. It breaks down like this:

We gain awareness of self.

We accept that we have the power to make choices about our own behavior.

We act with intention to achieve the desired impact.

We achieve our desired results.

> **Self-awareness can be taught to care givers throughout an organization.**

2. Compassionate Caring requires real connection with patients as unique people.

When we enter a patient's room, we use all of our clinical knowledge to do an assessment of each patient's clinical needs. That's one essential aspect of the connection care givers make in RBC organizations. The other essential aspect is to establish a caring connection. Compassionate care means sitting at eye level with patients, making eye contact, actively listening, adroitly seeking cues about what matters to them, and talking with patients and their families about their personal needs, concerns and expectations for their current episode of care. Through finding out how we can help patients to heal themselves as quickly and comfortably as possible we address the issues of safety as well as security.

> **The ability to connect with patients as unique people can be taught to care givers throughout an organization.**

3. Compassionate Caring means seeing through the patient's eyes.

The *Reigniting the Spirit of Caring* (*RSC*) workshop challenges our assumptions of what caring is. The workshop brings nurses, service support staff, doctors, allied health professionals, executives, board members, patients and family members together so that each can share his or her unique story of being the recipient of care (see page 524). When patients and families share their experiences, they invariably speak of needing to feel safe—not just clinically, but emotionally. It becomes clear in every *RSC* workshop that even the smallest act of authentic caring connection is recognized and appreciated by patients and their families—a touch, a word of encouragement, needed information. Through the inclusion of all constituents it becomes clear to everyone that, while the most powerful expression of RBC occurs at the point of care, every action taken by everyone in the organization affects what happens in the care giver/patient relationship. The *RSC* workshop offers participants an opportunity to see health care through the eyes of the patients and family members and to gain a greater appreciation for the contribution each person makes.

Every action taken by everyone in the organization affects what happens in the nurse-patient relationship.

> **The principles and practices of compassionate care can be taught to care givers throughout an organization.**

4. Compassionate Caring means conveying, "I am the one."

One of the most powerful things a care giver can do in establishing a therapeutic relationship is to "show up" mentally, emotionally and spiritually for his or her patients and families. And the most powerful way to show up in any situation is to declare, "I am the one." Tell your patients who you are, your role on the team, why you are with them, and what you intend to do. Tell them what they can count on you for. The essence of this connection is conveyed in the following:

I am your Primary Nurse and that means that I am the one who will be coordinating your care while you're here on this unit/service. I am the one who will talk with your other nurses, with your doctors, and with others who will provide services for you. I am the one who will find answers to your questions, make sure you get everything you need, and smooth the way for you in every transition you make while you're here.

This powerful language—along with the authentic devotion behind it—conveys to our patients and their families that we are there for them in every way imaginable. This is the essence of the therapeutic relationship and the full expression of professional nursing practice.

In a Relationship-Based Care Delivery model that focuses on a relationship in the moment rather than throughout the stay, the nurse might say, "I am your nurse for this shift or this period of time. I am the one who will ...."

While the therapeutic relationship takes form in an interpersonal exchange (typically it is born in conversation with patients and/or their families) it must take hold internally as well. The "I am the one" mentality must be evident in a care giver's ownership of time-management and resource decisions as well. The essence of that internal realization is:

I am the one who decides what I will do–and what I will not do–in order to provide the most clinically competent and compassionate care possible for my patients and their families.

The ability to "show up" mentally, emotionally and spiritually for patients and their families can be taught to care givers throughout an organization.

433

Professional relationships are different from social relationships.

> **The ability to "show up" mentally, emotionally and spiritually for patients and their families can be taught to care givers throughout an organization.**

5. Compassionate Caring means fostering healthy interpersonal relationships with colleagues.

Meg Wheatley says, "Relationship is the determiner of everything." Relationship-Based Care is about our relationships with one another as well as with the patients and families we care for. Patient and staff satisfaction is the hallmark of healthy interpersonal relationships among health care team members.

Professional relationships are different from social relationships. While it feels good to have friends at work, it is essential to have collegial/professional relationships among the members of the health care team. The purpose of work relationships is to create a culture of clinical competency and compassionate caring together. The core elements of healthy interpersonal relationships are:

- *trust*
- *mutual respect*
- *visible support*
- *open, honest communication*
- *appreciation*

The challenge in RBC is for each person to live these behaviors every day. It is easy to fall back into negative behavior, such as the 3Bs (bickering, backbiting and blaming). Education in assertive communication, appreciation and relationship skills can help team members focus on the 3Cs of commitment, caring and collaboration.

> **Behaviors to foster healthy interpersonal relationships can be taught to care givers throughout an organization.**

6. Education for RBC needs to be customized to the unique needs of your organization.

I am the one.

In designing your education plan, think in terms of what is needed in transition as well as what will be of benefit in the long term. Education is the foundation upon which learning organizations can build the next generation of excellence. Leaders and staff need educational experiences to explore and change mindsets, to gain new knowledge and skills and to develop collaborative relationships. Education is needed at the time of transition; continuing education is needed to meet ever changing competency requirements; and orientation to RBC needs to be an integral part of orientation for all employees. Education is the great equalizer.

Designing your educational program can be a creative and satisfying endeavor. Developing knowledge and skills for RBC (clinical and caring competencies) strengthens the capacity and confidence of staff members to implement and integrate RBC into their practice on the unit. It is a gift of caring—for the professionals providing care and service—and for every patient with whom they come into contact.

Caring Theory as an Ethical Guide to Administrative and Clinical Practices

—Jean Watson

Editors' note: *Originally published in* Nursing Administration Quarterly, *30(1):48-55. Used with permission.*

Caring and economics, and caring and administrative practices, are often considered in conflict with each other. One of the reasons for this conflict and dissonance is a separation of values of human caring as an underlying ethic and a moral foundation for practice. The dominant institutional values and commitments are informed and guided by economics, technology, medical science and administrative theory, instead of basic considerations of what it means to be human, to be vulnerable, to be ill, to be cured, to be cared for, to be healthy and to be healed.

These dominant business or economic models that are devoid of caring have short-term solutions to patient care needs and to the crisis of nursing shortage in the United States and elsewhere. They focus on beds and disease, body as physical object, technology, and products. In addressing the nursing shortage, they focus on incentives such as increasing enrollments, signing bonuses, tuition, relocation fees, etc., without addressing underlying dissatisfaction, for example, inability to practice own profession; dominance of medical-economic-technological-institutional foci over direct-care, person-centered, human-to human relationships and caring-healing processes and practices. This void in caring persists in spite of corporate rhetoric and slogans of "caring institutions." These dominant emphases and superficial, often trivial, catchphrases of *caring* are detours and barriers to practicing and achieving the work nurses love, and to what calls them into this ancient and noble profession in the first place. The result is a hostile environment that places dollars over human life and quality of caring-healing experiences for patients and practitioners alike. Thus, the lingering mood from nursing/nurses in the field: "Nurses love their work and hate their jobs."

If nurses leave organizations as fast as they are hired, money is wasted and hoped-for solutions are doomed for failure, as are patient care and satisfaction. What good is it to have an industrial model of treatment and cure/physical care when patients and practitioners alike are disenchanted and, even worse, worse off after hospitalization than before, owing to dissatisfaction, repeat hospitalization, medical errors, nursing recruitment, retention, etc.?

Numerous studies in the United States continue to document publicly that patient deaths are tied to lack of nurses. Recent crises related to safety concerns have brought renewed attention to nursing and physician practices and how to address the shortage and crises of care in acute care hospitals (Watson & Foster, 2003).

This dominant model has co-opted the language of industry and business, in that, rather than referring to the quality of caring and healing offered to whole human beings, what the hospitals increasingly mean is that they have the most advanced technology to diagnose and treat malfunctioning body parts. This is not the relational language of caring, but the language of the market. For example, patients are referred to as "consumers" or "end users," practitioners are "providers," nurses are "workers" (Quinn, 2003). This language conjures up an image of impersonal, functional exchange of fees for services or goods that requires no humanity or human relationship, no authentic caring connection, no mutuality, and no compassionate human service ethic, philosophy or value that guides the system.

A value-based, theory-guided approach to caring and administration helps to make visible that a caring model for professional nursing and system survival would meet needs of practitioners and patients alike. For example, as I have noted elsewhere,

Any profession that loses its values becomes heartless; any profession that becomes heartless becomes soulless. And any profession that becomes heartless and soulless, becomes [Worthless].

(Watson, 2005)

Thus, a shift toward theoretical practices guided by human caring values becomes an economic as well as human resource for nursing and systems alike. This shift includes the following:

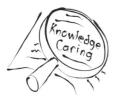

- *From economics to professional practice that is based on morality, ethics and values*

- *From mechanical cure approaches to spiritualizing of health and healing processes*

- *From rote, theoretical professional routines of nursing practice to professional actions consciously guided by intentional-caring theory*

- *From artificial "hospitality" environments to authentic healing environments*

- *From corporatization of health to public covenant for healthy citizenry*

- *From industrial product-line models of "managed care" to relationship-centered caring-healing partnerships, at multiple levels*

Such shifts acknowledge that caring is not a commodity to be bought and sold. Caring and economics, however, are not mutually exclusive, in that human caring is an essential resource. Cost-benefit and cost-effectiveness models can and must include human caring-healing—as a value-added resource, a foundational asset, as well as a more humane model to serve the whole.

In the dominant, but declining, model, caring-healing and human values have become a dwindling resource for systems and society alike. Such thinking fails to recognize human caring-healing values, ethics, knowledge, and practices of nurses (in particular) as an essential albeit underutilized resource; it fails to understand professional, theory-guided nurses as intentional, conscious, knowledge workers—professional experts in human caring and healing who can transform the entire culture. It is as if, as one of my physics colleagues said, "The health [read sick] care [read cure] system is using only one half of its brain." The other half of the model is waiting and longing to emerge for practitioners and the public alike.

This tension in the dominant approaches to hospitals and treatment is simultaneously juxtaposed against an accelerating public interest in complementary-alternative medicine, and an explosion of both public and professional interest in relationships between spirituality and health. These changing times now warrant, if not require, a reorientation—away from traditional hospital structures and patterns of care/cure with their routinized, industrial practices driven by economics, diagnosis, and treatment of acute disease and product-line management.

Health Care Economics and Human Caring: Resolving Moral Conflict

- Caring is not a commodity to be bought/sold.
- Caring and economics are not mutually exclusive.
- Synthesis of economics models must include caring (cost-benefit and cost-effectiveness analysis includes caring).

The evolving caring-healing practice environment is increasingly dependent on relationships, partnerships, negotiation, coordination, new forms of communication patterns, and authentic connections (Watson, 2003). The new emphasis is on a change of consciousness, a focused intentionality toward caring-healing relationships and modalities, and a shift toward a spiritualizing of health versus a limited medical view alone. Thus, new standards, principles, guidelines and models of excellence are required for advancing and sustaining professional relationship-centered caring practices.

It can be argued that these chaotic changes lead to uncertainty and confusion; however, when one interprets these complexities, it is clear those dominant practices and patterns are under fire from within and without, and something else is wanting to emerge out of the chaos. It is the responsibility of professionals and administrators alike to rethink conventional industrial models and work together for transformation from within. The will to make the changes necessary for renewal and transformation are dependent on human dimensions and skills, which arise from the human spirit, offering new visions, creativity, and possibilities that result in changing patterns, relationships, and depths of communication and culture. These changes involve worldview shifts that transcend professions, systems and institutional structures.

Emerging Theoretical-Ethical Model of Caring-Healing

This perspective incorporates life-generating and life-receiving processes of human caring and healing for the practitioners as well as the patients.

These emerging possibilities, longing to actualize, now have to be honored; they are now arising internally within hospital and nursing systems alike. Without attending to this emergence, practitioners become dispirited and the nursing shortage is accelerated, not diminished. The emerging model, which invites the human spirit back into the workplace, is based on caring-healing values and theoretical-philosophical and moral foundations. This orientation toward one's professional work adheres to an ethic of unitary being and becoming more human and humane, a model that honors the inner subjective experience of patients and practitioners alike. This emerging professional nursing practice model is overtly moving beyond the separate disease focus that defines the human. It is explicitly moving beyond a "clinicalizing" and "medicalizing" of the human condition, which reduces the person to the moral status of physical object. This new turn is toward a spiritualizing of human experience and requires a return to wholeness; unity of mind, body, and spirit; and acknowledging a human-environment energy field oneness, which affects, and is affected by, the human presence, the intentionality, consciousness, and practices of the practitioners (Watson, 2002).

This emerging model seeks to integrate inner healing and human caring processes with healing environments, no longer restricted to outer curing alone; this perspective incorporates life-generating and life-receiving processes of human caring and healing for the practitioners as well as the patients. The emerging model includes the transcendent as well as immanent view of human experience, attends to nonphysical phenomena as much as physical, and allows for human-environment energy field dynamics and processes. This emerging human caring values-guided ethic for professional practices happens to be consistent with what the public is seeking as well as with extant nursing theory. This convergence of change is an opportunity for an overt turn toward advancing nursing qua nursing professional practices and processes.(Watson, 1985, 1999a, 1999b). This turn is a moment in history and an occasion in time in which nursing can come of age and mature in its own hopeful paradigm for this era.

Watson's Theory of Human Caring

Recently, several hospitals in the United States have begun to use Watson's Theory of Human Caring (Watson, 1985; Watson, 1999a, 1999b) as a guide to change nursing practice—and ultimately the culture of hospital nursing and the hospital milieu—in seeking or sustaining Magnet status (see Watson's Web site: www.uchsc.edu/nursing/caring).

This theory involves making explicit that human caring and relationship-centered caring is a foundational ethic for healing practices; it honors the unity of the whole human being, while also attending to creating a healing environment. Caring-healing modalities and nursing arts are reintegrated as essentials to ensure attention to quality of life, inner healing experiences, subjective meaning, and caring practices, which affect patient outcomes and system successes alike. The theory places human-to-human caring as central to the professional nursing responsibilities and role and the moral foundation for the profession. Preserving human dignity, relationships and integrity through human caring is ultimately the measure by which patients evaluate their often "cure dominated experience" (Clark, 2004).

In this model, caring is acknowledged as transpersonal, in that it goes beyond the ego-oriented human; it involves the one caring as well as the one being cared for, and is mutual, intersubjective and reciprocal. The "caring moment" between the patient and nurse has a field of its own, which is greater than either one, and transcends both patient and nurse and becomes part of the life history of both, as well as of some larger, deeper, complex pattern of life (Watson, 1999a). The caring moment transcends the here and now and informs the life history of both patient and nurse beyond the caring

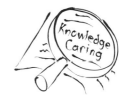

moment. The influence can be for better or for worse, depending on the nature of the relationship and the nature of caring. A caring moment involves the humanity of the nurse and potentiates healing. Healing occurs when the nurse connects with the spirit of the other; it involves listening, making one's presence felt and expressing emotions, as well as the instrumental acts of treatment, medication, procedures, etc.

But the (caring) consciousness, intentionality, mood, demeanor and presence of the nurse affect the human-environment energy field in the given moment, for better or for worse (Watson, 2002). Thus, the focus is on the person behind the patient and professional, as well as the caring relationship, the human consciousness field, generated by the nurse's very presence (Watson, 2002). In the Caring model, the practitioner's caring-healing consciousness is influencing and helping to shape the patient's health and healing experience as well as the practitioners" own experience in the moment.

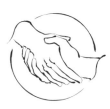

The following framework of transpersonal caring-healing highlights this model (Watson, 1999a, 1999b):

- *The whole caring-healing consciousness is contained within a single caring moment.*

- *Human caring and healing processes—or noncaring consciousness—of the practitioner is communicated to the one being cared for.*

- *Caring consciousness transcends time, space and physicality—that is, caring goes beyond the given moment and situation, and informs the future experiences of practitioner and patient.*

- *Caring-healing consciousness is dominant over physical illness and has the potential to help the patient access the healer within, or potentiates inner healing processes.*

- *One's (caring) intentionality and consciousness energetically affects the "whole field"; for example, thoughts that are positive, such as love, caring, joy, compassion, affection and forgiveness, have a higher frequency of energy. Likewise, thoughts that create emotions such as anger, hatred, jealousy and fear have low-frequency energy and therefore lower the*

> *frequency of the system (Watson, 1999a). "A system of higher frequency will soothe, calm, and refresh you because of the ... quality of ... your system" (Watson, 1999a, p. 112).*

Relevant Research on the Consequences of Caring-Noncaring

Relevant research points out the seriousness of a caring relationship. The presence and absence of caring can have either a positive or a negative consequence. This caring phenomenon is found to affect both patient and practitioner. For example, Halldorsdottir's classic research (1991) on levels of caring found that caring relationships ranged from what she called *biocidic*, or toxic, relationships between nurses and patients, to *biogenic*, which is congruent with transpersonal caring, in that a biogenic caring relationship is characterized by a life-giving and life-receiving relationship between both parties. The other levels in between these two extremes were referred to as *biostatic* caring or life-restraining, whereby the practitioner is cold, treating the other as a nuisance; or *biopassive*, which is life-neutral and characterized by apathy and a detached manner. The *bioactive* level was found to be the more classic nurse-patient relationship, whereby the nurse is kind, concerned and benevolent.

However, the deepest level of a caring relationship, the biogenic level, was related to authentic caring connection, whereby both were affected for life-giving experience. This biogenic level is consistent with transpersonal caring theory and occurs within any given caring moment (Watson 2005, 1999a, 1999b). However, this research also highlights the destructive, toxic, noncaring relationship. The biocidic level of noncaring can be an act of cruelty, leading to despair, anger, frustration, and nonhealing for both.

The research of Kristen Swanson (Swanson, 1999) likewise detected the positive and negative outcomes of caring-noncaring for both patients and nurses through her comprehensive meta-analysis of 130 studies on caring. For example, when patients experienced caring, the following consequences were reported:

- *Emotional-spiritual well-being (dignity, self-control, personhood)*
- *Physical lives enhanced, lives saved, increase in safety*
- *Decrease in costs*
- *Increase in trust relationships, comfort and family support*

When patients experienced noncaring, the following consequences were reported:

- *Humiliation, fear, lack of control*
- *Despair, helplessness, alienation, vulnerability*
- *Lingering bad memories*
- *Decreased healing*

These noncaring consequences from Swanson's 1999 work parallel Halldorsdottir's 1991 biocidic caring, which is actually harmful to patient and nurse alike and has negative outcomes for the system, including costs. These findings are also consistent with the transpersonal caring theory, helping to empirically validate the significance of theory-guided caring and patient and nurse outcomes.

Swanson's (1999) findings for patients were mirrored for nurses. For example, the following consequences were present when nurses were practicing caring:

- *Emotional-spiritual sense of accomplishment, satisfaction, purpose*
- *A sense of gratitude, fulfillment, wholeness, self-esteem*
- *Ability to live their own philosophy*
- *Greater respect for life, death*
- *Ability to be more reflective*
- *A love of nursing*
- *Desire for increased knowledge*

However, just as patients were negatively affected by non-caring, nurses who were not practicing caring reported the following:

- *Being hardened, oblivious, robot-like*
- *Feeling depressed, frightened*
- *Feeling worn down, etc.*

Once we awaken to the negative consequences of conventional approaches to health care, or models that do not honor caring and healing processes for the whole person, we realize the ethical and operational responsibilities administrators and leaders have to transform the system within.

Caring and Administrative Leadership: Responsibility of Nurse Administrator in The Caring Model

Nursing administrators as well as hospital managers and administrators have a significant role to play in transforming the medical system from one that is often biocidic to one that is biogenic. Nyberg (1998) was one of the early nursing administrators creating caring systems leading to Magnet designation, long before those systems were mainstream. Having had extensive leadership roles as a nursing administrator who early on was guided by caring theory, she developed a model of caring nursing administration that served to inform the entire health care system. The model is outlined in her book *Caring in Nursing Administration* (Nyberg, 1998). Her model incorporated the diversity of theories that inform caring administration in nursing leadership.

Nyberg Model of Caring Administration

If a nurse administrator were to take this model seriously, as many nursing leaders are doing today, the following leadership responsibilities are proposed:

- *Understanding and communicating caring as philosophy and ethic for organizational processes, structures and relationships*
- *Developing skills of caring behaviors, caring presence in formal-informal relationships with individuals and groups*

- *Being alert and responsive to situations for modeling, creating and articulating theoretical-philosophical ethics or caring with staff, colleagues*

- *Providing leadership in implementing and evaluating experimental models of caring based on theoretical-philosophical values*

- *Critiquing and helping to transform conventional practices by offering an inspired, informed, articulate vision for creating caring-healing systems*

- *Promoting and supporting research on caring and health/healing outcomes*

- *Pursuing relationships and data that document relationship between and among caring practice models and nurse retention, patient-nurse satisfaction, healing outcomes, and cost*

- *Becoming stewards of caring-economics-costs, by incorporating caring as a valuable economic resource and caring as a foundational, ethical variable in cost-benefit ratios*

- *Experimenting with new demonstration projects that showcase models of caring-healing excellence, new professional practice models (ex: "Nightingale Units," "Attending Nurse Caring/Attending Caring Team Models")*

Responsibility of the Nurse Administrator in Caring Model

- Understand and communicate caring as a philosophy/ethic for organizational processes and structures and relationships

- Develop skills of caring behaviors/presence in formal-informal relationships with individuals and groups

- Become a steward of caring-economics-costs

Nursing Administrator Responsibilities for Integrating Economics and Caring

- Being alert and responsive to situations for modeling, creating and articulating ethics of caring to staff, colleagues

- Implementing theoretical models of caring to critique and transform nursing practices

- Promoting research on caring and health/healing outcomes as well as nurse retention/satisfaction costs

The Attending Nurse Caring Model (ANCM) has been piloted at the Children's Hospital, Denver, CO (Watson & Foster, 2003). It was implemented as a research and advanced professional practice model for actualizing caring theory and evidence as a guide to advancing professional nursing practice. Furthermore, it allowed for more actualization of nursing as a mature caring and healing profession, not just as technical assistance to medical treatment and models of cure. The ANCM was designed to deliver and oversee a program of collaborative, comprehensive, continuous caring-healing nursing with its therapeutic practices for a group of identified patients/families on a pain-management, postsurgical unit.

The model is grounded in relationship-centered caring, which incorporates caring theory as a philosophical-ethical base that offers nurses a shared worldview and professional culture. It allows the emergence of a collective vision, whereby shared knowledge, values, goals, and advanced caring-healing arts and therapeutics extend nursing practices. This process seeks to generate a new pattern and structure for care delivery and administrative practices. A culture of shared knowledge and values serves as a guide to heartfelt caring practices that are grounded in both theory and evidence. This model translates theory and evidence into advanced nursing practices. It extends and advances professional caring practices and patterns, while expanding, supporting, and simultaneously sustaining independent and interdependent care goals.

The ANCM is both discipline-specific and transdisciplinary in its approach and experiences; for example, more recently this model has evolved to be renamed as the Attending Caring Team Model from Attending Nurse Caring Model, having been adopted by the full interdisciplinary team of this unit.

The original ANCM parallels an Attending Physician Model, except that the ANCM makes explicit that the professional nurse is "attending to" comprehensive (nursing-patient-family) caring-healing needs and practices along with the integration of medical treatments (and other interdisciplinary practices). The (redefined) Caring Attending Nurse/Team model is informed and guided by the ethics and theory of car-

The Attending Nurse Caring Model as an Exemplar of Caring Theory, and Clinical and Ethical Administrative Changes

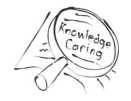

ing—and caring relationships—combined with best evidence, especially with respect to pain management of children.

In summary, this ethical, theory-guided professional practice model seeks to make explicit the caring relationship, the knowledge, values, philosophy, theory and therapeutics that guide advanced professional caring-healing practices in action. Finally, the ANCM creates a new pattern and structure for the delivery of professional nursing that transforms the practitioners themselves and conventional systems (Watson, 2005).

As a result of this initial project, the Attending Caring Team Model now serves as an inspired model for other units in the hospital. Additional developmental project activities are underway to expand the model within the Children's Hospital, Denver, CO.

Other National Initiatives of Caring Theory-Guided Practice Models

Other such models of caring theory-guided practices are underway in such systems as Denver Veterans Administration Hospital, Denver, CO; McKee Banner Medical Center, Loveland, CO; Elmhurst Hospital, NY; INOVA Health System, Fairfax, VA; Kendall Health, Miami, FL; Miami Baptist System, FL; Sarasota Memorial Hospital, FL; Winter Haven Hospital, FL; Resurrection Healthcare, Chicago, IL; Scripps Institute/ Hospital, La Jolla, CA; University of California Irvine Medical Center Hospital, Orange, CA; St. Joseph Hospital, Orange, CA; University of Arkansas Children's Hospital, Little Rock, AR; and Central Baptist Hospital, Lexington, KY, among others. Many of these named hospitals are already Magnet hospitals or are in the process of preparing to achieve Magnet status, using the caring ethic and theory as the underlying professional practice model.

These identified and named hospital systems serve only as some exemplars of hospitals today guided by an evolved ethic and theoretical-philosophical foundation of human caring as a means to transform practitioners and system alike.* Also, there are additional hospitals and care systems exploring this direction that have not been named, but have communicated with the author about their efforts in this direction. This

I apologize if I have inadvertently omitted a hospital or system that is informed by this philosophy and theory.

direction for caring theory-guided ethical practices is helping to more fully actualize nursing qua nursing in our contemporary institutions, educating and transforming nurses, other practitioners, and systems alike. These and many, many other nursing caring-focused administrators and practitioners, as well as all systems seeking to transform nursing from its ethical core, from the inside out, serve as inspirations of hope for the future of human caring-healing, health and the survival of this noble and ancient profession. For more information, see Watson's Web site: www.uchsc.edu/nursing/caring

References: Clark, J. (2004). An aging population with chronic disease compels new delivery systems focused on new structures and practices. *Nursing Administration Quarterly*, 28(2), 105-115.

Halldorsdottir, S. (1991). Five basic modes of being with another. In D. A. Gaut & M. Leininger (Eds.), *Caring: The compassionate healer* (pp. 37-49). New York: National League for Nursing.

Nyberg, J. (1998). *Caring in nursing administration*. Boulder, CO: University Press of Colorado.

Quinn, J. (2003). Revisioning the nursing shortage: A call to caring for healing the healthcare system. *Frontiers of Health Care Services Management*,19(2), 3-21.

Swanson, K. (1999). What is known about caring in nursing science? In A. S. Hinshaw, S. Feetham, & J. Shaver (Eds.), *Handbook of clinical nursing research* (pp. 31-60). Thousand Oaks, CA: Sage.

Watson, J. (1985). *Nursing. The philosophy and science of caring*. Boulder, CO: University Press of Colorado.

Watson, J. (1999a). *Nursing: Human science and human care*. Sudbury, MA: Jones & Bartlett.

Watson, J. (1999b). *Postmodern nursing and beyond*. New York: Elsevier.

Watson, J. (2002). Intentionality and caring-healing consciousness: A practice of transpersonal nursing. *Journal of Holistic Nursing Practice*, 16(3), 12-19.

Watson, J. (2005). *Caring science as sacred science*. Philadelphia: F. A. Davis.

Watson, J., & Foster, R. (2003). The attending nurse caring model. *Journal of Clinical Nursing*, 12, 360-365.

The Language of Engagement

—Rebecca Smith and Mary Koloroutis

The language of engagement is language that shows honor, respect and appreciation for others, and it is language that specifically invites individuals into a new way of being. The following four elements inspire the deep engagement of others.

Four Elements of Engagement

Honor

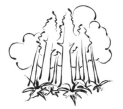

To honor someone is to recognize not only his or her achievements, but his or her very personhood. We honor others when we are authentic. The language of engagement is *real*—no seductive sales talk, no clichés, no buzz words, no jargon.

Show honor for those you wish to lead by finding a way to convey, "I understand and value what you do, and I see what's possible for this organization with your full engagement."

Respect

We believe that respect is inherently deserved—not just earned. Respect for self seamlessly translates into respect for others.

Respecting people's intelligence means providing them with meaningful information. Look at the subtleties between these two approaches: "We're doing this because it's for the best" versus "If we do this, our patients and their families will experience a higher quality of care." Both statements are true, but the first lacks meaningful information. We show respect for individuals when we consistently disclose our true intent, sharing information honestly and generously.

Appreciation

Appreciation has transformative power. It is a vital component in the language of engagement as well. If we approach people with a sense of appreciation uppermost in our minds, we are likely to see the good they are doing and to speak directly to it

Appreciation energizes those we wish to engage. We draw others in by helping them to see not only that their work is intrinsically valuable, but that we specifically value it. Appreciation engages the interest of individuals by pointing out to them, as specifically as possible, the value of their own contributions.

Invitation

Like respect, this aspect also has to do with giving pertinent information—this time, though, it's about providing information that is specific to the people we wish to engage. The invitation to "drop in any time" is very different from the invitation to a specific occasion at a specific time. The former may make us feel welcome, but only the latter makes us feel invited.

True invitation asks individuals to imagine themselves in the circumstances into which we're inviting them. We engage others by inviting them clearly and specifically into our visions for change. Once we have invited them in, we engage them by asking for their unique voice and contribution to a shared vision for change.

> Appreciation engages the interest of individuals by pointing out to them, as specifically as possible, the value of their own contributions.

Principles of Engagement

A number of identifiable principles are common to the language of engagement. This language:

- *gives meaningful information,*
- *addresses people directly,*
- *communicates clearly,*
- *honors the other person's viewpoint,*
- *shows authentic appreciation,*
- *shows kindness,*
- *asks rather than tells, and*
- *demonstrates a desire to listen.*

The language of disengagement shares common principles as well. This language:

- *offers mandates,*
- *sends the message, "We know what's best for you,"*
- *demonstrates a lack of understanding or desire to understand the world through the eyes of others,*
- *is dismissive in tone and/or content,*
- *tells rather than asks.*

In any professional communication in which your intention is to engage others, avoid language shortcuts. Notice whether your admonitions lack depth. *We have to, we should,* and *we can't* are mandates with no real information in them. They make engagement impossible as they provide nothing tangible to agree with or engage in.

Notice the difference as five disengaging phrases are transformed using the language of engagement.

Disengagement: *"Well, you're just going to have to work faster and smarter."*

Engagement: *"What will it take for us to find new ways to accomplish your priorities?"*

Disengagement: *"We can't keep doing things the way we did them before."*

Engagement: *"Thank you for the good work you've been doing. Now how can we work together creatively to make things even better for everyone going forward?"*

Disengagement: *"We'll be making some changes around here."*

Engagement: *"We're counting on your input to ensure that the changes we make will create the best care environment possible."*

Disengagement: *"We're finally going to get this unit up to snuff."*

Engagement: *"We're in a position to refine the best of what we're doing into something even better."*

Even subtle refinements of language can go a long way toward bringing honor, respect, appreciation and invitation to the forefront. Notice the language you use and respect the power in it. Most of us are careful in our prepared remarks to be consistently kind and respectful, but our "off the cuff" remarks count just as much. Deliberately using the language of engagement will put you on track to draw people into embracing the larger vision for change.

Establishing a System of Accountability: The Manager's Role

—Donna Wright

As I help clients develop competency and staff development systems for use in all departments, I am often asked, "How do we establish a culture of accountability?" Managers wonder, "What should I do if people do not comply with policies, rules or deadlines?" It's essential, of course, to have a clearly articulated change strategy, but what do we do when people just don't come along?

When considering solutions to this issue, managers tend to talk about discipline. We discuss ways to better articulate expectations with the staff members. We discuss action plans and what should take place during performance reviews. We discuss documentation of performance issues and the grievances that may follow the documentation of performance issues. All of these things are valuable to discuss, but they do not address the problem we really face as managers, as they don't address the issue *systemically.* Dealing with individuals who are not meeting standards or expectations is important, but it is like thinking about a single tree without considering the forest around it.

To better understand this issue, let's take a broader look at how accountability works in organizations. The following model illustrates the five essential elements that must be in place in order for any organizational change to be successful at the tactical, daily level. These elements are:

- *vision*
- *manager's clear articulation of expectations*
- *competency assessment*
- *quality improvement*
- *manager's response to staff performance*

Wright's Model of Accountability in Organizations

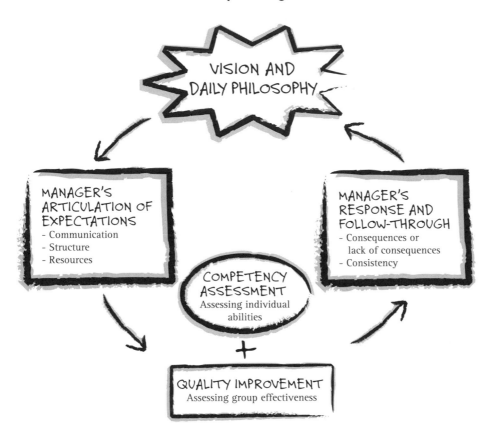

The Case for Establishing a System of Accountability

This model represents a system of accountability. It shows that when an organization's vision is articulated to staff members and staff then either meet the organization's expectations or not, managers then respond. The model is cyclical rather than linear because the response of managers to staff performance—their close, prompt attention to it or their ineffective or inconsistent response to it—then becomes (intentionally or not) a very real part of the culture of the organization. For this reason, it is essential that an organization safeguard this aspect of its functioning. Managers must respond purposefully and consistently to issues of staff performance, both positive and negative.

Let's examine each of the model's elements individually as it would be expressed in daily operations and practice:

Vision or daily philosophy can include anything from our mission statement, a policy, a memo that is posted on the bulletin board, or even an informal rule a group has created. It is a combination of our shared goal and the philosophy—be it stated or implied—that we live by in our daily practice.

Next, **managers articulate the vision** to the appropriate staff. We do this through memos and staff meetings, as well as through informal verbal communication. We also articulate the vision less directly, though no less significantly, through our allocation of resources and the structures that support our organization. For example, if we wanted people to use more handheld computers at work and verbalized this at meetings and through memos, but then did not provide any handheld devices, people wouldn't take the message we sent earlier very seriously.

The next step in the model deals with our ability to assess our performance. We do this through **competency assessment and quality improvement efforts**. We check people's current level of skill, and we examine outcomes through quality improvement and performance improvement efforts.

After we find out how we are doing, **managers respond**. Especially when performance is found to be less than adequate, it is in our response that we enhance or diminish our credibility as leaders. We respond with consequences or a lack of consequences, consistency or a lack of consistency. This step in the model is the most important because it actually has the power to inadvertently "rewrite" the vision and daily philosophy. No matter what we say we value, any actions we take in contradiction to our stated values will be perceived as infinitely more real than even the most clearly and vehemently articulated expectations. If we let people off the hook after they have failed to do something we've asked them to do, they will quite reasonably conclude that we will never hold them fully accountable, regardless of how many times we articulate a policy or expectation.

No matter what we say we value, any actions we take in contradiction to our stated values will be perceived as infinitely more real than even the most clearly and vehemently articulated expectations.

Most organizations struggle with this last element. We need to ask if our managers have the skills to consistently hold individuals accountable in our organizations—and if they do have the skills, whether they get proper backing when they exercise those skills. A manager's ability to respond appropriately and consistently is the number one competency deficit I find in most organizations. Managers do not always know how to be creative with consequences or to keep their efforts consistent.

Establishing a strong system of accountability may seem insurmountable, but in practice, the opposite is true. When individuals know what is expected of them and managers understand the five elements of the accountability model and how to apply those elements in daily practice, clarity replaces confusion and a stable environment is created within which creativity thrives.

The Most Essential Link in a System of Accountability

The most troublesome element of the accountability model for many seems to be "manager response and follow-through." When this is not carried out well, it can completely alter the vision. Sometimes we actually ignore this element, and our attentions are directed to other elements. For example: If staff members do not follow a policy, rather than holding them accountable for changing their behavior to fit the policy, we rewrite the policy to articulate a new expectation. The policy in this situation was not the problem. The staff's lack of commitment to the policy was the problem. When we as managers fail to hold individuals accountable, we create a culture in which the notion of accountability becomes meaningless.

If staff members are meeting their standards, effective managers make the time for reflection and celebration.

Effective managerial leadership, however, begins well before a staff member fails to perform. Most successful management follow-through starts when the vision is set and expectations are articulated. The articulated expectation itself sets a standard into place by which progress can be measured. If staff members are meeting their standards, effective managers make the time for reflection and celebration. If standards are not met, effective managers will make the time for reflection and inquiry into what it will take for us to reach the goal or standard to which we are committed.

As managers, we hope that when we create fair and reasonable policies, staff members will adhere to them. However, in almost every situation, a team member will test the boundaries of what the policy says. If managers then fail to enforce the policy, the team member will quickly share his or her experience with others—"Don't worry, everyone; I crossed the line and nothing happened." Soon we see more and more people stepping outside the articulated area of accountability, not because the vision was not clearly articulated, but because managers did not follow through on what they said they would do.

Many first-time managers in health care are in their leadership positions because of their superior clinical or service skills. Even the best clinicians do not automatically also have good management skills. They may not feel confident or even competent when it comes to holding people accountable. For this reason, it is extremely important that new managers understand their role expectations, engage in self-development and formal leadership development, and (when possible) work with a seasoned mentor. However, even seasoned managers often need formal leadership development. They have often learned what they know "by the seat of their pants," and sometimes the culture of limited accountability is so entrenched in the organization that managers have no idea how to change these long-standing patterns.

As with so much of what we ask people to do in organizations, the more we can involve individuals in setting the policies they will be asked to enforce, the more likely we are to get their committed participation. I suggest that when a new policy is written and ready to be officially placed in the policy manual, that we take the policy to the next managers' meeting. Tell the group, "We are about to make this policy public. In this policy, we say that 'abc' is the new standard; it is based on the latest evidence for safe care in 'xyz' conditions and when we implement this we are doing it with our full commitment to achieving it. Managers—What will it take to prepare staff members to meet this standard? How will you monitor it? *And are you ready to enforce it?*" It then falls to these managers to decide both how they will prepare staff members to meet the new standard and what will happen if an individual falls short. So many times managers hope the policy is so forcefully writ-

As with so much of what we ask people to do in organizations, the more we can involve individuals in setting the policies they will be asked to enforce, the more likely we are to get their committed participation.

ten that everyone will comply. I am sorry to say that there is almost always someone who will cross the line.

In the discussion that follows, the policy is carefully considered and often refined by those who will be asked to enforce it. Managers have more confidence in enforcing a policy they themselves have helped to shape. This also gives the management group the chance to discuss, practice and review potential responses to problems long before they arise. Some management groups have prepared case studies and/or exemplars, and have done role-play around these kinds of issues, all in preparation for being realistic, supportive and consistent in their response as managers.

Enforcing Accountability With Individual Staff Members: Secrets to Positive Disciplinary Action

Even if we are consistent in our actions as managers, there will still be employees who fall short of the articulated expectations. Following are some basic guidelines to help managers enforce accountability in these situations.

In every situation in which a staff member has fallen short of expectations, you must prepare a plan that will help the person to meet them.

This plan has a dual purpose: it helps us to actively assist the person in meeting the expectation and it also serves as documentation of our assistance in helping the staff member meet the expectation. The latter is important should we eventually determine that individual must either be reassigned or terminated.

There are two goals in every employee discipline situation: 1) solve the problem, and 2) maintain the relationship (Grote, 1995).

The key to success in any disciplinary situation is to strive for both of these goals at all times. Even if you have chosen termination as the appropriate solution, carry it out with dignity and treat the person with respect. Never let your emotions provoke an inappropriate response. (Also be aware, however, that in health care, managers easily fall into the care giver mode with employees in these situations. Managers are often so focused on maintaining the relationship that they ignore or overlook the problem of poor performance. It may help to remember that it is both respectful and caring to deal with their difficult situations directly, honestly and firmly. It is respectful to the individuals and to the team as a whole.)

Always get a second (and third) opinion.

One of the best things any manager can do is to ask another manager or human resources person to review their disciplinary plans of action. I encourage managers to get two other signatures on every disciplinary plan. Getting the input of other managers helps ensure that the plan is adequately supportive to the staff member and appropriate to the situation. This partnering can also provide legal support in instances where individuals being terminated take legal action. Seeking others to review and sign an action plan automatically starts a peer support process.

Carefully consider the likely consequences of all of your potential leadership responses.

As we look at the fifth element of the accountability model (manager response), apply the "If … then what?" question to any action you're considering. This is the smartest thing a manager can do to prepare for discipline situations. Ask yourself, "If I do this action, what would be the best and worst response I could expect?" Do this for every action you can think of, including the action of "taking no action." If you choose to "do nothing" in a situation, the person may like you, but you may lose the trust and respect of the rest of your team because of your poor follow-through. This exercise is an essential step in the success of any disciplinary process and in building overall team accountability.

> Managers are often so focused on maintaining the relationship that they ignore or overlook the problem of poor performance. It may help to remember that it is both respectful and caring to deal with their difficult situations directly, honestly and firmly.

A system of accountability supports the efficient functioning of any health care organization, but in a Relationship-Based Care (RBC) culture it is vital. In a culture in which individuals are asked to establish therapeutic relationships with patients and to make decisions about patient care, care givers must understand the full scope of what they are empowered to do

Accountability in Relationship-Based Care

on behalf of patients and their families. Knowing the limits of our authority, along with showing us what boundaries we are expected to operate within, can actually help us to better understand its scope.

Establishing RBC in your organization means moving to an RBC culture. It is essential to know what kinds of accountability culture you currently have created in your organization—to carefully consider both its positive and negative aspects. Since we "start where we are," you will bring your current accountability culture with you as you begin to implement any new changes. Being aware of the five elements of the accountability model and how they affect each other can help you make better choices in this transition and establish a culture of strong accountability in your organization.

It may help to remember that it is both respectful and caring to deal with their difficult situations directly, honestly and firmly. It is respectful to the individuals and to the team as a whole.

References and suggested readings: Grote, D. (1995). *Discipline without punishment: The proven strategy that turns problem employees into superior performers.* New York: American Management Association.

Levine, S. (2002). *The book of agreement: 10 essential elements for getting the results you want.* San Francisco: Berrett-Koehler.

Patterson, K., Grenny, J., McMillan, R. and Switzler, A. (2005). *Crucial confrontations: Tools for resolving broken promises, violated expectations, and bad behavior.* New York: McGraw-Hill.

Wright, D. (2005). *The ultimate guide to competency assessment in health care.* (3rd ed.). Minneapolis, MN: Creative Health Care Management.

Time as a Resource

—Colleen Person

Prior to the last 15 or 20 years, the fiscal aspects of health care were kept out of the hands of nurse managers. Staff involved in direct patient care at the unit level were even one more step removed from involvement in fiscal aspects of care delivery. The thinking was that the job of nursing was to care for patients and that the job of administration was to efficiently allocate the resources to make that possible. It is only in the last few decades that the people who actually use the resources on a daily basis are involved in making decisions about those resources. Nurse managers are now engaged in the budgetary processes and share this information with staff. Nonetheless, because this development is so recent, and because mindsets are sometimes slow to change, it is still common in health care to find that people do not see themselves as managers/ stewards of their own resources. Further, health care delivery models that are more task-based than Relationship-Based Care (RBC), do not so overtly encourage their practitioners to view their individual practices as a contribution to a larger whole.

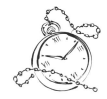

But RBC is different. Relationship-Based Care functions best in organizations in which individuals in every role keep a focus on their own contributions to the well-being of patients and their families. That means that individuals at all levels in the organization see themselves as part of something bigger than their individual practices. It means that individuals are empowered, and with that empowerment comes the responsibility for making decisions about the full range of what is possible within one's own practice.

In health care, when we think of our resources, we think of people and equipment. But if the way we think about our resources is limited to these two tangible areas, we're missing something vital. *Our most valuable resource—and the one resource that in an RBC organization we are most directly empowered to allocate—is our time.*

It takes individual reflection on practice, efficient teamwork, and innovative thinking to meet patient needs within the reality of finite resources.

Marie Manthey, founder of Creative Health Care Management (CHCM), spoke at the annual American Nurses Credentialing Center (ANCC) Magnet Conference in the fall of 2004.

In her speech she reminded us of how easy it is for nurses to get swept away with thoughts of there not being enough time to do "everything." Furthermore we hear again and again that we are to "do more with less." The anxiety that so often accompanies these realities comes from not realizing the control we each have over our own time; we rarely consider that it is possible to rethink or even redesign our own work. A mindset that creates a better sense of well-being in nurses is one in which *nurses allocate their time consciously, deciding not only what to do, but also what not to do.* These notions are both simple and radical. And while there is a fine line between doing-everything-you-can and consciously-deciding-what-you-will-and-will-not-do, it is essential to the well-being of nurses (and by extension, of course, of patients and their families) that they stand on the right side of that line.

In RBC organizations, we ask all care givers to take on this new time-as-a-resource mindset and to be as creative as possible in how they integrate it into their practice. We all need to reach for new ways to expand this concept every day. During a recent offering of our *Reigniting the Spirit of Caring* workshop, a patient-participant spoke of how her frustration mounted through the course of her hospital stay because every time her nurse left her room, she asked, "Is there anything else I can do for you?" She said that each time that happened she felt like she only had a second or two to think about it. Invariably she would think of something she wanted once the nurse was gone. She didn't feel good about using the call bell, so more often than not, she just went without whatever it was she wanted. At her suggestion, a number of practitioners have changed their practice. They now ask their patients *upon entering* their rooms to be thinking about anything else they might want or need—and then they ask near the end of their visit, "Did you think of anything else I can do for you?" Some have melded the principles of RBC and Resource-Driven Practice even further by saying to patients at the outset, "We're going to decide together how my time with you will be spent. I want to know what's important to you."

> A mindset that creates a better sense of well-being in nurses is one in which nurses allocate their time consciously, deciding not only what to do, but also what not to do.

While many may initially bristle at the seemingly cold notion that practice must be resource driven, the reality of resource-driven practice is that it can actually enhance our ability to be effective stewards of our time and talents. And clearly, once the notion of "time as a resource" is fleshed out for practitioners, they come to see not only the practical benefits of this new mindset, but the beauty of it as well. It allows staff to go home satisfied with what they *did* do.

So where does this time come from? In an RBC organization, a unit is not limited to doing things the "same way they've always been done." Unit Practice Councils (UPCs) are given the responsibility, authority and accountability to redesign many of their processes and practices to ensure that Registered Nurses and members of the patient care team have the time to work within the established principles of Relationship-Based Care. Further, practitioners are encouraged to add innovations of their own in order to create for themselves a "signature" RBC practice. To this end, communication and documentation procedures are streamlined as much as possible. While this can be a difficult sea to navigate, we have seen impressive restructuring efforts accomplished in organizations where commitments to both RBC and creative thinking are strong. When an organization formalizes its commitment to putting patients and their families first, we find that individuals look with new eyes at all that they do. Through creative thinking and meaningful dialogue with colleagues, innovative solutions invariably emerge.

It takes a big shift in mindset for each of us, regardless of role, to practice this kind of patient-centered, resource-driven care. Experience tells us that this is no simple transition. It takes individual reflection on practice, efficient teamwork and innovative thinking to meet patient needs within the reality of finite resources. It is essential for every organization that wishes to practice RBC to explore and change mindsets about resource management as needed. It is equally essential for each individual practitioner to personally embrace the reality of time as a resource and to proactively manage, every day, this most precious resource.

While many may initially bristle at the seemingly cold notion that practice must be resource-driven, the reality of resource-driven practice is that it can actually enhance our ability to be effective stewards of our time and talents.

Our most valuable resource is our time.

Competencies that Support Relationship-Based Care

—Donna Wright

Infusing your organization's competency assessment strategies with the principles of Relationship-Based Care (RBC) is an excellent way to reinforce and validate progress at the individual level. Competency strategies are a great way to articulate expectations, measure outcomes, and move teams and whole organizations toward Relationship-Based Care. In order to be successful in using competency assessment as part of your RBC implementation, you must be aware of the key factors of success of competency assessment. It is important to understand that it is not just about writing a competency and "checking everyone off."

To use competency assessment as a success strategy in implementing any new initiative, keep these key factors in mind:

- **Staff and manager collaboratively identify the competencies to be used in the implementation.** *This promotes joint ownership for the outcomes.*

- **Staff members are responsible for providing evidence of competency achievement.** *The manager or educator is not at the center of this process. Avoid getting into the "checker-off" role. Allow individuals to be accountable for providing evidence to the organization as it relates to their contribution to any initiative. This is a great strategy for promoting accountability.*

- **Use a variety of competency verification methods.** *The verification methods should match the type of competencies. Most organizations get in the rut of using two or three different verification methods. There are 11 categories of verification. Become familiar with all the methods. Be creative. It will enhance your overall success.*

- Give the staff member choices in selecting verification methods for the identified competencies. *I try to give two to four verification method choices for each competency identified. This incorporates adult learning principles into your competency process. You will also never find one method that will meet everyone's needs. Give people choices.*

Below is a sample of three competencies that reflect skills in the three key relationships in Relationship-Based Care:

- *relationship with the patient/family,*
- *relationship with your colleagues, and*
- *relationship with yourself.*

Competency	Verification Method (Select one verification method for each competency)
1) Demonstrates the ability to create a healthy therapeutic relationship with the patient/family.	• Submit an exemplar (a written or oral story) that shows how you created or developed a relationship with a patient or family members, even in difficult situations. • Submit a copy of a card or note from a patient or family member that reflects on your care. • Submit a copy of a section from a patient satisfaction survey that mentioned you by name in a positive way, reflecting your care or customer service.
2) Demonstrates the ability to establish and maintain healthy relationships with colleagues.	• Submit a written exemplar that shows how you used a value articulated on the "Commitment to My Co-worker©" card. • Submit three peer reviews that reflect your interactions with colleagues. (Suggestion for overall peer review process: The staff member distributes three peer review forms to peers of his or her choosing, and the manager sends out three peer review forms to randomly selected peers.)
3) Demonstrates the ability to care for self.	• Submit a receipt of some self-care activity that reflects a healthy self-care lifestyle. (e.g., receipt from a day at a spa, or monthly therapeutic massages, or photos from a day fishing.) • Complete a self-care inventory that provides a self-assessment of your self-care activities and identify two actions for self-care.

The competencies we select convey our organizational values to staff members When our competencies are written (or revised) with RBC in mind they become part of what helps to sustain focus on RBC within the organization throughout implementation and beyond.

Reference: Wright, D. (2005). *The ultimate guide to competency assessment in health care.* (3rd ed.). Minneapolis, MN: Creative Health Care Management.

Exuberance

—Jayne A. Felgen

Kay Redfield Jamison's book *Exuberance: The Passion for Life* begins with a reference to an Anglican prayer which petitions God to "Watch now those who weep this day; Rest your weary ones; Soothe your suffering ones." As she wryly points out, "The joyous tend to be left to their own devices, the exuberant ones even more so."

Many of us—especially in health care—tend to put the lion's share of our attention on soothing the sad, stuck and frustrated instead of deliberately harnessing the joyfully creative productivity of the exuberant among us.

We tend to write off the exuberant ones as pie-in-the-sky idealists or "Pollyannas." They are easy to dismiss, in part because we know they will not suffer personally because of our dismissal of them. (If we drop the exuberant ones, they bounce.)

But we miss a golden opportunity when we fail to take seriously the exuberant creators among us.

Their exuberance makes them fountains of ideas—some extraordinary, but many merely practical. Exuberance is not mania; it is an expression of the flow of positive energy through a human body. It is the energy that accompanies (and sometimes causes) the position of being actively for something rather than being positioned against it.

We tend to think that some people are naturally exuberant and that for others exuberance is not possible. But it is my experience (as one who is frequently exuberant, but not always so) that exuberance is not natural, but rather, it is practiced. If one's practiced habit is to focus on what is working well and therefore to position one's self to work for what is wanted, one will often, if not always, experience exuberance.

If it is one's practiced habit to focus on what is not working well and therefore to position one's self to work against what is not wanted, one will rarely if ever experience exuberance.

Exuberance comes and goes; it comes with focus on what is wanted and it goes with focus on what is not.

Exuberance is a powerful force, and while we may imagine that the great power of exuberance lies in its ability to help us persuade others to see things our way, its greatest power may in fact be in its ability to keep the exuberant ones themselves passionately focused on the task at hand. Emotional energies waver throughout the course of a long transformational project. When the project needs a shot of energy (well before anything actually becomes stalled) the exuberance of those leading the change can be reignited by a renewed focus on the group's past and current successes—from which it is only a small leap to deliberately focus on creating its desired future.

Be ever mindful of the power of exuberance. Train yourself to recognize it and to always express gratitude for it when you see it. And remember that even when its light is not visible, it is never far away.

Exuberance comes and goes; it comes with focus on what is wanted and it goes with focus on what is not.

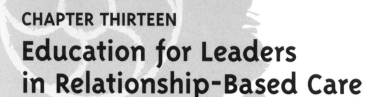

CHAPTER THIRTEEN
Education for Leaders in Relationship-Based Care

The *Relationship-Based Care Leader Practicum*: A Workshop for Leaders Who Want to "Know It in Their Bones"

—Mary Koloroutis

The *Relationship-Based Care (RBC) Leader Practicum* was created in response to the requests of RBC Project Leaders and executive team members who wanted to have a deeper knowledge of RBC so that they were more able to lead implementation efforts. As one participant put it, she wanted to "know it in her bones." The *Relationship-Based Care Leader Practicum* helps leaders to personally integrate the theories, principles and practices of RBC so that when they're leading it, they can put all of their energy into making it happen.

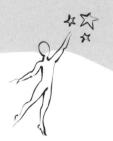

Who Should Take the Practicum

Project Leaders who have already begun RBC implementation have also helped us to develop a greater understanding of the importance of having a broad team of people who are deeply knowledgeable about RBC within the organization. For this reason, the *Relationship-Based Care Leader Practicum* works best when at least two to four other people in the organization attend with the RBC Project Leaders. The participant team, in addition to the selected "Project Leader," would ideally include:

- *an executive nurse leader*
- *an operational executive*
- *a chief medical officer*
- *a Staff Nurse leader and/or*
- *any other influential leader from any position within the organization who will be a champion for RBC, especially leaders of the results council*

This participant team will provide leadership for designing, implementing, sustaining and evolving Relationship-Based Care within their organization. While the assigned Project Leader guides the way, the aligned efforts of the Chief Nursing Officer, executive team and other key leaders are crucial to a successful implementation. When RBC gets integrated more broadly, it is stronger and more effective, and it is then less likely to be seen as pertaining to the nursing department alone or to a few select units.

We began offering the *Practicum* about a year after the book *Relationship-Based Care: A Model for Transforming Practice* was published. We have had organizations send participants who are about to begin RBC implementation as well as those who are in the thick of it. We've also had numerous participants from organizations that have had their curiosity piqued by the book. The *Practicum* has proven equally valuable (and equally appreciated) by individuals in each of these positions.

What It Is

The *Relationship-Based Care Leader Practicum* promises 5 days of immersion into RBC theory, practice, and implementation strategies and tools. This intensive 5-day program provides RBC Leaders with the clarity and competence essential for assembling a collaborative team of change leaders. The program blends a variety of experiential methodologies to develop competencies, integrate learning relative to RBC, and design customized strategies and outcomes for use in individual organizations. Experiential methodologies such as dialogue, circle, storytelling, reflection, Appreciative Inquiry and action learning facilitate active participation in the experience.

We have designed the *Practicum* to be 90% experiential and interactive and 10% presentation. (See "Accelerated Learning" page 381.) A comprehensive manual is provided with strategies, tools and resources that form the basis of discussions and exercises. As RBC works differently in every organizational culture, it is important for the majority of the application of the content of this workshop to be discussed and applied by the participants themselves. The facilitators of the workshop work with the participants to explore real-life examples of how support, coaching, inspiration, impending infrastructural changes, education and evidence of results will come into play once implementation has begun. This format helps an organization's leaders to make more informed decisions about what makes sense for them given their organization's unique culture.

The *Relationship-Based Care Leader Practicum* is divided into five main sections:

Day one *offers participants immersion into the knowledge and principles of Relationship-Based Care.*

Day two *offers theories, tools and strategies for transformational change.*

Day three *offers the basics of Project Management essential to RBC implementation.*

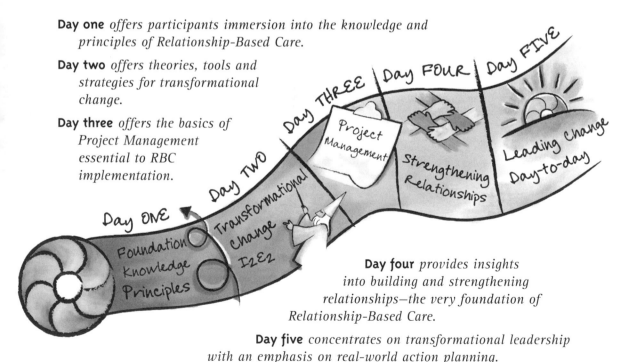

Day four *provides insights into building and strengthening relationships—the very foundation of Relationship-Based Care.*

Day five *concentrates on transformational leadership with an emphasis on real-world action planning.*

The *Relationship-Based Care Leader Practicum* provides participant leaders with a new way of thinking and being within their organizations. They gain insight and colleague support for intentionally modeling the values and behaviors of Relationship-Based Care in their leadership practices. One participant expressed her gain in insight in this way: *"Finally, the runway has lights!"*

Participants in the *Relationship-Based Care Leader Practicum* have reported that they've come away with:

- *a mental, emotional and spiritual recommitment to the values and beliefs that brought them into health care in the first place;*

- *a commitment to modeling the way in every action and interaction each day;*

- *a strong awareness of the three crucial relationships in Relationship-Based Care—self-awareness, care of patient and family, and healthy teamwork;*

- *a reservoir of specific strategies and actions for organizing and implementing Relationship-Based Care;*

- *a working knowledge of how to integrate RBC into existing organizational priorities and strategies for excellence;*

- *a true understanding of how Appreciative Inquiry (the practice of identifying past successes and building upon them) works to harness positive energies for change;*

- *a working knowledge of I_2E_2, a formula for comprehensive action planning and sustained implementation;*

- *an introduction to Human Dynamics, a course of study that helps individuals to better understand their own ways of being in the world and those of others;*

"Finally, the runway has lights!"

- *an appreciation of their own organization based on reflections of and learning from participants from other organizations; and*

- *an individual leadership action plan for leading and implementing Relationship-Based Care.*

An important byproduct of the experience is the strengthening and alignment of the team of people who will be leading Relationship-Based Care. When participants attend the *Practicum* as organizational teams, they are able to build a shared understanding and vision for RBC and work through strategies for maximizing its success in their organization. Participants work together in teams to prepare a presentation and engage in intensive dialogue with participants from other organizations to help them to articulate what RBC is, what it means to their organizational mission and vision, and how to make it come alive. The participants report that they leave with enhanced relationships, stronger alliances and a network of people with whom they can continue to collaborate and share ideas for integrating RBC into their organizations.

Relationship-Based Care is an inherently personal pursuit in which each individual is asked to make a deeply personal transformation. By immersing leaders into the formal contemplation of these topics, we invite them to begin the process of transformation to RBC from the inside out. Participants have reported that after the *Relationship-Based Care Leader Practicum*, they have changed the way they see their organizations, their individual roles and their relationships with those they serve as leaders.

"Getting Smarter": The Relationship-Based Care Core Curriculum for Executive Leaders and Unit Practice Council Members

—Jayne A. Felgen and Colleen Person

Preparing the Project Leadership Team to Lead

Every executive leadership team brings a wealth of educational background and experience to its organization, and every bit of that education and experience comes into play in leading the implementation of Relationship-Based Care (RBC). During the "getting smarter" phase, these leaders remember what's important about that previous learning, using it as a foundation for a deep conceptual and pragmatic understanding of Relationship-Based Care.

The "getting smarter" phase typically starts with the designated RBC Project Leadership team:

- *the executive sponsor*
- *the CNO (if he or she is not the executive sponsor)*
- *the Results Council leader and co-leader*
- *the RBC Project Leader*
- *all members of the Results Council*

Relationship-Based Care Leader Practicum

One strategy that we'd always recommend for this initial group is to take the *Relationship-Based Care Leader Practicum* (see page 468). This practicum is essential for the four designated RBC leaders and is recommended for as many of the Results Council members as possible, as well as all of the managers involved in the first wave of RBC implementation. Attendance at this practicum could either precede or follow the internal "getting smarter" phase, which includes an immersion into related books, articles and videos.

Recommended Reading and Viewing

Each member of the RBC Project Leadership team is requested to read and/or view the following books, articles, and videos:

- *Relationship-Based Care: A Model for Transforming Practice, Mary Koloroutis, editor*

- *The Practice of Primary Nursing, 2nd ed., Marie Manthey*

- *I_2E_2: Leading Lasting Change, Jayne Felgen*

- *A document of the RBC Principles as they have been developed and endorsed by the organization's CNO, nurse executive team and executives responsible for allied health professionals and service support staff.*

- *Articles related to the dimensions of RBC, paying special attention to:*

  a) *"Relationship-Based Care: From Concept to Reality," CHCM News, October 2005*

  b) *"The Patient as CEO: Passion In Practice," CHCM News, March 2000*

  c) *"Caring: Core Value, Currency and Commodity," Nursing Administration Quarterly, September 2003*

The Videos (3)

1. *"Patients Love Their Nurses"*

2. *"Healing Environments: Passion in Practice"*

3. *"Leadership for Relationship-Based Practice"*

The Moments of Excellence Video Series (4)

1. *"We All Need ... A Little Bit of Attitude"*

2. *"Celebrating Our Moments of Excellence"*

3. *"Breaking the Rules: The Secret to Making It Up as You Go"*

4. *"R+A+A: The Secret Formula for Making Communication and Delegation Easier"*

A customized RBC Implementation Guide is prepared for all of the constituent groups by the Creative Health Care Management (CHCM) Project Leader. The guide provides essential practical information, clarifies the responsibilities of all roles, outlines operational instructions and includes specific tools and tactics for all.

Recommended Education

The workshop *Leading an Empowered Organization* (*LEO*) (see page 483) is essential education training for everyone who will lead any aspect of the RBC change or who will be in a position of leadership on any unit in the organization on which RBC is in place. *Leading an Empowered Organization* ensures that individuals throughout the organization see their leadership roles the same way and have common language and tools. This ensures continuity of the way in which individuals are empowered within the organization to practice Relationship-Based Care.

A *Reigniting the Spirit of Caring* (*RSC*) workshop (see page 524) is also effective in preparing leaders to lead and practice within a culture of Relationship-Based Care. In fact, *RSC* has, on occasion, been selected to precede all of this work as it has great power to inspire unity in groups. This might be particularly valuable in organizations in which there is a new merger as it creates a shared experience, uniting everybody involved.

How and When the Learning Takes Place

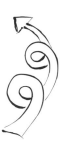

Although the curriculum itself remains largely consistent from organization to organization, the way in which the curriculum is presented and approached can vary. The education package can be designed by the project leadership team working in conjunction with the CHCM project leaders.

It sometimes happens that the RBC Project Leadership team participates in a one-day RBC workshop followed by a one-day orientation on the roles and function of the Results Council. Typically, each member of the RBC Project Leadership team is provided with the RBC curriculum reading materials and, depending upon their sense of urgency in terms of launching the implementation, they either have the luxury of creating a "book club" and exploring the individual chapters in-depth over time, or they may have an immersion program in which everyone consumes the materials quickly. That immersion or rapid-cycle program sometimes entails reading the RBC book and the articles prior to an all-day Results Council meeting. During this day, there is focused conversation about the concepts within the book and any immediately foreseen implications for the organization's implementation. Additionally, at an all-day meeting, the group views each of the videos after which the same focused dialogue takes place, identifying key concepts and exploring implications for RBC implementation.

Often these meetings work best when they are off-site, informal and catered, so that a focus on building the group's energy while having fun can prevent feeling overwhelmed. No matter what form it takes, however, the immersion program is essential as the first step no matter how urgent the implementation seems.

After the RBC immersion program, each member of the Results Council (and all managers of units involved in the first wave of RBC implementation) participates in a *LEO* workshop. The skills unique to *LEO* help individuals to lead change effectively because it gives the entire leadership body a shared experience, a common language, and concrete skills and behaviors that are unique to leading a change process. *Leading an Empowered Organization* prepares leaders to be acutely aware of the potential to get in the way of the empowerment process without even realizing it. It creates consciousness, allowing participants to walk away knowing precisely what to do and what not to do in order to lead a fully empowered staff. The shared experience is important because leaders can then also support each other in their quest to create a culture in which the word *empowerment* has real meaning in the organization.

When *Reigniting the Spirit of Caring* is selected by an organization as a way to inspire staff and managers, it is recommended that the Results Council attend the *RSC* workshop as soon as possible within the "getting smarter" process so that they can lead the way.

After the RBC Project Leadership team has completed its RBC immersion, this team must commit to keeping in touch with new information throughout the process of implementation. The RBC recommended reading list, however abbreviated, is already quite a commitment. However, it's important that this group understands that its work is not over. They need to find ways to continue their learning to lead initially, to sustain gains and to continually evolve the culture of RBC within the organization

---

There are leaders who are not intimately involved in RBC implementation, but must still be informed enough to fully support the project. In most organizations the Results Council will create an educational program for these individuals that generally includes reading the RBC book, reading the RBC Principles as adopted by their own organization, and attending a *LEO* workshop or at least a one-day *LEO* overview session.

In addition, periodic briefings with the RBC project leadership team and a CHCM consultant help the executive team and medical staff to link the project with the overall strategic mission, vision and values of the organization. This has proven useful in keeping these influential leaders linked to the organization's march toward a new culture. Getting to executive groups can be as tough as it is essential, because they may be on the periphery of the organization's move to RBC, and they are an exceptionally busy group. The bottom line is: This group has to know enough to be able to be fully supportive. These remaining executives and key medical staff

Preparing the Remaining Executive Team and Key Medical Staff Leaders for RBC Implementation

leaders have an open invitation to attend *LEO, RSC,* and the 5-day *Relationship-Based Care Leader Practicum*, and, while their participation in these opportunities for team immersion is not absolutely essential to the success of the implementation, it has proven its value time and again to both the leaders themselves and those who interact with them.

One of the most outstanding examples of expanding the depth of understanding of the full executive team occurred when a chief nurse attended a *Relationship-Based Care Leader Practicum* with the Chief Operations Officer, the Executive for Human Resources and two other key executive colleagues. This shared experience grounded each of them in a deep and personalized understanding of what RBC could provide in their organization. It fortified them as a team. They attended the *Relationship-Based Care Leader Practicum* after their RBC project team had attended, so while the Chief Operations Officer and fellow executives had previously been supportive, they now walked away unshakably committed to RBC—and to each other. In another instance, the Chief Nurse attended with the Chief Operations Officer and the Chief Medical Officer. Their experience paralleled the previous example and they left with clarity and a commitment as a team that exceeded their expectations.

The RBC leadership team should always be looking for ways, over time, to engage the remaining executive team members and key medical staff leaders in RBC-related information and education. This significant group must be kept in the loop as thoroughly and efficiently as possible.

Preparing Members of the Unit Practice Councils

Members of the Unit Practice Councils read and view the same materials that are offered to the RBC Leadership team. This group goes through the same preparation including the full-day meetings, the group immersion, and so forth, but it always follows the leadership team. The content and sequencing of learning activities for the UPCs is part of the customized organizational design.

While this group doesn't usually participate in the *LEO* workshop, it almost always participates in *Reigniting the Spirit of Caring* and/or *Leadership at the Point of Care.* Typically they would also have a one-day RBC Kick-off (see page 520), followed by an orientation on the roles and functions of the Unit Practice Council.

After this foundational work, many organizations ask CHCM to provide a *Work Complexity Assessment* (see page 263). This 2-day intervention engages the UPC members in examining their work environment, the complexity of patient care requirements, professional practice, delegation, potential within the unit, and current work allocation realities. This *WCA* and its related conversations inform the UPC regarding how best to translate the RBC principles into action plans specific to their units.

The volume of materials to be digested initially can seem overwhelming, and yet a systematic and consistent approach to getting all members on the same page at the same time is absolutely invaluable and saves time in the end. The process of transformation to RBC must be knowledge based.

The Five Conditions for Engaging in Change: The 5 Cs

—Jayne A. Felgen and Mary Koloroutis

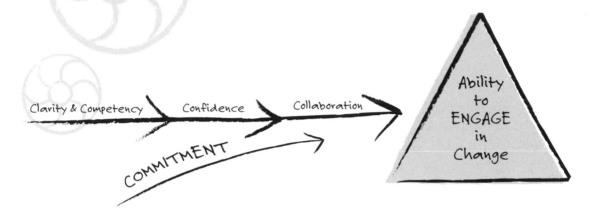

This model illustrates all of the elements that enable individuals to engage in change. While the model has five elements in it, the first two elements—clarity and competency—create sufficient momentum for the rest of the model to fall into place with relative ease. The other three elements—confidence, collaboration and commitment—are natural outgrowths of clarity and competency.

In the transformation of an organization's current culture to one of Relationship-Based Care (RBC), the change that individuals are asked to commit to is an intensely personal one. All are asked to interact in new ways with patients, each other and the organization itself. Because any change challenges us to "begin where we are," it is essential that we have a clear perception of where we are and where we want to go. In this model, having clarity means knowing yourself as a person, a leader, a colleague and a professional. It's about understanding your own thoughts and emotions as well as the ways you interact with others. It's about understanding you make a real difference and choosing to use yourself therapeutically.

When you are clear about the capacity and limitations of your role, as well as others' roles, you will be more effective. Clarity is knowing what systems of care delivery support or diminish our professional practice. To have clarity also means to know what RBC means to you and to your organization. This type of clarity happens through reflection, dialogue and collective learning. It happens through asking questions such as: What is Relationship-Based Care? Why is it important? What will it specifically look like and feel like inside our culture? What evidence is available to support our decisions? To have clarity means to embody your understanding of RBC and what it means to you and to the organization as a whole.

There are also three well-established competency domains for clinicians. These are the clinical/technical, interpersonal and critical thinking domains. While the clinical/technical domain tends to get the lion's share of our attention, *each domain is equally essential to strong professional practice.* In order for individuals to interact effectively with patients and each other, they must have strong interpersonal skills. In order for care givers to be efficient at the point of care, they must also be skilled critical thinkers—and even creative thinkers. We believe there is a fourth essential competency that arises from mastery of these three, and that is leadership. When the other three domains are equally developed and balanced, individuals emerge as influential leaders.

A natural outgrowth of knowing who you are and acknowledging your own competence is the development of confidence. Confidence provides the emotional foundation for exercising judgment and taking action. It improves our ability to build interpersonal relationships as we understand and value our own contribution and that of others. We recognize our talents and our limits. We know when to seek the expertise of others on behalf of our patients. We are clear about what we have to offer— what others can count on us for—and we therefore "show up," fully present and prepared to contribute as a full-fledged member of the team. This confidence emerges in both our personal and professional abilities and in our clarity regarding our own professional role.

In our own confidence, we inspire confidence in others. This confidence is one of the keys to effective collaboration.

> A natural outgrowth of knowing who you are and acknowledging your own competence is the development of confidence. Confidence provides the emotional foundation for exercising judgment and taking action.

True collaboration or partnership is based on mutual respect and trust. When individuals understand what they have to offer, feel competent and confident in their ability to accomplish the work, and respect the contributions of others, collaboration—the true collaboration of teamwork—thrives. And in health care, truly collaborative teamwork has been identified as the number one predictor of safe, high-quality care.

In our own confidence, we inspire confidence in others.

Undergirding the continuum from clarity and competency into confidence and collaboration is commitment. True commitment to accomplishing a shared goal is the highest level of ownership. Shared commitment creates a sense of unity and interdependence among team members. When we are committed to a common goal, committed to each other, and committed to the betterment of the organization, we work as One to create the changes we all desire.

Leading an Empowered Organization:
The Magic of *LEO*

—Leah Kinnaird

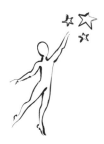

Leading an Empowered Organization (*LEO*) has an intriguing history. Its roots lie in a class for 13 nursing managers, first offered in the basement of Marie Manthey's home in September 1982. It has since grown to be an international movement shaping how people can be empowered within hierarchical structures, whether they be small groups like families or large groups like the National Health Service in the United Kingdom (UK) of 1.3 million people. *LEO* has been taught in nine countries, translated into five languages, and presented thousands of times as a 3-day workshop. It has withstood the test of time with relatively little change to the core framework. In fact, if anyone suggests *LEO* is old, I quickly respond, "So is the theory of gravity." *LEO* owes its staying power to its own extraordinary *power to empower.*

The debate about whether empowerment can exist in hierarchical organizations (which all health care and nearly all organizations are) is longstanding (Argyris, 1998). The magic of *LEO* is that it addresses how to work in decentralized ways within centralized organizations.

I remember the first time I made that statement to a group of facilitators. One participant's eyes got wide; she relaxed into her chair and exhaled a big breath that ruffled the hair on her forehead; then said, "Oh, I'm so glad I'm not going to be expected to reorganize the National Health Service." And that's the magic: to lead effectively in spite of the hierarchy. Instead of fighting the structure, we can be empowered to work within it with a judicious and practical approach.

My own experience with *LEO* began in 1987 when I attended the predecessor to *LEO*, Creative Health Care Management's *Leading Empowered Staff* (*LES*) seminar in Minneapolis. At that point I had attended many workshops on leadership and acquired considerable formal hours of credit in organizational development and counseling. I thought I knew a lot about leadership, but the *LES* experience gave me fresh insight. It helped me to put all of the management theory I had learned into actual practice. I came away inspired, with a set of tools that enabled me to create the kind of environment that had long been desired by the staff members I was leading. I learned how to give them all the information to do their jobs without my abandoning them or micromanaging them. The message spilled over to my personal life as well; I am probably a lot easier to live with since my experience with *LEO*. My primary learning has been a broader, more deeply integrated understanding of empowerment.

Many organizations have a history of talking about empowerment, but not "living" it. Simply put, it can be oppressive (the antithesis of empowering) to work in a centralized organization with layers of authority and a plethora of rules, regulations and documentation. Education is key to overcoming oppression, and the core concepts of the *LEO* workshop provide the political insight into the organization and the personal competencies to become someone who leads for empowerment.

In the UK, so many people have "been on the *LEO* course" that it is common to hear that a participant has been "*LEOed.*" In other words, the person has been inspired to change the way he or she leads. For that reason, I find it helpful to let the executive team know the core content that is going to be covered ahead of time, so that they can actively support the new spirit of enthusiasm and effectively model the approach to leading in the organization.

At times it is bewildering to those who work with someone who has been "*LEOed*" because they are so used to embedded behaviors of the former leadership style. In those situations, it is handy to say "You need to know I went to this workshop" as an opener, to say "Once I was one way; now I am this way." The results can be that dramatic.

Sustaining a culture of working in decentralized ways, being empowered, and creating an environment of empowerment can require occasional, well-timed follow-up sessions to help keep people on track. This can be done through formal

> The magic of LEO is that it addresses how to work in decentralized ways within centralized organizations.
>
> LEO is about the structure of organizations and teams— "the architecture of relationships."

reviews or through regular but informal gatherings where *LEO* principles are shared and group members can learn from each other. What we have learned through the expansive use of the *LEO* workshop is that once there is a language of leadership that the critical mass of employees understands, productivity and systematic improvements in processes occur faster.

We have also learned that the language of leadership transfers from culture to culture, which is a bit of a surprise considering the possible misinterpretations. We have hammered out definitions of responsibility, authority and accountability in German, Italian, Chinese, Portuguese and both British and American English through dialogue intended to clarify meaning and transfer the use of concepts. In the end, it is clear that *LEO* is about the structure of organizations and teams—or what we call "the architecture of relationships." Inspiring leaders to work as fully empowered team members within existing organizational structures drives straight to the heart of the mission of every organization that values exceptional care and service.

There are many ways for organizations to take part in *LEO*. Creative Health Care Management offers *LEO* as a 3-day workshop, for clients' employees as well as for the general public. A one-day *Shot in the Arm* workshop, available to organizations that have had *LEO* in-house, helps participants deepen their understanding of the content, reinforce behaviors they learned and strengthen the building efforts. The one-day *Executive Overview* session provides an overview of the key concepts for vice presidents, directors, coordinators, clinical specialists and representatives from staff development. Facilitator training and licensing are available to provide organizations flexibility.

Argyris, A. (1998). Empowerment: The emperor's new clothes. *Harvard Business Review*, 76(3): 98–105.

Responsibility, Authority and Accountability

—Marie Manthey

Decentralization of decision making is a hallmark of work environments that empower care givers to be true leaders at the point of care. The three elements that are necessary for role clarity and organizational effectiveness are exactly the same as the three elements necessary for personal growth to full maturity. These elements are: Responsibility, Authority and Accountability (R+A+A). These three concepts should be seen as legs on a three-legged stool: All are equally important. They also need to be clearly defined.

Care givers can work with confidence within established parameters when each individual understands his or her:

- *scope of Responsibility,*
- *level of Authority, and*
- *Accountability (ownership) for processes and outcomes of practice*

Responsibility: The Ability to Respond

Responsibility is the clear and specific allocation of duties in order to achieve desired results. Areas of responsibility need to be clearly allocated, so that everyone understands who is responsible for what and when. Generally speaking, responsibility for actions, functions or outcomes is defined by someone in an authority position.

For example, boards of directors give CEOs the responsibility to operate an institution according to the charter or mission defined by the board. This individual then decides (on the basis of available resources and his/her philosophy of management) how to divide up the specific functions and gives responsibility to individuals who agree to accept that responsibility. This line of responsibility can be clearly followed within the nursing department, from the nurse manager to the Staff Nurses specific to the responsibility for nursing care of patients. The nurse manager has the overall responsibility for the quality of care administered to all the patients on his/her unit, 24 hours a day, 7 days a week. The assignment of nurses to patients is the allocation of responsibility to a specific person for a particular period of time. Responsibility also comes from practice acts, job descriptions, delegation and self-assignment.

Managers often complain that some staff members do not 'have accountability': what they mean is that individuals haven't accepted responsibility.

Assignment of responsibility is a two-way process. Responsibility is visibly given and visibly accepted, meaning that if a manager has assigned a responsibility to a staff member, but the staff member has not clearly accepted the responsibility, responsibility has not been established. At best, responsibilities are clearly assigned and clearly accepted.

Authority: The Right to Take Action

Authority is the right to act and make decisions in the areas where one is given and accepts responsibility. It is vitally important that the level of authority delegated is commensurate with the scope of responsibility. Any disparity between these two elements will result in unhealthy situations for the workers, and will eventually create a toxic work environment. Just as clarity of responsibility is essential for healthy operations, so too is clarity of the levels of authority. The levels on the following page need to be understood and clearly articulated at the beginning of a decision-making process.

Accountability: The Retrospective Review of the Work Done and Decisions Made to Determine Whether or Not They Were Appropriate

While most of us think in terms of being accountable to others, in this model accountability begins when care givers review and reflect upon their own actions and decisions, and culminates with a personal assessment that helps them to determine the best actions to take in the future. It begins with a look back, and ends with a plan to build on what has worked well in the past while making whatever changes may be necessary to promote one's own best practice in the future.

It has been frequently stated that the role of the Clinical Nurse Manager (CNM) is the most important role in the hospital. He or she is responsible for the point of care "24/7" and facilitates achievement of the patient care delivery model, team collaboration and continuity of care. There is no question that leadership training is a requirement for such a position. Since leadership training is costly and a return on investment (ROI) often not calculated, executive support for these types of programs can be minimal. Collaboration among senior leaders, particularly between the Chief Nursing Officer (CNO) and the Chief Executive Officer (CEO), can make a positive difference for both program design and support. Moreover the inclusion of strategically-linked projects with ROI calculations can transform a "nice to have" 3-day leadership program into a "must have" 3-day program and can even spark the question as to when the next program will begin!

Levels of Authority:

Level 1: **Data/Information/Idea Gathering**

Authority to collect information/data and provide to another to make the final decision and determine what action will be taken.

Level 2: **Data/Information/Idea Gathering + Recommendations**

Authority to collect information, weigh the options and recommend actions to be taken to another who will make final decision.

Level 3: **Data/Information/Idea Gathering + Recommendations (Pause to communicate, clarify or negotiate) + Take Action**

Authority to apply critical thinking, weigh the options, recommend actions, negotiate the final decision. Includes pausing and collaborating with others before taking action.

Level 4: **Act + Inform others after taking action**

Authority to assess, decide and act. May follow up and inform another of the actions taken as required by the situation.

Developing High Performers with CEO Support and Involvement: The Clinical Nurse Manager Leadership Institute

—Lynda Olender

Clinical Nurse Manager Leadership Institute Program Overview

The program is designed to bridge the gap between the complex responsibilities of managers today with critical leadership skills needed to achieve unit level and organizational excellence. Additionally, the expectation is that the project will link to a strategic priority, be implemented at the unit level and achieve measurable outcomes. Graduation from the institute ends with a presentation from each participant and includes a cost-benefit versus cost-avoidance analysis for each project.

The training format is highly interactive and includes group work, role-play scenarios and sharing of personal stories and best practices. Involvement by and input from the CEO is crucial to the success of this program. Coaching and mentoring are also key components of the leadership institute and are integral to the participants' achievement of program objectives, particularly as related to strategically linked project identification, design and evaluation.

Editors' note: *Lynda Olender describes a leadership program for Clinical Nurse Managers developed in collaboration with the Chief Executive Officers (CEOs) of five medical centers with a network of VA hospitals. The CEO's input, as well as the CEO's role as program faculty, provides a model for developing and supporting excellent management practices within organizations. Additionally, as one of the primary stakeholders for this initiative, the CEO should be included in participant satisfaction measures.*

Program Design

Week I: Program Introduction and Personal Development Planning

Week one focuses on "self." Discussion related to personal development is through interactive exploration of Steven Covey's *Seven Habits of Highly Effective People* and by incorporating 360-degree evaluations into a personal development plan for each participant. Additionally, having the organization's network officer or CEO present in the introductory sessions sets the tone of the conference, establishes how important the conference is, and helps participants identify what their quality improvement project will be—and how the project will contribute to the individual's overall growth and development.

Week II: Interpersonal Effectiveness, Managing Human Capital and Related Business Skills

The second week is all about "other." A keynote speaker presents on the manager's obligation toward the public trust via "Law, Regulation, and Ethics in the Health Care Environment." An expert panel comprising, at least in part, the organization's own Human Resources department discusses and provides insight on common personnel and labor management issues. Interpersonal and business skills including conflict management, negotiation skills, health care economics, proficiency and report writing (including the presentation of data for reports) are also addressed. Additionally, CNMs are provided with workshops related to the design and implementation of performance-based interviewing. The managers also participate in a "Boot Camp" to develop and enhance fast feedback and coaching skills.

Week III: Transition to Relationship-Based Care (RBC) and the Collaborative Care Delivery Model

Preparation for a smooth transition to Relationship-Based Care (RBC) is a primary focus of week three. Experts in relationship-based scheduling present the concept of the Attending or Primary Nurses arranging their schedules to align with their patients' length of stay. Week three also features a workshop that teaches managers to redesign their units and to revisit RBC principles and their application to practice. Managers are challenged to stretch the concept of Relationship-Based Care to consider a collaborative care delivery model—one where physician and nurse admit and follow the same caseload of patients throughout their inpatient stay. This optimizes the likelihood for a seamless approach to the inpatient care for a select patient population.

Graduation of the participants occurs on the last night. "Best Practice" presentations of the aforementioned strategically-linked projects are made by the CNMs, and a graduation dinner with presentation of certificates is appropriately labeled "The Finale." Each project is presented in such a way that its content can easily be used in a poster session and serve as an outline for publication.

Organizational Facilitation and Oversight of the Program

Oversight by the CNO and Education Manager is a crucial element to the success of this program as it ensures continued review of program goals and objectives and just-in-time adjustment of intern-specific schedules and related didactic and experiential learning objectives.

Participants keep up to date with project progress. Each week and throughout the year, the project selected by each participant evolves, and input from the participant's mentor (in this case the CNO from each site) should be continuous from the inception of the project to its final presentation stage. Lastly, it is the mentor who encourages, guides and/or participates actively with the end in mind. This includes ensuring that measurable outcomes are possible and can be compared with baseline measures and that communication of the project via submission to a professional forum or journal is an expectation of the program.

Steps Toward Customizing the Program to Fit Your Organization

Assess learning needs of potential participants

Assess the learning needs of the nurse managers across the organization. Input should also be obtained from Nurse

Executives and Chief Executive Officers. The importance of taking time for the process of acquiring the information cannot be understated since it solicits buy-in, and the information gained proves invaluable when planning the curriculum. Since the cost of a 3-week program can be significant, face-to-face interviews for conducting needs assessments are preferable.

Solicit CEO involvement from the "get-go"

Plan for a CEO panel and have CEOs present their most innovative initiatives. Ask them to share what they perceive are the most critical areas where they believe the nurse managers can make the most positive difference. Facilitate the presentation of measures where opportunities are most needed. This may be related to quality initiatives (new or innovative solutions to regulatory mandates), cost factors (such as productivity, overtime, etc.) and patient and/or staff satisfaction goals.

Select the right participants

Each organization's Nurse Executive should interview the prospective candidates and select only those candidates who meet prescribed selection criteria to the planning committee. Although this program is targeted for current nurse managers, you may wish to extend training to assistant nurse managers and/or RNs in training for managerial positions. In addition to performance-based competency assessments, selection criteria should also include evidence of outstanding or highly satisfactory performance in clinical nursing practice, exemplary interpersonal relationships and highly satisfactory time and attendance.

Participants must also be interested in and committed to a leadership role as a nurse manager, motivated for continuous learning and professional development, willing to complete all requirements of the program (including the project), and be able to attend all 3 scheduled weeks of offerings.

Select the right faculty

One of the most notable aspects of this program is the inclusion of the organization's own experts as faculty when appropriate. Examples include the scheduling of the network director and a panel of CEOs and CNOs from the involved organizations to kick off the program.

It is wise to provide opportunities for leaders within the organization to share their expertise. For example, scheduling the Fiscal Officer and Human Resources personnel to present "Managing Human Capital" provides organization-specific information and sets a precedent for collaboration between manager and faculty down the road. Other examples include having contrasting presentations, such as having the organization's Equal Employment Opportunity Manager lead an exploration of "Interpersonal Effectiveness" and the facility's legal counsel (lawyer) discuss how interpersonal conflict can translate into arbitration and ultimately a court date if not handled correctly.

Examples of Program Outcome Measures

Upon successful completion of the program, participants will continue to develop, implement and evaluate project outcomes unique to the participant and his/her organization. Additionally, a forum for sharing and exporting projects should be facilitated, and poster presentations and publications should also be an outcome expectation. Examples of potential projects likely to be endorsed by the CEO and CNO are as follows:

- *increased patient satisfaction and reduction in staff turnover rates*
- *reduction of staff incivility and reduced staff-to-staff altercations*
- *increased OR productivity with decreased OR overtime utilization*
- *safe patient handling and use of lifting devices and reduced staff lifting injuries (and related worker's compensation claims)*
- *increased staff satisfaction and decreased staff absenteeism*
- *increased patient health education related to patients with congestive heart failure and reduced readmission rates*
- *reduction of unplanned clinic and ER visits for patients receiving telehealth services at home*

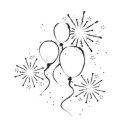

In summary, even the highest quality leadership programs will only bring long-term benefits if leaders make a conscious effort to integrate a specific return on investment prior to embarking on the program. Moreover the return on investment should be related to the organization's strategic goals. Additionally, the benefit of mentoring for each nurse manager can fuel continued progress in selected strategically linked projects that are beneficial to manager and organization alike. Lastly—the celebration of the project and related outcomes by all can set the tone for lasting success!

References: Department of Veterans Affairs. *The high performance model.* Updated June 23, 2005, retrieved February 22, 2006 from http://vaww. va.gov/hpdm/

Maguire, M., Spencer, K., & Sabatier, K. (2004). The nurse manager academy: An innovative approach to managerial competency development. *Nursing Leadership Forum,* 8(4), 133-137.

Mathena, K. A. (2002). Nursing manager leadership skills. *Journal of Nursing Administration,* 32(3), 136-142.

The Evolution of Nursing in the UK: A Commitment to Nationwide Nursing Leadership Development

—Gayle Garland

The Origins of Nursing in the UK

Before the modern age, nursing care in the United Kingdom (UK) was provided by nuns and other religious women, and in some cases by monks. The title "Sister" is still used in England today, especially by patients, to denote the person in charge of a ward. By the 1800s there was a need to supplement the capacity of religious communities in large cities to provide for the needs of the poor. A series of voluntary hospitals opened, funded by legacies, donations, subscriptions, and fund-raising events sponsored by philanthropists and political and industrial leaders. Only the poor were eligible for hospital care; the "better-off" were treated in their own homes.

Because of the generally poor conditions in hospitals and the exposure to disease, death and filth, hospital nursing in the early 1800s was considered low-status work. It was not uncommon that nursing attracted women who were considered too dishonest, slovenly or drunken for other occupations. There were no formal training programmes and nurses had similar status to common servants.

Hospital and nursing standards improved through the efforts of women such as Florence Nightingale. Born into a privileged family and privately educated, Nightingale was not content with the life of a gentlewoman. Choosing not to marry, she dedicated her life to a number of social causes including hospitals, public health and nursing. She was an accomplished observer and a prolific writer who used her social standing and connections to achieve her aims.

Nightingale argued that taking care of sick people in hospital was a skilled and important role. She and other like-minded women were instrumental in founding schools of nursing where "respectable" women were recruited to become trained nurses. Nightingale was very clear about the nature of nursing. The following quotation from *Notes on Nursing, What It Is and What It Is Not* shaped the origins of modern nursing internationally:

In watching disease, both in the private homes and in public hospitals, the thing which strikes the experienced observer most forcibly is this: that the symptoms or suffering generally considered to be inevitable … are very often not symptoms of the disease at all, but of something quite differ-ent—of the want of fresh air, or of warmth, or of quiet, or of cleanliness, or of … care in the administration of diet.

If the patient is cold, if a patient is feverish, if a patient is faint, if he is sick after taking food, if he has a bed-sore, it is the fault not of the disease but of the nursing.

I use the word nursing for want of a better. It has been limited to signify little more than the administration of medicines and the application of poultices. It ought to signify the proper use of fresh air, light, warmth, cleanliness, quiet and the proper selection and admin-istration of diet—all at the least expense of vital power to the patient. (Nightingale, 1859, pp. 6-7)

Nightingale went on to say that in addition to managing the "sanitary factors" (as she called them), professional nurses had the responsibility to observe the patients to notice changes in their condition. Managing sanitary factors and acting on obser-vation were identified as essential to professional nursing.

The final factor identified by Nightingale as essential to professional nursing was to "take charge" of her ward (or the home) to ensure that the patient did not suffer in her absence. She was informed that she had the responsibility for what hap-pened when she was not there, and was instructed to exercise her authority to tell others what to do. Though the word *man-agement* was not attached to this responsibility by Nightingale, it clearly aligns with the origins of management as a concept during the industrial revolution.

Increasingly, from the middle of the 19th century, people in Britain came to believe that public access to health care (not just for the people who could afford it) was part of the structure of civilized society. By the 1940s, the health services that existed were unfortunately uncoordinated, patchy and struggling for funds. The quality of services varied widely from town to town, and country areas were generally poorly served. Two world wars had left Britain's economy in tatters: Health needs were high and few people could afford to pay. If the country was to have a future, the population needed to be strong and healthy. The answer was to create the National Health Service (NHS) in 1948.

Different models of national provision were proposed, but eventually the model suggested by Aneurin Bevan was adopted. The following principles were to determine the future of health care in Britain, and continue to influence it today.

- *The NHS is financed virtually 100% from central taxation. (The rich therefore pay more than the poor for comparable benefits.)*

- *Everyone is eligible for care—even people temporarily residing in or visiting the country. Anybody could be referred to any hospital, local or more distant.*

- *Care was entirely free at the beginning, though prescription, dental and optometrist charges have been introduced since the founding of the NHS. Medical and hospital care remain entirely free without co-payment or any personal supplement (Geoffrey, 1998).*

Professionally trained nurses provided by the schools of nursing soon became a respected and effective part of the provision of health services even before the founding of the NHS. Nursing won its place beside the medical staff and administrators as essential to the running of hospitals. Nurses managed all aspects of the ward, often with a kind of military efficiency. This style of nursing was well suited to the early days of the National Health Service when money was tight, demand was high and standards were variable.

During the first waves of reform of the NHS (in the 1960s and '70s) it became clear that nursing had a strong role to play. Not only was nursing the largest workforce in the NHS; nurses were very important to the public. Nurses were well respected and seen to be aligned with the patients' best interests.

But nursing itself was in need of reform. Respect for the vocational heritage and apprenticeship training model were strong, but there was also a growing realization that nursing was failing to keep up with the times. Allied health professionals were all trained to degree level, as were teachers and other comparable groups. The complexities and demands of modern care, and the rising consumer awareness of the public, brought the traditional models of nursing into question. A national review of nursing led to a number of important changes. Hospital-based nursing schools were to close as nursing education moved into the universities. Nurses became able to prescribe medicines (in limited circumstances) and roles were revised and expanded.

There are those who would say that nursing lost its way on the road to modernization. Taking nursing training out of hospital schools meant that the close connection of nurses to *their* wards and *their* patients was lost. Less hands-on experience was provided in the university-based courses, and new graduates were seen as less capable than they should have been. Nurses trained under the old system were critical of the new ways, and hospitals had to invest in mentoring and orientation programmes that had been largely unnecessary in the past. Restructuring and outsourcing of support services meant that the "Sister" was no longer in control of the sanitary factors (as Nightingale called them); combine this with inadequate funding, and it was no wonder that infection rates rose, nutrition standards fell and patients started to grumble. Shortage of staff had become a problem across the service, including nursing. Waiting times for surgery went up, medical beds were full and patients stacked up in the emergency departments. Failures in care, though not many, had become a news item. Something had to change.

A Commitment to Nationwide Nursing Leadership Development

In addition to reforming its own house, nursing was seen as essential in the reform of the service as a whole. At least three national policy documents published over 20 years cited nursing as a key to the future of health care. I think Nightingale would have approved as she always saw professional nursing as having a role and responsibility to ensure that the patient got what was needed. She advocated that nursing should never be under the control of doctors or hospital administrators, but should stand independently as equal to the medical and management functions. It seems that the National Health Service was coming to the same conclusion, and it made the monumental decision to invest in the leadership development of nursing in a substantial way. Leadership development was seen as essential in enabling nurses to have the impact on health care that was needed, and to rekindle the clarity of role and quality of care the public deserved.

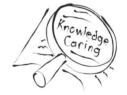

The Department of Health, through various governmental agencies, commissioned a wide range of leadership programmes for nurses starting in 1997. Programs were designed for nurses at all levels and roles across the service. The most ambitious undertaking of the national programme was to offer leadership development to nurses in first-level supervision and management roles. This decision was made in recognition that the quality of leadership at the first line affects the "feel and function" of the clinical area and the effectiveness of nursing staff, and therefore has a substantial influence on patient care.

National *Leading an Empowered Organization* (*LEO*) Programme

Over a 4-year span, 35,000 nurses and allied health professionals participated in the *LEO* programme. This mammoth undertaking was accomplished through the selection and preparation of facilitators from across the nation to train to deliver the programme. Each trainer committed to holding at least six workshops a year in their areas, and to attend refresher and development programmes. In the end, close to 400 facilitators were active all over the country helping people to learn leadership skills.

An independent evaluation of the programme was undertaken and the results were very positive. On the whole, participants enjoyed the experience and many reported a new enthusiasm for nursing and for the supervisory and management roles they were in. Many said that the programme had given them skills to tackle difficult issues such as poor communication and to improve their working relationships with others (Woolnough & Faugier, 2002).

The *LEO* programme remains a cornerstone of leadership development across the NHS. As of 2006, more than 100,000 health professionals, board members and support staff from the NHS have attended. One organization that is deeply committed to *LEO* and has put a substantial number of staff through the programme was praised by the British equivalent of Joint Commission for its excellence in leadership. As is always the challenge with development, it is hard to prove that participation in the programme has an impact on patient care. However, the nurses who have reported the strongest personal impact from attending the programme are convinced that they are making a difference to the quality of patient care (Woolnough and Faugier, 2002).

Leadership at the Point of Care

Following on from the success of *LEO*, it was decided that staff nurses should have the opportunity to develop their leadership skills. Leadership in this programme meant leading care rather than aspiring to a formal supervisory or management role. *Leadership at the Point of Care* was intended to prepare nurses in line with the ideals of Nightingale, that every nurse should be willing to take charge and work with others to ensure that patients' needs are met. This workshop focuses on helping Staff Nurses to clarify their role and contribution, to work effectively with others and to renew their commitment to providing care.

An independent evaluation of this programme also shows positive results. Nurses feel reenergized, motivated and valued, and learn skills that they apply to improve the patient experience. Each participant is asked to make a change that will positively impact care. The emphasis is on small actions within the direct control of staff. Some of these small changes have resulted in some of the most profound effects. One nurse decided that every visitor to a nursing home should be brought a cup of tea within 15 minutes of arrival. She expected that visitors would see it as a gracious gesture and no more. What happened is that the cup of tea provided an opportunity for visitors and nurses to talk, resulting in greater understanding on both sides and better care for the patient. Complaints dropped, satisfaction rose and all this at the price of a hot drink.

Summary

Florence Nightingale was convinced that it is the role of professional nurses to take charge, not being afraid to tell others what to do in the interests of the patient. She would no doubt approve of the national programmes of leadership development. Nightingale's nurses were also expected to take ownership of the patient experience, ensuring that ventilation, lighting, sanitation, food and quiet were abundant. She always saw nursing as having a role beyond service or compliance; she saw nurses as having a responsibility for ensuring that the patient was in the best situation to allow healing to occur.

The national leadership programmes were a public statement of commitment to nursing, to its contribution and importance, and to applying the talents of nurses to the public good. The British people remain as deeply committed to the principles that founded the health service as they were in 1948. Though the form and function of the health service will continue to evolve, I have no doubt that nurses are better prepared than ever before to have a profound and positive impact on that evolution.

References: Nightingale, F. (1859). *Notes on nursing.* London: Lippincott.

Geoffrey, R. (1998). *Short NHS history.*, National Health Service Retrieved June 20, 2006 History: From Cradle to Grave from http://www.nhshistory.net/short_history.htm

Woolnough, H., & Faugier, J. (2002). An evaluative study assessing the impact of the Leading an Empowered Organization programme. *NTresearch*, 7, 412-427.

CHAPTER FOURTEEN

Education for Professionals in Relationship-Based Care

Enhancing Nurses' Capacity for Compassionate Caring

—Kristen M. Swanson

Research provides ample evidence that caring matters (Swanson, 1999). It matters to those who provide caring, and it matters to the patients who receive it. We know that when nurses engage in caring practices they realize a stronger sense of accomplishment, better self-esteem, enhanced feelings of gratitude and purpose, higher respect for life, deeper satisfaction with their role, fuller awareness of living within their own values, and improvements in their skills, knowledge, connectedness and collegiality. Moreover, patients in receipt of excellent nurse care experience a deeper sense of relationship with their nurse and feel more relaxed, happy, trusting, grateful, safe and satisfied. Compassionate caring by nurses also leads to improvements in the patient's physical healing, sense of self-determination, confidence and mental attitude. Receipt of caring has been shown to increase the self-esteem, dignity and self-worth of patients, while offering them increased knowledge and coping capacity and enrichments in their personal development, quality of life and overall well-being.

Clearly, organizations that support compassionate caring stand to realize improvements in overall nurse, patient and family satisfaction. What, then, does it take to enhance the likelihood that compassionate caring will occur at the point of care? Is it possible that a unit could be staffed with the most capable and committed nurses and still find indicators of nurse and patient satisfaction lagging? What might be the culprit? As I discovered when writing a state of the science paper about caring, the gap between nurses' capacity for and commitment to caring and the actual occurrence of caring might well lie in an organization's failure to take into account any one of three conditions that enhance or diminish the likelihood that compassionate caring will be practiced by nurses at the bedside. These conditions may be directly related to the patient, nurse or organization (Swanson, 1999).

> Clearly, organizations that support compassionate caring stand to realize improvements in overall nurse, patient and family satisfaction. What, then, does it take to enhance the likelihood that compassionate caring will occur at the point of care?

As in any human relationship, the "players" and context matter. In the nurse-patient or nurse-family relationship, all bring to the equation personalities, life stories and expectations that shape the way their interactions unfold.

Three Conditions That Impact Caring

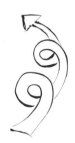

1. Starting at the level of patients and families, let us consider why some nurses might find it easier or more difficult to enter into caring interactions. Whether studying seasoned professionals or student novices, researchers have provided evidence that nurses are more likely to engage in caring practices with patients who are more cheerful, in greater need of nursing assistance and accepting of their own illnesses. Nurses are also more likely to enact caring practices with patients who are vulnerable, distressed, sicker and whose families are more engaged. Nurses are less likely to fully access their caring potential with patients and/or families who are verbally abusive, angry, combative,

unattractive, unwilling to communicate, resisting support, unusually demanding and in denial.

2. There are also things about the nurses themselves that enhance or diminish the likelihood that they will access their full capacity for caring. Be they personal or professional in origin, the demands, constraints and resources nurses bring to the point of care will shape the way their nurse-patient/family interactions unfold. Resources, in the form of life experiences (good upbringing, spiritual grounding, sensitizing encounters with death and illness), personal strengths (robust coping abilities, accurate self-appraising, effective self-caring practices, strong intuition, inner harmony, personal accountability), adequate knowledge (having witnessed excellent role models, been exposed to good book learning, being technologically savvy, having considerable practice experience) and a sense of congruence (agreeing with colleagues' care, truth-telling, practicing in accordance with one's own values, feeling respected) all serve to prime the nurses' likelihood of acting from a position of caring. On the other hand, constraints such as physical fatigue, unresolved conflicts with their own families or colleagues, repeated witnessing of untoward outcomes and an inability to get along with a given patient and/or family will all get in the way of adequate caring. Lastly, if there are too many competing home and work demands, nurses may find themselves "spread so thin" that they risk showing up at the point of care bereft of anything left to give.

3. The environmental context of care—be it viewed at the level of unit, hospital or society—also weighs in when it comes to the likelihood that nurses will act in a caring manner toward patients, families, colleagues or even themselves.

What follows are some solutions for eliminating, or even preventing, infrastructural, interpersonal, educational, administrative and environmental barriers to compassionate caring.

Well-designed infrastructure

A computerized, well-networked, readily accessible infrastructure combined with a well-conceived worksite layout and attention to occupational safety can eliminate wasted footsteps, strained backs, unnecessary phone calls, unanswered e-mails, and the endless search for meds, pillows and 4X4's. By freeing up time and energy, nurses can actually focus on people. Organizational policies, physical layouts and procedures can truly make or break the quality of nursing care. In a review of 14 separate qualitative studies published between 1987 and 1996, I found evidence that organizational conditions related to personnel and role expectations, resource availability, administrative support and the practice environment all influence caring practices.

Healthy relationships

When nurses work with a sense of community and teamwork with engaged, noncritical, nondemanding colleagues who communicate well and freely share information, the caring potential of the group is maximized. It is also helpful to have work clearly divided by roles and respectful, nonpolitical, nonhierarchical relationships with medical staff.

Comfort with technology

When nurses are comfortable and experienced with the use of complex equipment and the technology is fully functioning, upgraded, and readily accessible, it can be a great boon to practice. On the other hand, becoming focused on technology can serve as a way to retreat from human interaction, and if overly relied on, computer-generated printouts, waveforms and calculations can easily override a nurse's intuition and experience.

Becoming focused on technology can serve as a way to retreat from human interaction, and if overly relied on, computer-generated printouts, waveforms and calculations can easily override a nurse's intuition and experience.

Nurse executives and managers who relate to nurses in a caring, respectful manner beget nurses who relate to patients, families and each other in a caring manner.

Executive/managerial leadership

An organization's administration can play a key role in nurses' capacity to care. Firstly, nurse executives and hospital administrators who value patient and family-centered caring and recognize that nurses play a key role in keeping patients safe, will make sound financial decisions that put resources at the point of care. The magnificent studies of Linda Aiken and her colleagues (2002, 2003) have provided evidence that hospitals with reasonable patient-to-nurse ratios and a predominance of baccalaureate prepared nurses consistently realize better patient outcomes. The administration also plays a key role in creating opportunities for nurses' wisdom to be shared and their voices to be heard beyond their immediate units. Organizations with shared governance demonstrate trust in nurses and leverage their abilities to guide policies that will ultimately lead to better practice and improved outcomes for patients, families, clinicians and the organization as a whole. Lastly, "administrative style" can also directly influence caring at the bedside. Nurse executives and managers who relate to nurses in a caring, respectful manner beget nurses who relate to patients, families and each other in a caring manner. Specifically, by being available to nurses, noticing and rewarding compassionate caring by nurses, garnering resources to enable nurse caring, and advocating for nurses, nurse administrators support nurses to engage in caring practices.

Environment

Offering less than adequate care and compromising quality for quantity of care can only go on so long before nurses (individually or collectively) give up hope and lose their capacity to practice from a position of compassion, optimism and openness.

Last, but far from least, the environmental conditions under which nurses work matter. When nurses have unclear role expectations or are overworked, underpaid and undervalued, it is bound to have an adverse affect on their work, health and commitment to nursing. Being exhausted, witnessing poor care, navigating crowded or poorly planned work sites, dealing with missing or malfunctioning equipment, and being unable to access meds, supplies, medical backup, or another set of hands, all take their toll on nurses. Offering less than adequate care and compromising quality for quantity of care can only go on so long before nurses (individually or collectively) give up hope and lose their capacity to practice from a position of compassion, optimism and openness.

Engagement in optimal caring acts by capable, committed clinicians is ultimately dependent upon good stage setting. Just as good theater relies on the presence of capable and committed actors, a well-written script, an inventive creative director, an interested audience and a setting prepared with great deliberateness, so too does exquisite patient and family-centered care rely on the presence of compassionate, knowledgeable nurses; a well-conceived and resourced infrastructure; strong, creative administrative support; receptive patients and families; and a physical setting conducive to the unfolding of caring, healing relationships.

References: Aiken, L., Clarke, S., Cheung, R., Sloane, D., & Silber, J. (2003). Educational levels of hospital nurses and surgical patient mortality. *Journal of the American Medical Association, 290*, 1617-1623.

Aiken, L. H., Clarke, S. P., Sloane, D. M., Sochalski, J., & Silber, J. H. (2002). Hospital nurse staffing and patient mortality, nurse burnout, and job dissatisfaction. *Journal of the American Medical Association, 288*, 1987-1993.

Swanson, K. M. (1999). What's known about caring in nursing: A literary meta-analysis. In A. S. Hinshaw, J. Shaver, and S. Feetham (Eds.), *Handbook of clinical nursing research* (pp. 31-60). Thousand Oaks, CA: Sage Publications.

Exemplar: Coaching at Marion General Hospital

—Linda Pullins and Carolyn Kile

By 2000, Marion General Hospital (MGH) in Marion, OH, had set a clear vision of the hospital they wanted to become over the next 5 years. The vision:

Marion General Hospital—The hospital where patients want to come for care, and staff and physicians want to come to work.

The commitment was in place to change our work by "looking at each process through the eyes of the patients," and we held the strong belief that this would be accomplished through each member of the care team by establishing a therapeutic and meaningful relationship with the patient. We knew that this would be essential for the healing process.

We knew what we wanted to become, but we were struggling with the how. How would we accomplish what seemed to be a monumental feat? How would we change the environment for our patients? Where would we even begin?

The Situation at MGH in the Year 2000

After the hospital merged with a competitor, RNs were leaving at an alarming rate. This was especially true in the medical/surgical units. There were no nurse managers on these units and no experienced and dedicated charge nurses that did not have a patient assignment on their shift. One lone director was attempting to handle all aspects of operations and employee concerns. The numbers of actual minutes spent by RNs at the bedside were reported in one productivity study as *14 minutes in a 12-hour shift!* Morale was low, physician and patient complaints high, and agency usage costs had peaked at nearly two million dollars per year. Patient safety was of great concern, because the remaining staff switched to "survival mode" to cope with the rapidly increasing workload. Task completions were the only focus for much of the nursing staff. Communication suffered at all levels and care was fragmented.

Our plan to adopt an outcome-focused, patient-centered care model was our answer to our problems. But now who could help implement such a plan? The answer became "professional coaches at the bedside"—individuals who possessed knowledge and skills that could be imparted in a hands-on, just-in-time approach every day.

How the Coaching Program Took Shape

The CNO and the CEO met with 10 RNs from various departments in the hospital. Many of these RNs had left the bedside to work in departments outside of direct patient care, due to burnout, frustration and embarrassment with the care their organization was providing. This group pledged a one year commitment to reinventing and revitalizing the care environment by agreeing to coach RNs on the medical/surgical units with the new patient care model. The corresponding pledge from the CNO and CEO: Work in this new role for one year, and then return to your present job if the plan isn't working or there is dissatisfaction with the role. Leah Kinnaird, PhD of Creative Health Care Management and Ruth Hansten, PhD of Hansten Healthcare offered diverse topics in didactic sessions and provided much-needed, just-in-time feedback at key milestone times. Their commitment, enthusiasm and passion for the improvement of patient care processes were a guiding light for our nursing staff and leadership team.

Coaches were selected on their expertise in these areas:

- *Expert level of clinical competence*
- *Highly influential and respected by the staff and physicians*
- *High level of emotional intelligence and integrity*
- *Open, honest communication style*
- *Demonstrated belief in the Vision of the organization*
- *Ability to see the "big picture" and to drive the model to the bedside*

Making It Live in Daily Practice

What did it take every day to make our model a reality in the day-to-day operations of these medical/surgical units?

- *Executive and leadership support*
- *Specific expectations in the results to be achieved*
- *Defined measurement and monitoring tools*
- *Defined expectations for the coaching role with defined daily accomplishments*
- *The authority for the coaches to step into situations and make decisions on the spot*
- *A solid plan for continuous learning, ongoing feedback and celebration of successes*

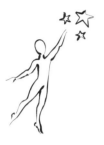

Integrating new behaviors was the key to our accomplishments.

While these may sound simple enough, integrating new behaviors was the key to our accomplishments. Every day started with a morning meeting. This was attended by the director of the medical/surgical unit, the coaching facilitator, the coaches and the CNO. Discussions were held about what went well the previous day and what didn't go so well. Role-play and brainstorming activities were used to reach potential solutions, daily report cards were reviewed, information for the Administrative Team was analyzed, a "parking lot" for items which needed future attention was created, and adjustments to the coaching program were made as improvements were realized.

In order for this program to succeed, we knew that the coaches must determine what they would measure as evidence of the success of the coaching program itself. They used daily logs and statistics from bedside changes, such as: 1) number of times care team members introduced themselves to the patients, 2) number of times the RN sat with the patient and discussed the patient's number one need, and 3) number of times members of the care team's name and/or patient's number one need was posted on the white board in the patient's room.

The coaches prepared clear expectations for the bedside care givers (see "A Day in the Life," page 514), and coaches' expectations were integrated into both the staff evaluations and Press Ganey patient feedback questions.

We also set up a system of measurements from other sources that would help us measure the effectiveness of the program on a larger scale. We looked at the financial impact of decrease in shift overtime for RNs. We looked at the quality of work life for staff as evidenced in RN recruitment and retention. The impact on clinical quality was evidenced by a decrease in medication errors and improved completion of the patient's Health Profile. Customer service was impacted as patient satisfaction scores improved. And we saw evidence that the work life of the staff improved as scores on Employer of Choice and Internal Report Cards recorded improvement also (see page 629).

Just as important as the above was the fact that the coaches worked side by side with the staff on a daily basis. Eighty percent of their time was spent observing for coaching opportunities on the unit at the bedside. Observing shift report and assignment making, and speaking with other care givers and physicians throughout the shift gave them an insight into strategies they could develop to improve each RN's practice. This was usually accomplished by role modeling the new behaviors, asking questions, providing information about clinical research and "converting" old habits and behaviors one RN at a time.

Success Creates Buy-In

The coaches were successful because they were able to show RNs what was in it for them if they would make some changes to their daily work patterns. But this was not without challenge. Many RNs felt that they already provided good care and had resistance to working with a coach. An early win for the coaches was when the call light frequency diminished—something that was noticed pretty quickly. But how?

The coaches worked with the staff to set an expectation with each patient on how often the patient wanted someone to stop in and check on him or her. When the staff took on this practice, patients felt safe, secure and seen. Once patients felt that nurses were reaching out to them, they felt less need to reach out to nurses via the call lights!

Another "aha" moment occurred when the RNs began to see value in sitting at the bedside for 3 to 5 minutes and establishing a plan with the patient. The RNs quickly discovered that this made their day much more efficient and focused. The patient helped them focus on what was important, instead of on everything that could possibly be accomplished. The RNs felt more connected to their patients and quickly grew to believe that "establishing a relationship is essential to healing."

Continuous learning was also high on the priority list for this model. Basic tenets missing in our care delivery had included appropriate delegation and good evaluation through critical thinking and problem solving. We started with a didactic class on the Nurse Practice Act in our state, leading to additional classes in and hands-on practice with delegation, assignment making, critical thinking and follow-up.

Credibility further improved for the coaches when each RN developed an individual practice plan for continued growth. The coaches met with every RN on the medical/surgical units to accomplish this. It proved to be a huge step in renewing the passion in their profession. It also proved to be invaluable in identifying RNs who could not commit to the model or think about new ways to practice for their patients. These issues were handled by positional leaders (not the coaches) and resulted in some RNs eventually leaving the system.

The coaches also identified system issues that were affecting patient safety, clinical quality or operational excellence. As a result of their work, an Admissions Nurse was added to the organization to improve the information and the flow of patients coming to an already busy nursing unit. This RN travels to the Emergency Department and to the medical/surgical units completing nearly 40% of unplanned admission profiles and care plans, thus making it much easier for the medical/surgical nurse to accept the new patient. Working with physicians on better communication resulted in a resource for each unit entitled "Top 10 Reasons to Call a Doc," outlining what to have ready when calling a physician about a patient need.

The success of this new model is reflected in the change in our Press Ganey Patient Satisfaction score over four years (see right). Like any major change, it is often difficult to see the continual improvement on a daily or even quarterly basis. Measurements and celebrations are critical to knowing where you are and where you need to go next. Detailed tracking indicators that influence the bedside RN's adoption of this model are key. If you were to ask our coaches about their work and their success, they would tell you that:

- *Changes must be behaviorally focused at the individual practitioner level,*

- *Changes can only be made one person at a time,*

- *Other departments (besides Nursing) need to adopt this model to change a culture, and*

- *It requires ongoing commitment and belief to stay focused and energized.*

Evidence of the Program's Success

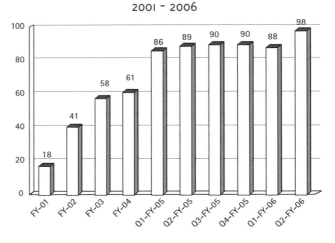

Marion General Hospital
Overall Inpatient
Press Ganey Patient Satisfaction Scores
2001 – 2006

Our results speak for themselves. We are a better nursing organization and we provide better care for our patients. We have nurses pounding on our doors to work with us. Our patient, physician and staff satisfaction scores are at an all-time high. We are fiscally sound. We are proud of our accomplishments and know that we can go on to do even greater things in our future.

> **The RNs felt more connected to their patients and quickly grew to believe that "establishing a relationship is essential to healing".**

A DAY IN THE LIFE OF AN RN
What Does An Outcomes-Based Care Shift Look Like?

After Report

☐ *RN will meet with LPN/NA/NT to give them initial direction and discuss plan for the day, outcomes/focus for each patient*

☐ *Planning includes "CHECKPOINTS" and specific agreed upon times to evaluate outcomes*

☐ *LPNs are included in planning and DO NOT FUNCTION INDEPENDENTLY*

☐ *The RN is accountable for the patients in his/her assignment*

☐ *The NA/NT worksheet will be utilized on all Med/Surg units*

Introduction to Patients

☐ *Introduction to patients*
This includes your name, role, and who else is involved with the patient's care; "I am X, the RN who will be coordinating your care for the next X hours."

☐ *Focused interview*
With each patient or family, 3-5 minutes at bedside, sitting, with eye contact, to discuss priorities, patient's number one need/goal for your shift, plan for the day (this is your connection with patients)

Throughout the Shift

☐ *Think critically*
Use your logical, creative, intuitive and analytical mental processes in all you do; use critical thinking in resolving patient care and team problems

☐ *Communicate the plan*
Planned outcomes are shared with the members of the health care team (social worker, case management, physicians) at care conferences, rounding with physicians; ALL RNs WILL ATTEND

CARE CONFERENCES TO DISCUSS THEIR PATIENT'S PLAN OF CARE

☐ *Checkpoints*
Continue so that periodic inspection and corrective action, positive feedback are included; REVIEW THE 4 Ps: PURPOSE, PICTURE, PLAN, AND PART FOR EACH PATIENT

☐ *End of shift feedback among team members occurs*
The RN requests feedback from each team member; things that did not "go well" are reviewed for ideas for the future

☐ *Celebrate the results*

Outcomes-Based Care Delivery Model

- *Think critically*
- *Plan and report outcomes, short and long-term*
- *Partner with patient/family in planning outcomes at their bedside*
- *Discuss planned outcomes with everyone on your team*
- *Evaluate progress and plan at checkpoints*

Behavioral Expectations

- *Focus on the patient as the primary customer*
- *Maintain accountability for the actions and communications*
- *Commit to work as a team*
- *Trust the work of your peers*
- *Support unit decisions*
- *Take risks and get involved*
- *Be a role model for others*
- *Be patient with the process and focus on the outcome*
- *Contribute to problem identification and resolution*

A Labor and Management Partnership to Support Registered Nurses: Remembering Our Common Purpose

—Jayne A. Felgen

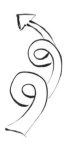

At the worst point in their relationship, labor and management for a coalition of health care facilities on the East Coast of the United States were nearing a stalemate. Individuals on both sides staked out positions and stood their ground rather than looking for shared interests. As both sides ultimately began to focus on their shared interest, *creating the healthiest and most supportive work environments possible for their registered nurses*, they forged a partnership based on the principles of interest-based bargaining. The two partners essentially agreed upon a new way of being together to serve their constituencies (RNs, hospitals, and ultimately, the patients and families they serve) more effectively.

By the time Creative Health Care Management (CHCM) entered the scene, the union/management partnership was 5 years old, and both labor and management had made significant inroads in improving their relationship and were working toward true collaboration. The labor-management partners were in the completion stages of the first four initiatives of their shared project, focusing on team self-scheduling, quality improvement, Nurse of Distinction Awards, and flex scheduling (12-hour shifts).

We joined them to address the fifth and final initiative, the Nurse Leadership Project (NLP), which focuses on relationships, morale and retention. They determined that evidence of the success of this final initiative would be:

- *improved staff morale and*
- *reduced registered nurse (RN) turnover.*

Our proposal focused on improving the morale of the nursing staff through improving relationships. We proposed the ultimate goal be one of improving care and service to patients and families because that is the shared interest for all parties involved. We based our proposal on evidence that:

- *nurses get their greatest reward in caring for patients,*

- *nurses stay in an organization because they feel connected to their colleagues, and*

- *when nurses feel connected to each other while caring for patients, their morale is high.*

We customized *Leadership at the Point of Care* (see page 424), for this partnership. The *LPC* workshop identifies the leadership qualities inherent in each individual while identifying the leadership skills and knowledge required for professional nursing practice. It was originally designed for use in the United Kingdom through a collaborative process for the National Health Service (NHS) between CHCM, the Royal College of Nursing and the University of Leeds (page 495).

Leadership at the Point of Care is based on the belief that there are five conditions necessary for people to engage in and accomplish substantive changes in practice. When the following conditions are in place, the progress for change is steady, problem solving is creative and proactive, and desired results are achieved (see page 480).

Clarity—*individuals must be clear about their mission and purpose, professional role requirements (including responsibility, authority and accountability), and the essential elements of a care delivery system that support professional practice. Clarity about who we are as care givers—a deep self-knowing—is fundamental to establishing therapeutic relationships with patients and healthy relationships with team members and to acquiring the competencies for professional practice.*

Competence—*clinical competence includes establishing and managing healthy interpersonal relationships and applying creative and critical thinking skills. When individuals are competent in technical knowledge and skills, interpersonal knowledge and skills, and critical and creative thinking skills, they are in a position to develop as leaders in their role.*

Confidence—*when individuals know what they are expected to contribute and when they have the knowledge and skills to make that contribution, they feel confident. Confidence provides the emotional foundation for exercising judgment and taking action.*

Collaboration—*organizational change requires people to work together to achieve a common goal. When individuals come to the interaction with real clarity about their purpose, role and contribution, having the competence to contribute fully and feeling confident in their abilities, collaboration and teamwork thrive.*

Commitment—*this is the undergirding of organizational change. Deep commitment is the inevitable outcome when a group of individuals has clarity about their shared purpose, the skills to achieve that purpose, confidence in the value of their own contributions and a sense of community that comes from working in collaboration with others to achieve a meaningful goal.*

When evaluating the program, RNs frequently cited "having chief nurses and clinical managers developing a vision for meaningful practice alongside Staff Nurses" as being highly valuable to them.

During the initial stages of the Nurse Leadership Project, many participants described their hospitals' culture as hierarchical, with a clear division between managers, administrators and clinical staff. For this reason, the *LPC* workshop was specifically designed so that RNs worked with their nurse managers and chief nursing officers to experientially discover the common thread connecting them. When evaluating the program, RNs frequently cited "having chief nurses and clinical managers developing a vision for meaningful practice alongside Staff Nurses" as being highly valuable to them.

We were thrilled with the results of the *Leadership at the Point of Care* workshops offered for the Nursing Leadership Project. There was statistically significant improvement in all 13 key indicators. The results affirmed that caring for patients and families is the most important aspect of nurses' work and that their relationships with colleagues are why they stay. (The results are explained in more detail on page 645. John Nelson of Healthcare Environments, Inc., describes the method used to measure the effectiveness of the *LPC* workshop and the results achieved.)

This program culminated in the creation of action plans. Participants created plans for substantive changes affecting patients, families and their relationships with colleagues on their own units. A few weeks after the end of the initial *LPC* workshop, participants presented these refined action plans in collaboration with colleagues at a one-day World Café (see page 391) follow-up session. The purpose of this day was to demonstrate their accountability for their plans, to inspire them to continue with their changes and to allow them time to learn from each other. Combining knowledge and skills acquired in the *LPC* workshop with the action-planning activity refocused the RN participants on why they chose health care, validated their desire for a purpose-filled practice, and helped them to more consistently provide the care experience patients and families seek.

Leadership at the Point of Care provided individuals in this health care system with the initial inspiration and infrastructure necessary to move forward together. This was a great beginning! However, we know from experience that deep sustainable cultural change requires an overarching vision and strategy with a focus on:

- *continuous inspiration,*
- *a well-designed and aligned infrastructure,*
- *ongoing education, and*
- *the collection of evidence that demonstrates successes that will inspire further improvement and continually stimulate new growth.*

We are excited to continue our work with this unique partnership. In the second phase, we are supporting ongoing inspiration and education with an emphasis on the design and implementation of the infrastructure necessary to accomplish substantive and sustainable change in practice and relationships.

The Unit Practice Council "Kick-off" Day

—Susan Wessel and Colleen Person

The success of Relationship-Based Care (RBC) is largely in the hands of the staff that comprise Unit Practice Councils (UPCs) (see page 214), so giving them the responsibility to plan how RBC will come to life on their units is essential. We recommend an official "Kick-off" meeting to get UPC members inspired and to provide them with essential education and direction.

Unit Practice Councils typically come together after the Results Council has established their structure and approved the RBC Principles for the organization (see page 182). Kick-off Day is often the first time UPC members will have met as defined groups. In some situations, however, they may have attended an inspirational program, such as a *Reigniting the Spirit of Caring* workshop, before Kick-off Day. If so, this will have enabled them to develop a vision for RBC for their unit, giving them a head start.

The list of invitations to Kick-off Day should include all members of the Unit Practice Council for "Wave 1" of implementation (usually three to four nursing units) along with their managers and the RBC project leader or co-leaders. Another Kick-off Day should be held in 4 or 5 months when the second wave of units is ready to begin. The agenda is somewhat dependent upon the staff's previous education and exposure to the vision for Relationship-Based Care. The agenda is developed to meet the specific learning needs of each group. For example, if this is their first exposure to the concept of staff empowerment, the group may need content on "responsibility, authority and accountability" (see page 486) and group process.

> Unit Practice Councils typically come together after the Results Council has established their structure and approved the RBC Principles for the organization

Two sample agendas are presented here to give you ideas for your own organization. It is ideal to have the CNO or an RBC project leader present the organization's vision for RBC and its link with the mission and values. Managers should also attend the Kick-off Day so that everyone hears the same expectations. The Kick-off Day should end with the first scheduled meeting of the new UPC group. You will want to decide if the manager should sit in on the first meeting for support, or if his or her presence will inhibit the group from coming into their own. This can vary with the culture of each organization and even with each unit.

UPC Kick-off Day Agenda (Sample A)

Welcome and Introductions

"Organizational Vision"—link to Relationship-Based Care

Appreciative Inquiry Assessment Findings

UPC Members' Intentions and Visions from Reigniting the Spirit of Caring Workshop

Dimensions of Relationship-Based Care: Implications for the UPCs

Video: "Leadership for Relationship-Based Care," Marie Manthey's Presentation at the Sacramento, CA, Magnet Conference, 2004

Hospital-Specific RBC Model:

- *Infrastructure, Roles and Responsibilities*

- *The RBC Principles*

- *Introduction to the UPC Implementation Guide*

Individual Meeting of the UPCs With Their Managers

Questions and Wrap-up

UPC Kick-off Day Agenda (Sample B)

Advance Reading: Implementation Guide for Relationship-Based Care *with Hospital-Specific Principles*

Introductions: Focus on Talents and Strengths You Bring to the Group

Hospital Journey Toward Relationship-Based Care, Link to Mission and Vision

Overview of Dimensions of Relationship-Based Care

Individual and Collective Visions

UPC Process for RBC Design—Implementation Guide

Principles of RBC; Timeline for Implementation

Meeting Process—Roles, Minutes, Communication, Consensus Decisions

Questions, Discussion

First Meeting of Individual Unit Practice Councils Without Manager

Managers Meet with RBC Project Leader and CHCM Consultant

Adjourn

Finally, we'd like to offer some key points for successful Kick-off Days:

- *Remember that the overall goal of Kick-off Day is for UPC members to gain the commitment, information and tools they need to begin their work—leading their colleagues in implementation to Relationship-Based Care.*

- *The agenda should have staff involvement through group activities and dialogue, especially during the visioning exercise.*

- *Schedule something inspirational to build excitement, such as the video/DVD "Patients Love Their Nurses" and some appreciative storytelling.*

- *Check in periodically during this first UPC meeting, and at the same time encourage the group members to begin establishing leadership as a group and gain independence.*

By the end of a Kick-off Day the UPC members are excited and proud of the initial decisions they've made as a unified team. The momentum they've established carries them through their initial work sessions and provides a great beginning to RBC planning at the unit level.

Reigniting the Spirit of Caring: Inspiring through Connection

—*Mary Koloroutis*

The simple act of touching someone is a powerful way to begin healing loneliness and isolation.

—*Dean Ornish*

Reigniting the Spirit of Caring (*RSC*) is a 3-day workshop that has been presented to thousands of hospital staff and managers throughout the country. The three areas of focus in *RSC* are:

1) caring for self (body/mind/spirit),
2) caring for colleagues (collegial behaviors) and
3) caring for patient's families.

Through experiential learning, new awareness emerges which affirms—or changes—behavior.

In groups of usually 25 to 30 participants, *RSC* brings individuals from all areas of the organization into the same forum to reflect and discuss what matters most in our work—our human relationships with self, each other, and most importantly, the patients and families we serve. While the curriculum was originally designed with direct care givers in mind, the workshop's content has great significance for everyone in the organization.

Reigniting the Spirit of Caring is an experiential workshop using dialogue, reflection and "deep listening" to foster greater understanding of what it means to care for and heal patients not just at the point of care, but at every level and in every department in the organization.

I am often asked "What is the magic in *Reigniting the Spirit of Caring*?" Participants are always keenly aware that something significant is happening, but they can't always put their finger on what it is. *Reigniting the Spirit of Caring* is profoundly moving for most of the participants. It is intimate in some ways that parallel the connection and intimacy of patient/care giver relationships. It creates new understanding between the participants and is a source of inspiration as participants recognize and validate the meaning of their work in caring for and serving patients and families. But most simply put, the magic that happens is in the connection between participants. A common bond emerges—one born of shared meaning—that they carry with them into the workplace. It helps strengthen their focus and creates in them a more powerful resolve to provide compassionate and humane care. They are nurtured and inspired through connection which is healing and life affirming.

In the feedback from every session, themes like these invariably emerge:

> *I feel more connected to my co-workers and the organization as a whole—I have a greater sense of being part of something bigger than I am—part of a mini-universe in which all is poised to help me do what I feel deeply called to do.*

> *You helped me to remember why I went into health care in the first place.*

> *I feel like I have "permission" to take as good care of myself as I do of my patients.*

> *I feel like the organization really understands what I do here. I am amazed that the leaders are supporting my learning and growth in such a meaningful way. I feel valued.*

> *I am not alone in what I feel or the problems I face. I take great comfort in that.*

Simply put, the magic that happens is in the connection between participants. A common bond emerges—one born of shared meaning—that they carry with them into the workplace.

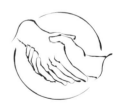

The collegiality of the diverse groups drawn together for these workshops creates a bond between individuals from vastly different roles and levels in the organization. This fosters greater understanding across lines, which serves to dissolve lines in the minds of the participants. *Reigniting the Spirit of Caring* inspires participants to engage in their work of caring for patients and families with a sense of joy, meaning and purpose.

Exemplar: *Reigniting the Spirit of Caring* at Centra Health

—Cheryl Burnette, Susan Bullock and Michelle Cabell

Centra Health's CNO, Golden Bethune, had a vision to enhance professional nursing practice within the organization and the community. Her vision led to collaboration with Marie Manthey, Jayne Felgen and Creative Health Care Management (CHCM) to provide the workshop *Reigniting the Spirit of Caring* (*RSC*) for all professional nursing staff.

Nursing leadership at Centra Health (Lynchburg, VA), recognizing the value of educating nurses in Relationship-Based Care (RBC), started offering *Reigniting the Spirit of Caring* in June 2004. Three of our registered nurses were trained and licensed to facilitate the workshop. Initially two classes a month were held at a local country club. Over the course of the last 18 months, we have trusted *RSC* to reignite the spirit of caring in 564 nurses representing over 41% of our nursing staff.

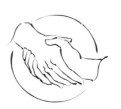

As is encouraged in *RSC* facilitator training, we added several items of our own to customize *RSC* for our culture. We added movement and dance as reinforcement of "care of self" which is one of *RSC*'s three primary focuses. In the storytelling breakout sessions, we added a dimension by asking each group to draw a symbol representing a common theme or story that emerged from their group storytelling. The use of the symbols to share their stories of extraordinary care deepened the meaning of this experience for the participants.

On the last day of the workshop, we ask participants to write a letter to themselves. We ask guiding questions related

Reigniting the Spirit of Caring Follow-Up Survey

Since attending Reigniting the Spirit of Caring, have you used any of the tools in your work?

    1. Commitment to Co-Worker

    2. Circle of Influence, Circle of Concern

    3. Transformational Leadership Cycle

    4. Ideas for best practice.

    5. Other

Can you give an example of how you used an RSC tool?

Did RSC cause you to think differently about how you do your job?

    1. Yes

    2. No

    3. Not sure

    If yes, please offer an example

Has your RSC experience helped you to identify any work processes (QI or PI) which could be improved?

    1. Yes

    2. No

If yes, please offer an example

Has your experience with RSC inspired you to take steps toward initiating a process improvement?

    1. Yes

    2. No

If so, please offer an example

How does your work environment support your using the skills you learned in RSC?

What are you doing differently since RSC?

to changes they will make in their practice and the evidence that will demonstrate this change. This letter is designed to serve as a reminder and hold them accountable for their own intentions. In 3 months, this letter, along with a CD of photos of their 3-day experience and the major tenets of the *RSC* workshop, is mailed to them. To encourage participants to stay in touch with one another, a roster is also included. Personal notes of positive affirmations from others in the group are also added to support *RSC*'s "care of colleagues" theme.

In addition, we collected anecdotes from nursing leadership concerning the behaviors of participants who had made a dramatic change in their professional demeanor. It was also very important to us to demonstrate and capture a positive change over time in a more formalized and systematic way. We determined the next step was to gather data at approximately 9 months from the participants that demonstrated an actual change in behavior in their practice in their own units.

We designed a survey to gather this data, which is available on our online education system. Each participant was asked questions about changes in his or her practice and personal transformation from thinking to doing to outcomes.

Our initial results from those responding indicate that nurses in our organization now think differently about how they do their jobs. They offered comments about their *RSC* experience such as:

- *"It helped me to bridge gaps between the units."*

- *"Meeting staff from other units puts a personal face to the unit so that it's not just the Pulmonary Unit anymore, it's Debbie."*

- *"I have kept my Commitment to Co-workers card in my pocket to remind me of my responsibility to my colleagues."*

- *"I am now spending five minutes at the bedside with my patients."*

- *"I assisted in writing the pain protocol for Emergency Room patients."*

- *"On our unit we have developed a CNA orientation manual."*

- *"I am currently working on a policy to initiate an infiltration and phlebitis scale."*

- *"I really try hard to build strong working relationships with my co-workers including nurses, other nursing personnel, patients, families, physicians, etc. I encourage others to address problems with the appropriate individuals and get the problem solved quickly."*

- *"I try to help out every time I am needed, not just fellow RNs but to all others as well."*

- *"I spend quality time listening to my patients."*

- *"I feel increased compassion and patience .... it reignited my practice."*

- *"It gave me motivation to do my job better."*

- *"RSC was a "Booster Shot" for appreciation of our work environment."*

- *"We are encouraged to be autonomous in our practice and to do projects that will improve the quality of care our patients receive."*

Some care givers affirm that they are consistently spending 5 minutes at the bedside, avoiding gossip, improving their attitudes when precepting students, being more assertive, caring for themselves more, and thinking more about the patient as a unique individual.

The participants report that they see that individuals throughout the organization are working together as a whole—not in competition with each other. These comments reflect that nurses are doing something differently in their work as a result of their participation in the *Reigniting the Spirit of Caring* workshops. Some care givers affirm that they are consistently spending 5 minutes at the bedside, avoiding gossip, improving their attitudes when precepting students, being more assertive, caring for themselves more, and thinking more about the patient as a unique individual.

Some 30% of the nurses attending have also identified work processes that could be improved and have taken steps themselves to initiate the improvements. These responses include patient waiting time studies, new procedural pain protocol for NG tube placement, urinary catheter placement, RN and CNA orientation, as well as patient flow in the Cardiac Rehabilitation Unit.

At Centra, 66% of the nurses now say that their working environment supports the skills that they have learned in the

RSC workshop. This is reflected in the great support of the professional nursing staff by the unit managers.

Approximately 50% of the nurses, surveyed 9 months after completing *RSC*, have indeed used the Commitment to My Co-worker information and 20% are already actively using the "best practices" shared.

We are seeing an increase in nurses applying to advance on our clinical ladder. We are also seeing large numbers of staff becoming certified in their specialties. In fact our Women and Children's division coordinated study groups and had 21 nurses achieve certification in their specialty at one time. We are seeing bedside nursing staff publishing and not only applying to, but speaking at, national and state conferences.

The organization as a whole has also achieved some measurable successes since our participation in *Reigniting the Spirit of Caring.* We are proud to say that we achieved ANCC Magnet designation in August 2005. We have received the AACN Beacon Award for both our Cardiovascular Recovery and Medical Intensive Care Units. For the third time, we are in the top 100 hospitals in the country for cardiac care according to Solucient[1]. Centra Health has been honored with the VHA Leadership Award for its entry "The Road Toward World Class AMI Care." The award is given to VHA member organizations that demonstrate innovation and dedication in the delivery of health care. Press Ganey, a national health care survey research firm, tabulated patient satisfaction scores for our pain management in the top 2% at the Virginia Baptist Hospital campus and the top 8% at the Lynchburg General Hospital campus.

Reigniting the Spirit of Caring was the beginning of something great at Centra Health. It changed our thinking, it changed how we see each other, and it helped a creative, professional nursing staff with the focus of "excellent care every time" to catapult our organization into ranking within the top 2% of all nursing staffs in the country. We know that implementing the *RSC* workshop with the vision of our nursing leadership team has helped us achieve our exemplary status.

> The organization as a whole has also achieved some measurable successes since our participation in Reigniting the Spirit of Caring. We are proud to say that we achieved ANCC Magnet designation in August 2005.

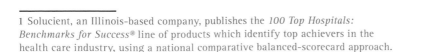

---

1 Solucient, an Illinois-based company, publishes the *100 Top Hospitals: Benchmarks for Success®* line of products which identify top achievers in the health care industry, using a national comparative balanced-scorecard approach.

CHAPTER FIFTEEN
Education for Colleagueship

Editors' note: *Adapted from* The Human Side of Medicine: Learning What It's Like to Be a Physician and What It's Like to Be a Patient, *Chapter 14: Language and Communication (2002), by Laurence A. Savett Published by Greenwood Publishing Group. Used with permission.*

Language and Communication for Relationship-Based Care

—Laurence A. Savett

Mutual understanding facilitates genuine collaboration. Only when we "speak the same language" can we truly be allied. Seeking to fully understand those with whom we communicate prevents our conversations from becoming confrontational, patronizing or full of jargon.

Most of us have experienced superb interactions in which we have successfully communicated facts, opinions, consistency, reliability, accessibility and commitment. But there are potential barriers to communication. The concept of "language barrier" applies not only to the difference between the native language of the patient and of the physician and nurse; it can also refer to barriers between those who share a common language.

One of the hallmarks of Relationship-Based Care is superior communication between patients and care givers. This superior communication requires us to be ever conscious of the many nuances peculiar to the patient/care giver relationship. As care givers we must learn to:

- *read "between the lines,"*

- *be aware of misunderstandings, and*

- *listen for cues for what's not being said.*

By *reading between the lines*, we enhance our understanding of what the patient means. Here are two examples of how physicians may notice opportunities to engage in meaningful conversation with patients:

- *The unexpected question from an 80-year-old patient, "What's my cholesterol?" was her way of asking, "How much longer do I have? How's my heart?"*

- *When a patient with widespread cancer asked, "How long do I have to live?" the physician realized she was not looking for a numerical answer. Instead the physician saw the opportunity to discuss the patient's goals and values, and to address what the patient really wanted to know: "Will I have uncontrollable pain? What will the remaining time be like?"*

When patients become silent, we often have to control the urge to fill the silence quickly with a comment, an assurance, or another question. But patients pause for various reasons: to deal with painful thoughts, to stifle tears or other signs of emotions, or to think about what they are going to say next. Often what a patient says immediately after a period of silence has great significance and to interrupt a silence is as inappropriate as interrupting a narration. Silence may allow the patient and us time to reflect on what has been said—and left unsaid.

Words can harm. We may describe a patient as "difficult," "manipulative," "hysterical," "noncompliant," or "a hypochondriac," and a family as "dysfunctional." Careless and pejorative language clouds precise thinking. A word can't ever completely define patients or their families—not even after we know more about their story, motivations, points of view, reasons for behavior and values.

As nurses and physicians, we especially need to choose our words carefully. What we say may mean something entirely different from what we intend for the listener to hear, because it's unclear, because the listener is tense, or because the listener doesn't understand our language—even if we're both speaking English.

Words can harm. We may describe a patient as "difficult," "manipulative," "hysterical," "noncompliant," or "a hypochondriac," and a family as "dysfunctional." Careless and pejorative language clouds precise thinking.

Here are some examples of what's said versus what's heard:

> • *When a physician told a 27-year-old man, a heavy drinker, "Your liver tests are abnormal," the patient concluded that he had irreversible and fatal liver disease. The physician needed to explain that the abnormalities were reversible, and he needed to say it more than once.*
>
> • *"You have hypertension" was a statement of trivial importance to the physician, because high blood pressure is so common. However, one patient took it to mean imminent stroke and the transition from perfect health to a flawed body.*

Any patient's question becomes an opportunity to engage in discussion and explore issues. Good physicians and nurses read between the lines and ask themselves, "What does my patient's question mean?"

Even the way we address patients carries weight. Greeting an adult patient for the first time with "Hi, Harry" initiates a different quality of interaction from, "How do you do, Mr. Swenson." The first greeting lacks the respect and deference due any adult with whom we are not already acquainted. Many will prefer to be addressed more informally by their first name, but that's their call, not ours.

When patients or families become angry, we need to ask ourselves, "What does my patient's anger mean?" Patients may be angry for various reasons, and misunderstanding is the most likely of them. Patients may also be experiencing depression, recalling a prior unpleasant interaction with a physician, feeling frustrated with the "system," feeling frustrated with an illness that isn't going well, or grappling with unrevealed psychological issues.

Here are some lessons I've learned about language and communication:

Sit. Don't minimize the importance of body language. Sitting when one talks with a patient is an important gesture. Is doesn't matter if the conversation is less than a minute long; patients see this as a commitment to them and them alone, a gesture that conveys, "You are all I have on my mind now."

When patients or families become angry, we need to ask ourselves, "What does my patient's anger mean?" Patients may be angry for various reasons, and misunderstanding is the most likely of them.

Less than a minute sitting has the impact of five minutes standing. Five minutes standing seems as if "you've got one foot out the door."

Talk with patients as equals. Don't talk down. Talk in a conversational tone. Don't shout.

Set the context. In order to explain things to patients, provide a context and start where the patient is. Ask, "What have you already been told about your illness?"

Make no assumptions about the patient's level of knowledge. Even if the patient is a professional colleague, state the assumptions about the illness, clarify them if necessary, and be certain of agreement about their validity.

Explore the patient's beliefs and values, because they will invariably have to be integrated into decisions about the patient's treatment and overall care.

Recognize that a long conversation is often better than a short one. In the midst of a patient's long hospitalization for liver disease, a nonmalignant ovarian tumor, and many surgical complications, I spoke with her and her husband for an hour. During this time, I reviewed the entire hospitalization, how we had gotten to where we were (she was still seriously ill); inquired about prior crises they had faced and their strengths during those times; expressed hope for a quick recovery; assured them of my commitment to do all I could; and recognized the uncertainties in the patient's care. We could not have addressed all these issues in a brief time, nor could a few short conversations have explored them in depth.

Recognize that a confrontation signals a need for a longer conversation. In that subsequent encounter, one can uncover invalid assumptions, and defuse hidden and unrecognized frustrations and distrust (see page 361). Encourage the patient to speak freely. Declare clearly, "I want you to know that there is nothing we can't talk about. And if you don't understand what I have said or if you disagree, you should let me know." Acknowledge the patient's fears with "You wouldn't be human if you weren't apprehensive." Ask any patient, "What about this surgery (or illness) concerns (or frightens) you the most?"

Negotiate. I propose a diagnosis and suggest a remedy, and then the patient and I refine it. I ask, "Does this sound reasonable to you?" and allow the conversation to evolve. I never

Provide a context and start where the patient is.

Never forget that patients are expert.

forget that patients are expert and have firsthand knowledge about their symptoms, reaction to certain drugs, and the impact of life's events on their health. I reason out loud, in order that together we can decide if the decisions are appropriate.

Acknowledge uncertainty.

Acknowledge reality. "You'll be okay" may be an appropriate assessment, but it's inadequate in some situations. To the patient who was recovering from a heart attack and had real fears about the future, I said, "I know that what will reassure you the most is first getting two weeks and then two months of good health behind you."

Recognize that not all questions have answers. Acknowledge uncertainty. Most people can handle the uncertainty.

Developing a warm communication style takes practice. When what we say to a patient is misunderstood, the reflective nurse or physician will ask:

- *Why didn't this work?*

- *What can I learn so that next time I'll say it better?*

The way we communicate defines a great deal of our interactions with patients and their families. Therefore the power of the language we use is not to be underestimated. In forming nurturing of our therapeutic relationships with patients, we must be as conscious as possible in our patient and family interactions about what we say and how we say it. We actively pursue mutual understanding—not merely so that we can escape the unpleasantness of misunderstanding—but because we honor and value human relationships.

Less than a minute sitting has the impact of five minutes standing.

Physicians, Nurses and Patients: What Each Brings to the Therapeutic Relationship

—Laurence A. Savett

In every encounter with patients, we need to understand what each brings to the relationship, however brief or extended.

Patients bring their needs

Besides professional expertise, they need:

- **someone who listens.** *Sometimes the patient needs neither answer nor remedy, but simply someone who listens with respect and without interruption. A patient told me, "When I have a physician who listens, it's magic."*

- **to understand.** *The patient may be hearing things for the first time and need time to understand what the physician and nurse already comprehend.*

- **to be understood.** *A nursing home resident who had long-standing unexplained abdominal pain said, "Thank you for spending the time with me. It doesn't solve anything, but I appreciate the fact that you try to understand me."*

- **to be validated.** *Patients may already have figured out that their symptoms are not serious, but they need the reassurance from someone with a credential. A patient may be grieving over the loss of a spouse, and need to be reassured that she is not going crazy. "You didn't minimize," one patient told me. "You believed in me," said another.*

- **moral support.** *"You have a 90% chance of improvement with this surgery" is information only.*

What Patients Bring to Therapeutic Relationships

Editors' note: *Portions of this article have been adapted from* The Human Side of Medicine: Learning What It's Like to Be a Patient and What It's Like to Be a Physician (2002), *by Laurence A. Savett. Published by Greenwood Publishing Group. Used with permission.*

"We'll do everything we can to make this turn out well" is support.

- **context.** *When a radiologist told my patient that "you have many small changes on the brain MRI," he and his wife called in panic, concerned that this was the beginning of Alzheimer's disease. I was able to provide context and reassurance that the changes were not significant.*

- **a prognosis—a prediction of how things will turn out.** *They need to hear: "There's a better than 90% chance that this therapy will cure your lymphoma, though we'll keep track of it for years to come." "Within six weeks of therapy, your shoulder will be back to normal." After such an explanation, a patient told me, "If you know how it's going to turn out, that it's going to get better, you can handle a lot more." Otherwise, patients' worst fantasies may take over.*

- **consistency.** *More than one explanation from different sources is confusing and adds to the anxiety of a serious illness. Patients want an integrated story and consistent explanation and advice.*

- **an advocate and a sense that the nurse and the physician care.** *Patients need to feel safe anywhere in the system. Whether in the hospital, a nursing home, the physician's office or at home, patients need to feel that there is a plan of care, access to someone in charge, and attention to all their needs. Anatole Broyard writes, "The doctor [and, I would add, the nurse] is the patient's only family in a foreign country" (Broyard, 1992).*

> Patients need to feel safe anywhere in the system.

Patients bring their fears, often undeclared

What to physicians and nurses may be a self-limited illness with a good prognosis—abdominal pain from gastroenteritis, for instance—may mean to the patient that he has cancer. It's up to the physician or the nurse to discover those fears of discomfort, uncertainty and outcome. I ask, "What about this illness worries you the most?" Here are some examples in which patients feared the worst:

- *Though he had known about his hypertension for five years, a 45-year-old man finally consulted a physician. He feared that he might be at risk for stroke, after he learned of his friend's stroke.*

- *In her mid-twenties, a social worker, the wife of a physician-in-training, developed a severe sore throat and swollen lymph nodes in her neck. She was concerned that she might have leukemia, and was relieved when her physician, not her husband, told her, "You have mononucleosis."*

Some patients fear being dependent on family members and friends or on a physician who may underestimate the seriousness of their illness. A patient with cancer of the pancreas told me, "You don't get top-notch care unless the doctors think you're top-notch sick."

Some patients fear being too narrowly defined as a sick person. Long ago I stopped referring to patients as "diabetics;" instead, each is "a person with diabetes." I am careful to make that point directly to the patient when I say, "Your diabetes does not define you."

Patients bring their experiences with nurses and physicians

If they have had encounters that turned out well, then their expectations will be similar for the current one, and they will, more likely than not, be at ease. But if their experiences have been unpleasant or inconsistent, if their prior physicians and nurses have been moody, unavailable and incomprehensible, then it will be no wonder that they may be tentative, suspicious and argumentative.

They bring their strengths, their values and their resources

They bring the ways they have met adversity and the strategies they have used to solve their problems. They bring the experiences and examples of family and friends. "When my mother was ill with cancer, she handled it in an admirable way by ...." Many bring their philosophies of life and the lessons from their religion.

They bring their biases, positive and negative

They may have positive or negative expectations about an ethnic group, race, gender or manner of dress. A dislike based

Patients bring the ways they have met adversity and the strategies they have used to solve their problems. They bring the experiences and examples of family and friends.

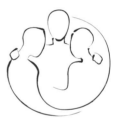

539

on prejudice may not last once the relationship is enriched with time, but the initial encounter may be overpowered by such impressions.

They bring their unstated agenda

"I'm here for an examination before my knee surgery" may disguise the concern that "this means I'm beginning to fall apart and that I'm getting older." A simple question from the physician or nurse like "What does this surgery mean to you?" can expose these fears.

They bring their goals and expectations

"I want to be completely healed" may be the unspoken goal, or it may be "I just want to make it to my daughter's wedding. Then I'll be content."

What Physicians and Nurses Bring to Therapeutic Relationships

Physicians and nurses bring their technical expertise and humanity

They bring their sensitivity to the patient's needs and fears.

They bring their professional experience

After all, the reason patients find themselves under a nurse's and physician's care is because nurses and physicians are experienced in dealing with the patient's illness in ways the patient is not. They bring their own special professional strengths, which may be both technical and humanistic.

They bring their own prejudices

Though physicians and nurses ought to be prejudice-free, many are not. At the very least, though, they need to recognize their prejudices and neutralize them during the patient encounters.

When the patient and the family are upset, the nurses' and physicians' calm demeanor, reassurance and attention to detail can help defuse the disarray and uncertainty.

They bring consistency

They are not "hot" one day and "cold" the next. Though the patient may be volatile and labile in his behavior from one encounter to the next, nurses and physicians need to be consistent and trustworthy. "I am the same. I will never lie to you.

I will not abandon you" are the unspoken reassuring messages of this consistency.

They bring equanimity at a difficult time

When the patient and the family are upset, the nurses' and physicians' calm demeanor, reassurance and attention to detail can help defuse the disarray and uncertainty.

They bring what they have learned from their own life

Like the patient, there is more to their life than the time spent in professional encounters.

They bring their own values

Physicians and nurses bring the sum of their personal family, religious, community and professional values, among which are altruism, a respect for the patient as an individual and a commitment to discovering and honoring the patient's needs.

And they bring their own fears

Physicians and nurses bring their fear of death, fear of making a mistake and fear of failure.

The linchpin of the therapeutic relationship is mutual understanding. As we form patient/care giver relationships, we need to have realistic expectations about what most patients bring to the relationship, while still actively discovering the uniqueness of each patient.

In each encounter, physicians and nurses need to reflect on what it's like for the patient. Self-reflection doesn't hurt either. With real empathy, nurses and physicians can ask themselves, "What would this be like for me if I were in the same situation?" Recognizing the complex dimensions of our relationships with patients enhances our effectiveness in caring for them and enriches our careers.

In each encounter, physicians and nurses need to reflect on what it's like for the patient.

> The linchpin of the therapeutic relationship is mutual understanding.

References: Savett, L. (2002). *The human side of medicine: Learning what it's like to be a patient and what it's like to be a physician.* Westport, CT: Greenwood Publishing Group.

Broyard, A. (1992). *Intoxicated by my illness.* New York: Fawcett Columbine.

The Importance of Nurse-Physician Communication to Safe Patient Care

—Sandra Hoffman and Michael Leonard

> Medicine and nursing are irrevocably tied together for the care and cure of patients.

Although from country to country health care varies in its uses of technology, resources and culture, its essence remains the same; medicine and nursing are irrevocably tied together for the care and cure of patients (Zwarenstein & Reeves, 2002). However, the two disciplines have a long history of education and role socialization that has lent itself to a parallel and indirect, rather than a collaborative and direct, way of communicating and providing care to patients. A lack of teamwork and communication—specifically poor nurse-physician communication—has been identified as a key factor in errors that have resulted in patient harm. In a review of more than 2,400 Sentinel Events in which 73% mortality resulted, the analysis cited communication failures as a root cause of errors that have resulted in patient harm in over 70% of the cases (Joint Commission on Accreditation of Healthcare Organizations, 2004a, 2004b). In an analysis of 47 cases of perinatal death or permanent disability reported to the Joint Commission under the Sentinel Event Policy, communication issues again topped the list of identified root causes at 72%, with 55% of the organizations citing organizational culture as a barrier to effective communication and teamwork. Some of the barriers in organizational culture were:

- *hierarchy and intimidation*
- *failure to function as a team*
- *failure to follow the chain of communication*

Cultures exist in many health care settings today that have not changed appreciably with regard to the hierarchies and perceived power differences between the two professions. Ineffective "respectful workplace or code of conduct policies," peer review processes and hospital "physician as customer" philosophies have sometimes resulted in reluctance or even barriers to addressing disruptive physician behavior or response issues. The result is often a culture where nurses hesitate to speak up or to be appropriately assertive when they are concerned about the well-being of a patient or see something happening that may place the patient at significant risk. Efforts to improve health care safety and quality are dependent on respectful, effective work relationships. If leadership does not strongly support respectful, collaborative work between nurses, physicians and other members of the care team, both the safety and quality of patient care will be compromised.

Barriers to Professional Collaboration

Author Suzanne Gordon (2005) found in her interviews with nurses that their most common complaints were:

- *Physicians do not understand what role nurses play in the health care system,*

- *Physicians misunderstand who nurses serve,*

- *Physicians do not value the knowledge and skill that nurses have amassed during their careers, and*

- *Physicians fail to appreciate that collaborative, cooperative, collegial relationships between nurses and physicians are central to quality patient care.*

Further, the complex structure and function of health care delivery may serve as a barrier to nurses and physicians getting to know each other. Interactions often consist of brief encounters in patient care areas, rather than teamwork that helps build valuable relationships and improve care. In these settings there is no second chance to collaborate effectively, and a given interaction may leave lasting positive or negative impressions on those involved or on those who witness a particular nurse-physician interaction (Lindeke & Seickert n.d.). The volume of these fleeting professional encounters may be increasing, due in part to both primary care and specialty physicians spending less time on hospital wards than they once did (LeTourneau, 2004); physicians frequently having patients on multiple floors; and changing nurse work agreements or scheduling. The ability of the nurse to get to know patients or physicians is often adversely impacted by staffing practices that do not emphasize the importance of continuity of care (such as a Primary Nursing care model), or continuity may be disrupted because of staffing shortages. Patients may be seen in large physician group practices, and patients may not know or be known by their physicians. In the hospital setting, the result may be that the nurse knows more about the patient's story than does the busy physician who responds to information and requests, perhaps without appreciating the full context. In this setting effective nurse-physician relationships, respect and trust are essential for safe care.

In an American Association of Critical Care Nurses research report (2004) about health care providers titled *Silence Kills: The Seven Crucial Conversations for Health Care*, it was reported that all too often well-intentioned people in health care institutions choose not to speak up when they're concerned with the behavior, decisions or actions of a colleague. In an *Institute for Safe Medication Practices* (Smetzer & Cohen, 2005) survey of more than 2,000 hospital health care providers (1,565 nurses, 354 pharmacists, 176 others):

> All too often well-intentioned people in health care institutions choose not to speak up when they're concerned with the behavior, decisions or actions of a colleague.

- *88% of respondents in the previous year encountered condescending language or voice intonation*

- *87% encountered impatience with questions*

- *79% encountered a reluctance or refusal to answer questions or phone calls*

- *48% reported being subjected to strong verbal abuse*

- *43% reported being subjected to threatening body language*

> Given what is known about communication and medical error, it is clear that ensuring excellent nurse-physician communication and collaboration is imperative for safe care and quality outcomes.

According to respondents, physicians and others, prescribers (i.e., pharmacists, nurses, supervisors) engaged in intimidating behaviors more frequently than other health care providers. Respondents also made it abundantly clear that intimidating behaviors were not attributable to physicians and prescribers alone; they encountered a surprising degree of intimidation among other health care providers as well. Almost half (49%) of all respondents reported that their past experiences with intimidation altered the way they handle order clarifications or questions about medication orders. Given this landscape and what is known about communication and medical error, it is clear that ensuring excellent nurse-physician communication and collaboration is imperative for safe care and quality outcomes. "Psychological safety" has been described as the degree to which people perceive their work environment as conducive to taking interpersonal risks such that they believe if they make a mistake others will not penalize or think less of them for it (Edmondson, 2002). It must always "feel safe" to voice a concern and advocate on behalf of a patient; otherwise we risk compromising the care of that patient.

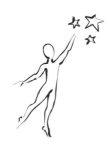

Application to Practice

Organizational leaders are accountable for acknowledging issues relating to nurse-physician communication and collaboration which may adversely affect patient care, and for creating and sustaining cultures that value the contributions of both to achieving optimal patient outcomes and safety. Leaders create and sustain a culture by role modeling the behaviors in the culture, the mechanisms used to deal with critical organizational incidents, and rewarding desired behaviors while sanctioning culturally destructive behaviors (Arford, 2005).

Research carried out at fourteen hospitals which have achieved Magnet designation from the American Nurses Credentialing Center (ANCC) have indicated that healthy collaborative relationships between nurses and physicians were not only possible, but were directly linked to optimal patient outcomes (Kramer & Schmalenburg, 2003). Ineffective nurse-physician communication has been linked to medication errors, patient injuries and patient deaths (Kohn, Corrigan, & Donaldson, 2000; Page, 2004; Baggs, Schmitt, Mushlin, Mitchell, Eldredge, Oakes, et al., 999). How doctors and nurses work together can have a significant impact on anyone who is sick and vulnerable and in need of care.

Ineffective nurse-physician communication has been linked to medication errors, patient injuries and patient deaths.

The importance of the human aspect of error prevention has been identified as key to keeping patients safe. Crew Resource Management (CRM) techniques borrowed from the aviation industry has offered valuable lessons for medical care (Leonard, Graham, & Bonacum, 2004). CRM techniques that focus on teamwork, communication, flattening hierarchies, managing error, creating situational awareness, and decision making offer valuable tools and processes that can be customized to the health care environment. Creating a cultural change that emphasizes communication, teamwork and safety first must be visibly, tangibly and actively supported by nursing, physician and administrative leaders, and in most organizations, this requires changing "business as usual." Our patients' lives depend on it.

References: American Association of Critical Care Nurses and VitalSmarts. (2004). *Silence kills: The seven crucial conversations.* Retrieved Feb 15, 2006 from www.silencekills.com.

Arford, P. (2005). Nurse-physician communication: An organizational account-ability. *Nursing Economics,* 23, 2.

Baggs, J., Schmitt, M., Mushlin, A., Mitchell, P., Eldredge, D. Oakes, D., et al. (1999). Association between nurse-physician collaboration and patient outcomes in three intensive care units. *Critical Care Medicine,* 27:1991-1998.

Edmondson, A. (2002). *Managing the risk of learning: Psychological safety in work teams.* Retrieved from www.hbs.edu/research/facpubs/workingpapers/papers2/0102/02-062.pdf Feb 05, 2006

Gordon, S. (2005*). Nursing against the odds: How health care cost cutting, media stereotypes, and medical hubris undermine nurses and patient care.* Ithaca, NY: Cornell University Press.

Joint Commission on Accreditation of Healthcare Organizations. (2004a, July 21). Preventing infant death and injury during delivery. *Sentinel Event Alert Issue* 30, 14 – 15.

Joint Commission on Accreditation of Healthcare Organizations. (2004b, June 29). Sentinel event statistics, Retrieved June 29, 2004, from www.jcaho.org/accredited+organizations/ambulatory+care/sentinel+events/sentinel+event+statistics.htm

Kohn, L., Corrigan, M., & Donaldson, M. (2000). *To err is human: Building a safer health system.* Committee on Quality of Health Care in America, Institute of Medicine, Washington, DC: National Academy Press.

Kramer, M., & Schmalenburg, C. (2003). Securing "good" nurse-physician rela-tionships. *Nursing Management,* 34(7), 34-38.

Leonard, M., Graham, S., & Bonacum, D. (2004). The human factor: The critical importance of effective teamwork and communication in providing safe care. *Quality and Safety in Health Care,* 13 (Suppl. 1), 85-90.

LeTourneau, B. (2004). Physicians and nurses: Friends or foes? *Journal of Healthcare Management,* 49(1), 12-14.

Lindeke, L., & Seickert, A. (n.d.). Nurse-physician workplace collaboration. *Online Journal of Issues in Nursing,* Vol 10, No. 1, Manuscript 4. www.nursing-world.org/ojin/topic26/tpc26_4.htm

Page, A. (2004). *Keeping patients safe: Transforming the work environment of nurses.* Committee on the Work Environment for Nurses and Patient Safety, Institute of Medicine. Washington, DC: National Academy Press.

Smetzer, J., & Cohen, M. (2005). Intimidation: Practitioners speak up about this unresolved problem. *Joint Commission Journal on Quality and Patient Safety,* 31(10), 594-599.

Zwarenstein, M. B. and Reeves, S. (2002, May). Working together but apart: Barriers and routes to nurse-physician collaboration. *Joint Commission Forum,* 28:5, 242-247.

Structures to Improve
Patient Safety and Care

—Sandra Hoffman

In my roles as both a clinical specialist and obstetrical nurse manager, I have worked to influence the culture of care with a mindset that "patient safety is everything." Because of this focus, I've been successful at creating structures and processes to improve patient safety and quality of care. Key to this success is the fostering of collaboration that can only happen in a culture in which efficient, professional, barrier-free communication between nurses and physicians happens reliably.

Patient safety is everything.

In order for such a culture to exist, a commitment to barrier-free communication must become an organizational norm. Visible support from administrative, medical and nursing leadership is essential for this to live in day-to-day practice. To this end, it is necessary for organizations to create structures which promote a culture where patient safety is a primary focus of the physician-nurse relationship. These structures can help create cultural parameters which free nurses and physicians to collaborate as effectively as possible within well-established, fully understood, mutually agreed upon guidelines.

Joint nurse/physician practice committees exist to establish standards for practice based on the most current and best evidence. These groups promote communication and greater understanding between nurses and physicians about practice. Collaboratively developed orders, pathways and protocols/guidelines help to promote nursing practice autonomy and excellence as they provide evidence-based, mutually agreed upon parameters established by physicians, nurses and other health professionals. This is a powerful way to affect day-to-day care by maximizing all care givers' contributions.

Joint Nurse/Physician Practice Committees

Joint nurse/physician practice committees have been identified as one of the structures designated by the National Joint Practice Commission (NJPC) as necessary for collaborative practice (National Joint Practice Commission, 1981).

These committees (typically comprising nurses, physicians and other health care providers focused on clinical care improvements, safety initiatives or quality review) can examine practices and make recommendations for practice refinements for individual units, service lines or across the whole organization. An excellent example of this is the Allina Pregnancy Care Council, a group of nurse and physician leaders representing obstetrics from 10 facilities in the Allina Health System, which has met for over 15 years with the goal of developing evidence- and standards-based practice resources and improving safety and quality of care to childbearing families.

Interdisciplinary Rounding

Interdisciplinary rounding can be as simple as the nurse accompanying the physician during patient rounds, but at its best, invites all members of the care team to collaborate as often as possible on behalf of the patient.

Interdisciplinary rounding can be as simple as the nurse accompanying the physician during patient rounds, but at its best, a culture in which interdisciplinary rounding is the norm invites all members of the care team to collaborate as often as possible on behalf of the patient.

Issues facing patients and their families are rarely limited to the clinical/medical realm. Input from the full range of service providers—nurses, physicians, anesthesiologists, social workers, pastoral care professionals, etc.—can help identify when patients are at risk or in need of services that often go undiscussed or unnoticed in a less collaborative culture. Interdisciplinary communication may also help prevent delays in care, failure to diagnose or treat in time, or conflict over care decisions and the subsequent need to access the medical chain of command and/or communication. Daily interdisciplinary unit review and/or debriefings of select medical records can also help team performance by educating all care providers regarding lessons learned from near misses or incidents resulting in patient harm (Knox, Simpson, Rice, & Townsend, 2003). Inclusion of the Clinical Manager in rounding activities promotes increased awareness of barriers to safety and organizational or systems issues to be addressed.

While daily full-team interdisciplinary rounding may be the ideal, it is also, in most busy organizations, more than can reasonably be expected. At minimum, however, any unit can identify 1) ways to notify nurses when their patients' physicians arrive, and 2) methods for physicians to ask for the nurse who is caring for the patient he or she will be seeing. The use of white boards with nurses' names often makes it easier for physicians to know who is caring for the patient and supports the practice of finding them and discussing the plan of care. There is great potential to both improve care and avoid rework in the form of pages and phone calls to clarify care issues.

Formalized daily or weekly rounds are also effective ways to ensure that essential communication and collaboration occur, especially for patients with complex conditions, multiple physician providers and/or extended lengths of stay. Interdisciplinary rounding has been identified as a structure that promotes collegial and collaborative nurse-physician relationships (Schmalenburg et al., 2005).

> At minimum, any unit can identify ways to notify nurses when their patients' physicians arrive, and methods for physicians to ask for the nurse who is caring for the patient he or she will be seeing.

Care Coordination

Patients, nurses and physicians benefit any time advanced planning for a patient's care or hospitalization occurs. This is especially important when unique medical, cultural or religious circumstances exist.

Obstetrics is a specialty where care coordination works well, as hospitalization nearly always becomes part of the patient's experience at some point. Physicians or others may identify patients with unique or complex needs to a nurse in the hospital who can do the research or advanced planning necessary to create a written plan for care during the hospital stay that will assist direct care providers in providing safe, sensitive and appropriate care. Care coordination may be a function of certain nurses on a unit on an as-needed basis or can be an actual role filled by a designated individual. Clinical nurse specialists or nurses in leadership positions help provide this service in many settings.

Multidisciplinary Quality Review Committees

When carefully reviewed, near misses and good catches provide a rich source of information about error, and tend to be easier for providers to discuss than a bad outcome.

In Multidisciplinary Quality Review Committees, nurses, physicians and others learn together by examining recent cases. Cases may be selected for review for either of two reasons: 1) quality indicators agreed upon by nurses and physicians can drive the case selection, or 2) nurses, physicians and other care givers can submit a "request for review" through an established protocol, also agreed upon by nurses and physicians. Multidisciplinary quality or peer review groups that are open are the most successful at stimulating teamwork and joint learning. Providers whose cases are being reviewed are invited to the review, and attendance is voluntary. In such a system, over time, the need to have closed medical peer review is rare. Being careful to always focus the discussion on providing optimal care for the patient in the bed keeps the tone positive and helps create a safe environment for learning.

As I began in my role as nurse manager in a larger tertiary perinatal center, I instituted a system of Concurrent Quality Screening. This involved placing a peer-protected quality screening tool with each patient's chart which reflected the clinical quality indicators or data needed for process improvements. The information collected with this tool was then used for quality review or as a source of data which may not have been present in, or easily retrievable from, the medical record (for example, information the nurse or physician wants known about systems, processes or people that would not otherwise be available to assist improvement efforts). This system facilitated awareness and communication among nurses and between nurses and physicians regarding areas of high importance for patient care and safety.

The information set to be collected in the screens was determined by nurses and physicians together, and the process of selection itself built a clearer understanding of the indicators and their importance for everyone involved. This system of concurrent screening has worked well to obtain information for process improvements such as labor epidural safety or timeliness of cesarean birth, as data is gathered in "real time" versus through retrospective chart review. This is a nonthreatening way to identify "near misses" or "good catches" that are not technically incidents reported on safety (incident) reports. It is important that some kind of blameless tracking of this information occur for the purpose of identifying trends or organizational opportunities for improvement. With the implementation of electronic medical records, systems could be built in to identify and report those same cases from data already entered.

As a manager, it was useful for me to know immediately if there were any concerns in care. It was not unusual for a nurse or physician to bring me the screen personally, or I might find a screen requiring prompt attention on my desk. This facilitated excellent teamwork, provided opportunities for service recovery, helped prevent potential interpersonal or care problems, and provided an impetus to address issues that could adversely affect patient care immediately so that they did not become sentinel events, areas of significant dissatisfaction or potential liability risks.

Critical Event Review (CER) / Near Miss or Good Catch Case Reviews

Typically a series of "near misses" precedes an event that ultimately results in patient harm or a sentinel event. When carefully reviewed, near misses and good catches provide a rich source of information about error, and tend to be easier for providers to discuss than a bad outcome. However, near misses may remain invisible if a clear organizational value and expectation to report them is not communicated by medical and nursing leaders. Critical Event Review (CER), also known as "root cause or causal analysis," incorporates human factor and other system components into the detailed analysis of near misses, and can also be used for "good catches" or "sentinel events."

In CER, health care team members participate in a peer-protected, nonpunitive analysis of an event to identify the contributing system factors and other process of care issues that contributed to the outcome. It is necessary for the organization to provide skilled facilitators for participation in this process, and timely review is preferable while facts are fresh in the minds of the care providers involved. Action plans are developed to prevent similar occurrences, or learnings from excellent care can be reinforced and disseminated.

Multidisciplinary case-based learning from near misses, sentinel events or situations demonstrating excellence is one of the more powerful ways to promote teamwork and good care, and is often identified by nurses and physicians as a preferred mode for learning.

Learning from near misses, sentinel events or situations demonstrating excellence is one of the more powerful ways to promote teamwork and good care.

Notification or Consultation Guidelines

Nursing staff may observe high-risk patient situations evolving in hospitals where resident physicians, midwives and family practice doctors provide specialty care (i.e., obstetrics) or where procedures or surgery are done for patient populations with unique or specialized needs (i.e., pediatrics). If nurses see that patient needs are not being met, or they feel that patients are at risk and the primary medical provider is not responding to the concern, the nurse remains responsible to address and resolve the issue, and if necessary, to climb the medical "Chain of Communication and/or Command" to ensure the patient's safety. In these situations, interdisciplinary conflict may result. Creating collaboratively developed guidelines that describe when communication or consultation with a specialist should occur is a proactive strategy to ensure that a nurse's fear of conflict (or even retribution) will not get in the way of patient safety.

As structures that promote collaboration and communication become part of everyday practice, the benefit to patient care increases.

An example of this would be creating an organizational guideline that all hospitalized children and their families have consultation with a pediatrician. Another example would be the establishment of mutually agreed upon high-risk clinical conditions under which a resident, midwife or family practice physician should notify or consult with an obstetrician.

As structures that promote collaboration and communication become part of everyday practice, the benefit to patient care increases. When systems and processes that promote safety become part of the "way we work," people then feel free to work within them creatively and know there is a place to address issues or concerns and to proactively problem solve for safe, quality patient care.

References: Knox, G., Simpson, E., Rice, K., & Townsend, K. (2003, Fall). High reliability perinatal units: Further observations and a suggested plan for action. *Journal of Healthcare Risk Management, 23,* 17-21.

National Joint Practice Commission. (1981). *Guidelines for establishing joint or collaborative practice in hospitals.* Chicago: Neeley Printing.

Schmalenburg, C., Kramer, M., King, C., Krugman, M., Lund, C., Poduska, D., & Rapp, D. (2005). Excellence through evidence, securing collegial/collaborative nurse-physician relationships, Part 2. *Journal of Nursing Administration* 35, 507-514.

A View From a Patient: Attitude, the Big "A"

—John O. Hardiman

In August, I developed intense chest pain that extended between my shoulder blades along with severe respiratory distress. I called my doctor and he told me to go to the emergency room of Eliza Coffee Memorial Hospital (ECM) in Florence, AL and he would meet me there. The next day I had a cardiac catheterization and 3 days later I had an aortic valve replacement and then spent 5 days in the cardiac care facilities before being discharged.

This hospital stay exposed me to some of the finest nursing care I have ever seen and, as a result, I wrote a letter to the administration expressing my admiration for the nursing staff. Why did I consider this care was the best? Because it met the patient's needs and was gently and promptly delivered with kindness and courtesy by caring professional people who obviously knew and paid attention to what they were doing. Of course, in the intensive care units the quantity of nursing care I received was more than could possibly be delivered to the average hospital patient, but every patient deserves high-quality nursing care even if it is smaller doses. **Attitude**, the big "A," makes high-quality care possible. Let's look at some examples.

When my wife and I rushed across town and got to ECM, we were scared, anxious and confused. I was so busy breathing; we got out of our car in the drive in front of the endoscopy entrance instead of the ER entrance. We took the keys out, but in our haste did not turn off the flashers, headlights or even shut the doors to the car as we dashed in the endoscopy entrance. I got in the hall but couldn't go any further. A nurse came by, saw I was in trouble, and got a wheelchair and took me to the ER. Later in the ER when I was hooked up to oxygen, IVs, monitors, etc., someone reminded us that our car was in the wrong place. Marc, one of the nurses in the ER, calmly told my wife to just stay with me and he would take care of the car as he was going off duty. Later he came back, gave the keys to my wife and explained that the battery was dead when he

Editors' note: *This "patient's perspective" provides important insights on the power of "Attitude" and presence in caring. Presented at a* Reigniting the Spirit of Caring *workshop at Eliza Coffee Medical Center.*

tried to start the car. He had gotten some jumper cables and started the car, took it to the parking garage and parked it under a light close to the security guard and cleared it with the security guard so if my wife had any trouble with getting it started, the guard would help her. That really demonstrates the helpful Attitude of being willing to help a good nurse should have. We appreciate it.

A good nurse is a professional and must have the competence and skill expected of a professional. A nurse should look and act like a professional. It is not enough for a nurse to be educated in chemistry, pharmacology, anatomy and all those things taught in nursing school. Yes, nurses have to know those things, and they must keep up with changes in pharmaceuticals, new equipment, and nursing practices, etc. However, even that is not all it takes to be a good nurse. It takes the right Attitude, a good "A."

> Good nurses treat patients like they would like their favorite grandmother or grandfather treated.

To be a good nurse requires someone who is considerate and who understands that patients are people in trouble. Generally patients are anxious, weak, sick, often confused and need not only medical support but emotional support by someone who can convince them that he or she has a genuine regard for the patient's well-being. Some patients are very difficult to "put up with." A good nurse will find a way to "put up with them" anyway. My nurses did. They had the right Attitude.

Good nurses treat patients like they would their favorite grandmother or grandfather. They shouldn't say, "Hey Joe, how you doing?" to a 60-year old pneumonia patient. They should say, "Mr. Jones, how are you today?" I think it is disrespectful for people I don't know to call me by my first name and I don't like it. Most of my generation seems to feel the same. I became a "Mister" before most of my nurses were born, when I first registered to vote in a state election. I happen to have some other titles, but if someone doesn't know them, "Mister" is still appropriate. You may not agree, but remember, it is the opinion of the recipient that determines if something is respectful or not. My nurses were respectful. Why? "Attitude" is why.

When someone is going to do something to a patient, I think that person should tell the patient what and usually why. "Mr. Smith, I need to give you a shot for your infection" is a lot better than "Roll up your sleeve." My nurses kept me informed and were always courteous about it. The big "A."

If you tell a patient you will go check to see if there is something that can be done about her back pain (or anything else), GO DO IT. Then immediately take care of the patient. Don't go off and get sidetracked with another chore and a half-hour later remember that poor Mrs. Brown is writhing in pain because she didn't get her analgesic. My nurses were prompt, and did what they said they would. They had the right stuff—the right Attitude.

The nurses I had were very attentive to my needs. After the cardiac catheterization, I was not supposed to bend my right leg but I had a frequent cough from the anesthesia endotracheal tube. Every time I coughed, I would reflexively double up my right leg. Almost immediately, this warm friendly voice would say, "You need to keep your leg straight," and at the same time gentle hands would push my leg back down on the mattress. This happened many, many times and each time it got the same prompt response from the nurse. Even though it must have been extremely frustrating to her for the constant repetition, there never was any indication of frustration in the tone of her voice or in any of her actions. Many things occur with a nurse's duties that are frustrating, stressful and irritating, but remember a patient's day may also have been filled with frustration, stress, irritation, fear and pain. With the right Attitude, good nurses will avoid showing irritation to a patient no matter how difficult that might be.

I couldn't eat. I understand that is a common occurrence with cardiac patients. I had no appetite, and just didn't want any food. My nurses offered again and again to get whatever I wanted, but I just didn't want anything. The nurses encouraged me, but not to the point that I became resentful. It must take a lot of understanding, practice and tact to develop the ability to walk that narrow path. My nurses had that art down pat.

The nurses talked to me and listened to me when I wanted to talk. I know they were not really interested in knowing the dumb things I had done in my life, but, in paying attention to my ramblings, they gave me more encouragement than they will ever know. They shared with me. For example, I know that two of them live near Collinwood, Tennessee, and one and her husband attended the University of Arkansas. These things helped me feel less like just a body lying on a bed in a strange place and more like a person in a place where people

The nurses talked to me and listened to me when I wanted to talk. I know they were not really interested in knowing the dumb things I had done in my life, but, in paying attention to my ramblings, they gave me more encouragement than they will ever know.

cared about me and I had some friends. Just a few seconds of chitchat can mean a lot to a lonely, bored patient.

I was encouraged to walk. At the same time it was carefully pointed out to me that I should not overdo any exertion. When I did walk–using a walker–the nurse was six inches away from my left arm and gave me her total attention. I knew I was in safe, caring hands and I walked around secure in the knowledge that she would not let anything bad happen to me.

When walking down the hospital halls it is easy to forget that behind some of those closed doors are people who are scared and nervous and may be trying to rest. I remember in my previous hospitalization after a very restless night, I had just finally dozed off in sleep when two nurses passed in the hall and, talking in loud voices about how someone kept pulling out her IV, woke me up. That just about ruined my day. That did not happen in my stay at ECM. ECM nurses have the right Attitude.

While I was walking one time, someone walked past and, in a gesture of encouragement, patted me in the middle of my back. It had been only 4 days from the time of my open chest surgery and this pat hurt very badly. While it was done so suddenly the nurse could not have prevented it, good nurses must understand the patient's condition and do their best to protect the patient from situations that might produce distress.

Some of us do not have the gift of the considerate and caring Attitude that good nurses have. We are a product of our heredity and environment and we all are different. However, if a nurse is not naturally gifted with that Attitude, and cannot learn and develop that Attitude, he or she can never be really good in giving nursing care to people. My nurses had that considerate and caring Attitude.

The number one goal of a good nurse is to give the best of care to the patient. Good nurses must be capable, competent, considerate, and caring. They must protect the patient from harm. They must have an Attitude of sincere regard for the patient's well-being, both physical and emotional, and that hopefully earns from the patient the confidence and trust that will sustain the patient during the stressful time of illness. That is what my nurses did and I am grateful to each one of them. I hope you will do the same with each and every one of your patients.

I wish the best for each of you and hope God will bless you and your big Attitude.

CHAPTER SIXTEEN

Crosswalks Between Relationship-Based Care and Professional Organizations

We have included this section on Crosswalks between Relationship-Based Care and various professional organizations as a way to assist you in identifying how Relationship-Based Care can help you achieve standards and goals for your organization as a whole. Clearly, this is not a section to "curl up by the fire" and read. It is a reference section to help you understand and connect the principles and concepts in RBC with the Code of Nursing Ethics, some specifics standards from the Joint Commission, the Forces of Magnet, the American Organization of Nurse Executives Guiding Principles for Patient Care Delivery, and the Institute of Medicine's Standards for Keeping Patients Safe. Our hope in including this section is to save you some work in researching these connections yourself.

Introduction to the Crosswalks

Crosswalk Between the Code of Ethics for Nurses and Relationship-Based Care

—Susan Wessel and Mary Koloroutis

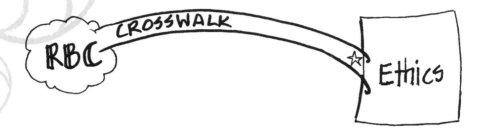

The long ethical tradition within nursing has been a source of professional pride for most nurses. Our ethical heritage began with the Nightingale Pledge in 1893, which is understood as the first nursing Code of Ethics. As the Code of Ethics evolved over the years, it's always been fundamentally based on key ethical principles. These principles include doing no harm, benefiting others, loyalty, truthfulness, social justice, and in later years, autonomy of the patient and the nurse (American Nurses Association, 2001).

Relationship-Based Care (RBC) supports and promotes adherence to the nine elements in the Code of Ethics for Nurses. The principles of RBC provide a foundation for nurses to practice in a highly professional and ethical manner.

The crosswalk below links the American Nurses Association's Code of Ethics for Nurses with principles and concepts of Relationship-Based Care.

Provision from the Code of Ethics	Relationship-Based Care Principles and Concepts
The nurse, in all professional relationships, practices with compassion and respect for the inherent dignity, worth and uniqueness of every individual, unrestricted by considerations of social or economic status, personal attributes or the nature of health problems.	**Principles:** Culturally responsive patient care is provided in a caring, therapeutic environment. Care is attentive to body, mind and spirit. **Concepts:** Patient advocacy, focus on the patient's most important goals and concerns for care, knowledge-based care
The nurse's primary commitment is to the patient, whether an individual, family, group or community.	**Principles:** The registered nurse is responsible for establishing a therapeutic relationship and an individualized plan of care. It is expected that the patients and/or families will know the name of their Primary/attending Nurse. As the nurse-patient relationship is established, the insight gained into what matters most to specific patients must be communicated appropriately to other members of the team to ensure care needs and outcomes are met. The manager maintains a clear focus on the purpose of the work—caring for patients and families—and articulates expectations for performance and competency. **Concepts:** Six professional nursing practice roles, clinical and emotional safety, empowerment of patient and family
The nurse promotes, advocates for, and strives to protect the health, safety and rights of the patient.	**Principle:** Patient advocacy, patient safety and patient education are high values and are consistently demonstrated in practice. **Concepts:** Patient advocacy, focus on the patient's most important goals and concerns for care, nurse as guide, nurse as leader
The nurse is responsible and accountable for individual nursing practice and determines the appropriate delegation of tasks consistent with the nurse's obligation to provide optimum patient care.	**Principles:** The RN has full authority for determining the kind and amount of nursing care a patient will receive, the work that care requires, how much of that work requires the attention and time of the RN and how much can be delegated to other care givers. The RN has the responsibility, authority and accountability to coordinate communication between the patient and family and members of the interdisciplinary team. **Concepts:** Articulated expectations, principles of delegation, Commitment to My Co-workers, three realms of nursing practice, four essential functions of nursing practice
The nurse owes the same duties to self as to others, including the responsibility to preserve integrity and safety, to maintain competence and to continue personal and professional growth.	**Principles:** The manager creates an environment supportive of professional nursing practice where RNs are autonomous decision makers and creative problem solvers. **Concepts:** Self-knowing, 5 Cs (clarity, competency, confidence, collaboration and commitment), personal and professional development, staff empowerment, self-care, care for colleagues, four domains of competency, novice to expert theory of competence

Provision from the Code of Ethics	Relationship-Based Care Principles and Concepts
The nurse participates in establishing, maintaining and improving health care environments and conditions of employment conducive to the provision of quality health care and consistent with the values of the profession through individual and collective action.	**Principles:** Leaders and staff work together to assure that patients and families have what they need in a timely manner by simplifying work processes to achieve desired outcomes. Patients and families experience exceptional cooperation among all members of the health care team who treat them and each other with dignity, respect and sensitivity. Caring and healing practices are visible in relationships, clinical interventions and the physical setting. **Concepts:** Decentralized decision making, unit practice councils, caring leader behaviors, healthy, nondefensive communication, Commitment to Co-Workers
The nurse participates in the advancement of the profession through contributions to practice, education, administration, and knowledge development.	**Concepts:** Nurse as leader, evidence-based practice, characteristics of a profession, nurse as teacher
The nurse collaborates with other health professionals and the public in promoting community, national, and international efforts to meet health needs.	**Concepts:** Nurse as collaborator, nurse as healer, nurse as leader, interdependent practice
The profession of nursing, as represented by associations and their members, is responsible for articulating nursing values, for maintaining the integrity of the profession and its practice, and for shaping social policy.	**Concepts:** Characteristics of a profession, ANA Social Policy Statement, social responsibility/contract, voice of agency, staff empowerment (R+A+A), realms of nursing practice, professional rights and responsibilities

Provisions from the Code of Ethics reprinted with permission from American Nurses Association, *Code of ethics for nurses with interpretive statement* (2001). Silver Springs, MD: Author

Reference: American Nurses Association. (2003). *Nursing: A social policy statement.* Washington, DC: Author.

Koloroutis, M. (ed.). (2004). *Relationship-Based Care: A Model for Transforming Practice.* Minneapolis, MN: Creative Health Care Management

Crosswalk Between the American Nurses Credentialing Center Forces of Magnetism and Relationship-Based Care

—Alice Weydt

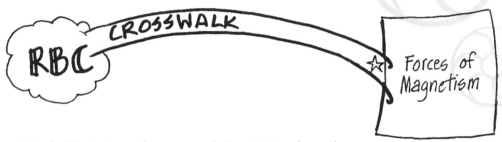

The original Magnet study occurred in 1981 when the American Academy of Nursing established a task force to study the nursing shortage. Of more than 150 hospitals studied, there were 41 hospitals not experiencing a nursing shortage. Hospital characteristics that attracted and retained these nurses were identified. These organizations were able to create work environments that nurses found professionally and personally rewarding. Since then, the American Nurses Credentialing Center (ANCC) has identified 14 characteristics, or Forces of Magnetism, which serve as a road map for organizations to create environments that reward, retain, and attract staff. The Magnet Recognition Program™ is not prescriptive in how systems or structures are to be organized, but rather asks for evidence about how administration, professional practice and professional development contribute to quality patient outcomes. The Forces of Magnetism correlate to patient and staff satisfaction because there are positive perceptions about the quality of care.

Magnet status results when systems are in place that support professional nursing practice. Magnet asks for evidence that demonstrates that the nurse leader at the executive level fosters a culture where a competent workforce not only contributes to the quality improvements but owns the outcomes of the practice. Complex patient care issues with primary and secondary diagnoses that require sophisticated professional nursing interventions create the need for flexible, responsive and timely decision making systems that foster responsibility, accountability and autonomy at the point of care. Meeting Magnet standards by incorporating Relationship-Based Care (RBC) principles into the organizational fabric ensures that collaboration between members of the nursing staff and the interdisciplinary team meet patient and family needs in a timely manner because work processes have been simplified to achieve desired outcomes. Using these principles means that meeting Magnet standards is not in addition to what is being done but rather is the outcome of satisfied staff providing quality care that meets, if not exceeds, the expectations of patients and their families.

The Magnet Recognition Program is administered by the American Nurses Credentialing Center (ANCC), which is a subsidiary of the American Nurses Association (ANA). Rigorous documentation is required to be considered for a site visit. When that requirement is met, Magnet appraisers from the American Nurses Credentialing Center meet with direct care staff during a scheduled visit to validate the documentation. Magnet designation is a highly coveted award that is bestowed upon the organization. It indicates the existence of a professional environment that supports growth and development of the nursing staff and excellence in nursing service and patient care.

The Magnet Recognition Program acknowledges that professional nursing practice makes a difference in the lives of the patients and families being served. The following crosswalk demonstrates how the Forces of Magnetism and the Principles of Relationship-Based Care are synchronistic. Magnet recognition is an outcome of practice principles that are inherent in the infrastructure of Relationship-Based Care.

Forces of Magnetism	Relationship-Based Care Principles and Concepts
Quality of Nursing Leadership: Nursing Leaders are perceived as knowledgeable, strong risk-takers who follow an articulated philosophy in the day-to-day operations of the nursing department. Nursing leaders also convey a strong sense of advocacy and support on behalf of the staff. Results of quality leadership are evident in nursing practice at the patient's bedside.	Leaders inspire a shared vision, collective purpose, and real change at all levels of the organization. Nursing leaders create an environment of appreciation, caring and healing. They have a vision of what is important and are committed to making the vision live in relationships with patients at the bedside. Relationship-Based Care is the "core business." The nurse leaders create an environment in which caring relationships happen. Caring leaders influence caring interactions with patients and families by virtue of their own caring interactions with staff.
Organizational Structure: Organizations are characterized as flat, rather than tall, structures in which unit-based decision making prevails. Nursing departments are decentralized, with a strong nursing representation evident in the organization committee structure. The nursing leader serves at the executive level of the organization, and the Chief Nursing Officer reports to the executive level.	The infrastructure of the organization is decentralized with clear responsibility, authority and accountability to support empowerment. The principles of RBC for the organization emerge from the Appreciative Inquiry processes that engage staff from disciplines and departments throughout the organization, including nursing. The CNO, as the champion for RBC, articulates the intent of RBC to the executive team and board. The CNO also has the responsibility for the development of the principles of the care delivery model which incorporates the professional nursing role. The nurse manager provides leadership at the unit level. Based on the RBC principles Unit Practice Councils develop unit-specific plans with input from 100% of the staff on the unit.
Management Style: Organization and nursing administrators use a participative management style, incorporating feedback from staff at all levels of the organization. Feedback is characterized as encouraged and valued. Nurses serving in leadership positions are visible, accessible, and committed to communicating effectively with staff.	Nurse leaders provide the inspiration, infrastructure, resources for education and the processes for evidence-based practice to guide nursing practice. The success of their efforts is dependent on the quality of the relationships that leaders have with one another as well as with the staff they lead. Nurse leaders lead with purpose, model the way, and maintain clear and unrelenting focus on care to serve patients and families. Nurse leaders create the environment whereby the principles of Relationship-Based Care can be lived in daily practice. They articulate clear expectations for patient care and professional performance, inspire and encourage staff to learn and develop, serve as coach and mentor and consistently demonstrate respect for all members of the team.
Personnel Policies and Programs: Salaries and benefits are characterized as competitive. Rotating shifts arc minimized, and creative, and flexible staffing models are used. Personnel polices are created with staff involvement, and significant administrative and clinical promotional opportunities exist.	The infrastructure supports retention and promotes employee satisfaction. Recruitment is focused on matching the employee to the organizational culture. Care is resource driven. Staffing levels, skill mix, staffing schedules and patient assignments are based on what is best for the patient. The competency domains of clinical skills, interpersonal skills, critical thinking and leadership at the point of care are reflected in job descriptions. The organization supports competency development through education, time and resources so employees continually develop new skills and knowledge.
Professional Models of Care: Models of care are used that give nurses the responsibility and authority for the provision of patient care. Nurses are accountable for their own practice and are the coordinators of care.	RBC is based on nursing theories and models, e.g.: Jean Watson's Theory of Human Caring, Kristen Swanson's Five Caring Processes, and Sharon Dingman's Caring Model. Relationship-Based Care is a care delivery model that may be interdisciplinary (including nursing) or nursing only. Classic principles in three of the elements of an RBC Nursing Care Delivery Model are: 1. The professional nurse (Primary Nurse) makes decisions about patient care based on an individualized therapeutic relationship and plan of care. 2. Staff scheduling, assignments, and delegation are driven by continuity of care and relationships of professional nurses and practice partners with the patient and family. 3. The Professional Nurse coordinates communication with the patient/family, the nursing team, the physician and the interdisciplinary team. 4. The manager creates an environment of professional nursing practice where RNs are autonomous decision makers and creative problem solvers.

Forces of Magnetism	Relationship-Based Care Principles and Concepts
Quality of Care: Nurses perceive that they are providing high-quality care to their patients. Providing quality care is seen as an organizational priority as well, and nurses serving in leadership positions are viewed as responsible for developing the environment in which high quality care can be provided.	Patient advocacy, patient safety and patient education are of high value and are consistently demonstrated in practice. Relationship-Based Care focuses on strengthening the interpersonal skills of the hospital staff. A therapeutic relationship between patients, families and a Professional Nurse is core to quality of care. Quality care occurs in environments where the standard within the health care team is to: • Respect and affirm each other's unique scope of practice • Work interdependently to care for and serve the patient and family • Work together to create a culture of learning, mutual support, and creative problem solving, recognizing that everyone has a valuable contribution to make
Quality Improvement: Quality improvement activities are viewed as educational. Staff nurses participate in the quality improvement process and perceive the process as one that improves the quality of care delivered within the organization.	Inspiration, Infrastructure, Education and Evidence are the four elements of Creative Health Care Management's (CHCM's) formula for transformational change. Outcome measurements related to patient satisfaction, staff satisfaction and quality of care monitors are integral to an RBC implementation. Leaders and staff are involved in defining the measurements and using qualitative and quantitative data at the unit/practice level to improve practice in a continuous cycle of learning.
Consultation and Resources: Adequate consultation and other human resources are available. Knowledgeable experts, particularly advanced practice nurses, are available and used. In addition, peer support is given within and outside the nursing division.	Consultation, internal and external, is integral to the development of Relationship-Based Care. Relationship-Based Care is a framework for organizational transformation in which everyone's contribution is valued and valuable. Collegial relationships are integral to Relationship-Based Care. Interdependence and collaboration among members of the health care team is a major focus.
Autonomy: Nurses are permitted and expected to practice autonomously, consistent with professional standards. Independent judgment is expected o be exercised within the context of a multidisciplinary approach to patient care.	Primary Nurses have the responsibility, authority, accountability to make decisions about the nursing care their patients receive based on the individualized therapeutic relationships, the nursing process and the plan of care. The Primary Nurse also determines which work requires his or her own time and attention, and which work can be delegated to other care providers. Care is collaborative and interdisciplinary.
Community and the Health Care Organization: Organizations that are best able to recruit and retain nurses also maintain a strong community presence. A community presence is seen in a variety of ongoing, long-term programs. These outreach programs result in the organization being perceived as a strong, positive, and productive corporate citizen.	The overarching aspect of RBC is a commitment from the boardroom to the bedside. Patient care is the core business. Relationships within the organization and connections with the community, including academic institutions, are fostered.
Nurses as Teachers: Nurses are permitted and expected to incorporate teaching in all aspects of their practice. Teaching is one activity that reportedly gives nurses a great deal of professional satisfaction.	In RBC the professional nurse fulfills six practice roles: sentry, healer, guide, teacher, collaborator and leader. As a guide the nurse leads or directs another's way through unfamiliar circumstances and uses his/her knowledge to enable the patients and family's passage. As a teacher, the nurse imparts knowledge to facilitate the patient and family's capacity to continue recovery and care for themselves. The professional nurse teaches and mentors staff, patients and families as they learn approaches to either improve health status or expand knowledge and expertise.

Forces of Magnetism	Relationship–Based Care Principles and Concepts
Image of Nursing: Nurses are viewed as integral to the organization's ability to provide patient care services. The services provided by nurses are characterized as essential by other members of the health care team.	Through the "voice of agency" nurses articulate their contribution to health care to patients and their families, the interdisciplinary team and the community.
Interdisciplinary Relationships: Interdisciplinary relationships are characterized as positive. A sense of mutual respect is exhibited among all disciplines.	The behaviors articulated in CHCM's Commitment to My Co-workers card which guide all relationships, including interdisciplinary, are: trust, mutual respect, consistent and visible support, and open, honest communication. Honoring the dignity and worth of each person is fundamental to RBC. It is understood that teamwork is the most significant predictor of quality; and that teamwork and collaborative practice are essential to delivering safe, ethical, efficient care.
Professional Development: Significant emphasis is placed on orientation, in-service education, continuing education, formal education, and career development. Personal and professional growth and development are valued. In addition, opportunities for competency-based clinical advancement exist, along with the resources to maintain competency.	RBC is predicated upon a commitment to continuous organizational learning based on the framework of Inspiration, Infrastructure, Education and Evidence. Through the decentralized processes individuals and groups are engaged in professional development as well as interdisciplinary collaboration, critical thinking and mutual problem-solving. Competency assessment, development and advancement are an ongoing process.

Forces of Magnetism reprinted with permission from the American Nurses Credentialing Center (ANCC).
The Magnet Recognition Program® and ANCC Magnet Recognition® names and logos are registered trademarks of the American Nurses Credentialing Center. Magnet™ is a trademark of the American Nurses Credentialing Center. American Nurses Credentialing Center (ANCC) is a subsidiary of the American Nurses Association (ANA). All rights reserved.

Reference: American Nurses Credentialing Center. (2005). *Magnet Recognition Program® Application Manual 2005.* Silver Spring, MD: American Nurses Credentialing Center

Koloroutis, M. (Ed.). (2004). *Relationship-based care: A model for transforming practice.* Minneapolis, MN: Creative Health Care Management.

Crosswalk Between Relationship-Based Care and the American Organization of Nurse Executives' Seven Guiding Principles for Patient Care Delivery

—Jayne A. Felgen, Alice Weydt and Mary Koloroutis

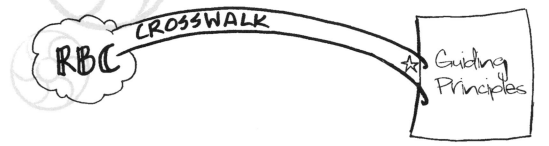

The passion of nursing is found in caring relationships. These relationships bridge the isolation and vulnerability of disability, infirmity, poverty and age. Quantifying caring has been elusive and nurses have been driven away from this because of external pressures such as fiscal constraints, regulations and current emphasis given to data-driven outcomes reflecting a medical model.

The importance of relationships and caring processes has long been known to nurses. Nurses realize that technology and data are extremely important, but without the ability to relate the experience in the patient's terms, the process is mechanical and impersonal. It is through the relationships that nurses develop with patients and families that hope is instilled and concern for outcomes is communicated. To practice nursing as if it is only a science, without the art of healing practices, leads to dissatisfied nurses and a negative experience for patients and families. It is encouraging to see that the importance of therapeutic relationships is once again gaining recognition and seen as essential to care and healing as technology and data.

Relationship-Based Care principles and concepts guide practice and delineate the role of the registered nurse. The constructs of Relationship-Based Care are consistent with important statements from professional nursing organizations, such as the American Organization of Nurse Executives' (AONE's) Seven Principles for Patient Care Delivery. The crosswalk below demonstrates how AONE's Guiding Principles and Relationship-Based Care principles and concepts relate to each other and reinforce caring processes as essential to professional nursing practice.

AONE Guiding Principles for Patient Care Delivery	Relationship-Based Care Principles and Concepts
The Core of Nursing is Knowledge and Caring. The actual work that nurses do will change, but core values will remain.	• The therapeutic nurse-patient relationship is the cornerstone of Professional Nursing Practice and a fundamental element of Relationship-Based Care. • There is universal agreement among nurses that their relationship with patients and patient families is a sacred privileged trust. • Nurses voice a fierce commitment to the values of caring, advocacy, collaboration, safety and seeking what is in the best interest of the patients and families they serve. • Knowledge-based caring is the core or essence of nursing practice and is expressed through the therapeutic relationship between the nurse and patient/family.
Care is User-Based. Care will be directed in partnership with the patient/client or population needs and will be respectful of the diversity of the health belief models of all users.	• The registered nurse assesses and determines the patient's needs through listening to the patient's/family's personal story, formalized interviews, and review of records. The patient's number one concern for this episode of care is identified and his/her definition of desired caring behaviors is determined. • The professional registered nurse develops and implements an individualized plan of nursing care with the patient and family, based on patient and family requests and concerns. • Culturally responsive patient care is provided in a caring and healing environment. • Care is attentive to mind/body/spirit. • The patient and family are actively involved in their care and experience a relationship with their nurse. • Professional nursing practice is built on interdependent relationships.
Knowledge is Access-Based. The knowledge base of the nurse will shift from "knowing" a specific body of knowledge to "knowing how to access" the evolving knowledge base to support the needs of those for whom care is managed.	• Knowledge-based caring is the core or essence of nursing practice and is expressed through the therapeutic relationship between the nurse and patient/family. • The RN proactively seeks information and provides information to others involved in the care of the patient and family. • Professional Nursing Practice requires ongoing development to sustain proficiency in practice. • The boundaries of nursing practice, as in all health care disciplines, change with the changing needs and requirements of the patients they serve. • Competency levels are determined on both the individual and the clinical situation. • The responsibility and accountability for continuous learning is shared by the nurse and the organization. • Nurses are responsible for accessing knowledge and skills required to attain and maintain proficiency in their practice. • The organization is responsible for promoting and supporting continuous learning and providing opportunities for growth.

AONE Guiding Principles for Patient Care Delivery	Relationship-Based Care Principles and Concepts
Knowledge is Synthesized. The processing of accessed knowledge will shift the work of the nurse from critical thinking to "critical synthesis." Synthesis occurs as care is coordinated across multiple levels/disciplines/settings.	• Registered nurses are accountable for planning, delivering or delegating, coordinating, evaluating and modifying the patient care and for effectively communicating the plan of care with attention to the continuity across shifts and settings of care. • Six practice roles provide a framework for critical thinking and integration of R+A+A in leading, coordinating and integrating patient care requirements. Role of Sentry. The nurse continuously assesses, monitors, and intervenes for the patient to prevent complications, promote healing and optimize safe outcomes. Role of Healer The nurse establishes a therapeutic relationship with the patient and family, ensuring they receive physical, emotional and spiritual care based on an assessment of their needs. Role of Guide: The nurse helps the patient and family by translating pertinent information and processes, by clarifying and explaining procedures and by making certain that the patient and family understand what to expect, ensuring they are informed enough to make decisions about their care. Role of Teacher: The nurse teaches the patient and family how to safely care for themselves within the health care setting and upon discharge. Role of Collaborator: The nurse works with each member of the health care team to ensure they receive and provide pertinent information regarding the patient and family and to coordinate the patient's plan of care. Role of Leader: The nurse advocates for the patient and family, provides supervision and leadership to other members of the care team and identifies and initiates changes that will improve the quality of care for patients and families.
Relationships of Care. Our knowledge and the care provided are grounded in the relationships with our patients/clients/populations. The relationship will be multidisciplinary and include the full societal scope of generations, diversity and interdependency.	• Professional Nursing exists to provide compassionate care to individuals and their loved ones. • The therapeutic nurse-patient relationship is the cornerstone of Professional Nursing Practice and a fundamental element of Relationship-Based Care. • Nurses help patients and their families maintain health, attain healing and experience a peaceful and dignified death. Nurses bring to this noble pursuit a profound understanding of the human condition. • Nursing has a relationship with society based on a social contract that delineates professional rights and responsibilities and mechanisms for public accountability. • The social accountability for nursing is demonstrated in three distinct realms of nursing practice: delegated, independent and interdependent. • Professional Nursing Practice is built on interdependent relationships. • Nurses, physicians and other health care professionals share the common purpose of caring for patients and families. • The Professional Nurse plays a key role in creating collaborative relationships among members of the health care team that promote coordinated care and service for patients and families.
The "Virtual" and the "Presence" Relationship of Care. Relationships will be dramatically changed by the increased application of technology, causing us to further define the relationship context as being "virtual" or "physical presence" and knowing when each is required.	• It is important for nurses and all other members of the health care team to understand and articulate their boundaries and to provide care within ever expanding/changing boundaries to most effectively meet the needs of patients and families. • Influential leaders in nursing must maintain a strong vision of nursing as an evolving discipline and determine how to best serve the needs of patients in an ever changing health care environment.
Managing the Journey. The work of the nurse in the future will be to partner with the patient/client to manage their journey in accordance with their needs and desires and available resources.	• The new mindset for nursing staff is to move away from thinking about their work as being driven by tasks and routines to thinking about their work as being driven by prioritized caring based on the needs and desires of the patients and families they serve and available resources. • The new mindset shifts from "taking time" for each patient to "being with" each patient and mutually determining the aspects of care which are most important, productive and satisfying.

AONE Guiding Principles used with permission.

Reference: American Organization of Nurse Executives. (2005). AONE guiding principles for future care delivery toolkit. Retrieved January 4, 2007, from http://www.aone.org/aone/resource/guidingprinciples.html

Koloroutis, M. (Ed.). (2004). *Relationship-based care: A model for transforming practice.* Minneapolis, MN: Creative Health Care Management.

Crosswalk Between Institute of Medicine Standards for Keeping Patients Safe and Relationship-Based Care

—Susan Wessel

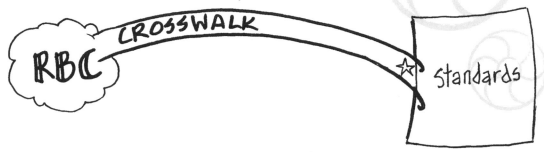

The 2004 report by the Institute of Medicine (IOM) entitled "Keeping Patients Safe: Transforming the Work Environment of Nurses" has an interesting background. The underlying study was requested by the U.S. Department of Health and Human Services' Agency for Healthcare Research and Quality (AHRQ). The agency asked the IOM to identify key aspects of the work environment for nurses that likely have an impact on patient safety and potential improvements in health care working conditions that would likely increase patient safety (IOM, 2004).

The findings and recommendations in the report are insightful and comprehensive. There is a welcome recognition that many practices in hospitals are based on complex and interacting pressures on health care organizations. These pressures create incentives that impact both the social and physical systems.

The IOM report on the work environment of nurses begins by reviewing the body of evidence on the direct impact that nurses have on better patient outcomes. It also highlights the damaging effects of reengineering initiatives in recent decades and their lasting impact. The authors found many serious threats to patient safety in the typical work environment of nurses. These threats fell in four categories:

1. Frequent failure to follow management practices necessary for safety
2. Unsafe workforce deployment
3. Unsafe work and workspace design, and
4. Punitive cultures that hinder the reporting and prevention of errors

IOM Recommendations

The IOM recommendations cite the "need for bundles of mutually reinforcing patient safety defenses in nurses' work environments" (IOM, 2004, p. 7). The IOM calls for multiple reinforcing changes in all organizational components: 1) leadership and management, 2) the workforce, 3) work processes, and 4) organizational culture. They emphasize that a piecemeal approach won't be successful because all the recommended actions form an important component of the whole.

A very high-level overview of the recommended changes will be presented here along with the potential impact of Relationship-Based Care (RBC) on their achievement. As you'll see, Relationship-Based Care provides a wonderful platform for meeting these IOM recommendations. The recommendations are rich with detail and substantiation as to their importance. The reader is encouraged to take advantage of the source report.

IOM Standards for Keeping Patients Safe	Relationship-Based Care Principles and Concepts
Governing Boards That Focus on Safety: • Are knowledgeable about the link between management practices and patient safety. • Emphasize patient safety to the same extent as financial and productivity goals. The standards call for executive leaders to educate their board and all levels of management about the link between management practices and safety. The balance of emphasis in safety and financial goals should be evident in public reports to stakeholders.	Relationship-Based Care is positioned as the mechanism to achieve not only the organization's mission but also its quality and safety goals. Board education is encouraged about RBC being the core business. This emphasis helps board members see financial results as an outcome of quality care rather than an end in itself. Patient safety is potentiated by RBC; the mechanisms for this are continuity of care, interdisciplinary collaboration, and the accountable RN understanding the patient and his or her goals in depth.

IOM Standards for Keeping Patients Safe	Relationship-Based Care Principles and Concepts
Leadership and Evidence-Based Management Structures and Processes: • Provide ongoing vigilance in balancing efficiency and patient safety • Demonstrate and promote trust in and by nursing staff • Actively manage the process of change • Engage nursing staff in nonhierarchical decision making and work design • Establish the organization as a "learning organization" The detail of this recommendation emphasizes the need for nurse leaders at all levels of management facilitating the direct input of the direct care nursing staff into decisions. The need for trust and communication with nursing staff is included. The IOM sees the need for transformational leaders skilled at managing change.	Relationship-Based Care involves managing organization-wide change in culture and patient delivery system through active involvement and empowerment of staff. The change methodology used, I_2E_2, produces well-planned and sustainable changes at the strategic, operational and tactical levels. Unit Practice Council (UPC) and Results Council structures for implementing RBC build mutual trust and break down barriers between management and staff. Education is an important and ongoing part of RBC implementation both at the staff and leadership levels.
Effective Nursing Leadership: • Participates in executive decision making • Represents nursing staff to management • Achieves effective communication between nurses and other clinical leadership • Facilitates input from direct-care nursing staff into decision making • Commands organizational resources for nursing knowledge acquisition and clinical decision making	The principles taught in *Leading an Empowered Organization* (*LEO*) promote ownership of leaders regarding their role in decisions and in establishing decentralized systems for staff decision making. Effective communication is emphasized as a tool to build trust and solve problems effectively. The role of managers in developing the skills and competence of staff is reinforced. During implementation of RBC the nurse executive has an important role in bringing forth RBC to the organization and educating both other executives and the board on its role in meeting the organization's vision for excellence.
Adequate Staffing: • Is established by sound methodologies as determined by nursing staff • Provides mechanisms to accommodate unplanned variations in patient care workload • Enables nursing staff to regulate nursing unit work flow • Is consistent with best available evidence on safe staffing thresholds The study that formed the basis of these recommendations placed special emphasis on nursing work hours and nursing workload as requested by AHRQ. The current evidence base for the role of RN staffing on better patient outcomes formed the basis for their recommendations. Conclusions are very specific on recommended hours of care in nursing homes and ICUs. They recommend the development of national standards by the Department of Health and Human Services for collecting and publishing staffing recommendations to the public.	While RBC does not prescribe specific staffing levels, it does maximize the time of nurses at the bedside and the best use of LPNs and nursing assistants. A Work Complexity Assessment documents how much of the work in individual nursing units must by done by RNs and how much can be delegated to others. It helps staff see the advantages of staffing through pairs and partners in using their time most efficiently and in potentiating teamwork and closer observation of patients. The principles of resource-driven staffing decisions help nurses prioritize care with the needs of patients at the uppermost priority. We help staff set criteria for assignments that consider patient complexity, staff skills and ability and continuity of care as high priorities rather than the geography of the patient on the floor. The empowerment of staff to make decisions at the point of care is foundational to RBC, and this encourages staff to exercise their authority in the best interest of the patients.
Organizational Support for Ongoing Learning and Decision Support: • Uses preceptors for novice nurses • Provides ongoing educational support and resources to nursing staff • Provides training in new technology • Provides decision support at the point of care. The authors emphasize the importance of investment in ongoing employee learning and advocate that a defined percentage of the nursing payroll be budgeted for ongoing education. This budget should support experienced staff to precept new nurses, an annual education plan for each nurse, and dissemination to individual staff of clinical learning tools such as algorithms and pathways.	Specific resources are focused on staff competence during the implementation of Relationship-Based Care. Staff often needs additional education on delegation, working as healthy teammates, critical thinking and group process. Four levels of staff competence are attended to including: interpersonal skills, clinical/technical skills, critical/creative thinking and leadership. The specific design of assignments on each unit includes provisions for novice nurses to be mentored and supported by experienced nurses.

IOM Standards for Keeping Patients Safe	Relationship-Based Care Principles and Concepts
Mechanisms That Promote Interdisciplinary Collaboration: • Use interdisciplinary practice mechanisms, such as interdisciplinary patient care rounds • Provide formal education and training in interdisciplinary collaboration for all health care providers.	Relationship-Based Care is generally implemented in multiple disciplines and is used to enhance communication and unification of effort around the patient's most important priorities. The plans for RBC are most effective when key members of other disciplines are invited to meetings of the Unit Practice Council (UPC) as appropriate. There is special emphasis on communication with physicians during planning and implementation. The role of the Primary Nurse as coordinator and communicator with other disciplines is a core RBC Principle.
Work Design That Promotes Safety: • Defends against fatigue and unsafe and inefficient work design • Tackles medication administration, hand washing, documentation and other high-priority practices. The research behind these recommendations cites the effects of fatigue on slowed reaction time, lapses of attention to detail, errors of omission, compromised problem solving, reduced motivation and decreased energy for successful completion of required tasks. The authors are specific in their recommendations. The IOM seeks regulations that prohibit staff from working more than 12 hours in a 24-hour period or more than 60 hours in 7 days. There is also rich information on the impact of distractions and noise during medication administration. They quantify the time nurses spend walking the halls, on non-nursing tasks and particularly on documentation. The IOM entreats various regulatory organizations to reduce mandatory documentation and encourages leaders to use appropriate personnel for non-nursing duties.	RBC does not recommend specific work hours or days, but does encourage a healthy work environment and staff input into scheduling practices that will enhance continuity of care. We applaud such strong recommendations that are evidence-based and support safe patient care. The results of work complexity assessment help staff understand appropriate delegation and the importance of using RN time for those things that require professional judgment. Leaders get a detailed report that helps them plan the appropriate skill mix for individual units.
Organizational Culture That Continuously Strengthens Patient Safety: • Regularly reviews organizational success in achieving formally specified safety objectives • Fosters a fair and just error-reporting, analysis and feedback system • Trains and rewards workers for safety. The IOM examined other industries that created safety-conscious cultures and significantly reduced their errors. They found pervasive employee engagement and attitudes around continuous improvement of safety practices. These organizations recognize that most errors are the result of systemic organizational defects in work processes, not blameworthy individuals, and their leaders support staff and foster continuous learning. The IOM concluded that creating a fair and just culture in responding to errors reduces workers' fear and reluctance to report errors or near misses.	In the curriculum of the *LEO* workshop, we teach managers about the importance of avoiding a culture of punishment and encouraging staff to learn from mistakes. Taking risks, generally on behalf of patients, can only be fostered in such an environment. The objective analysis of systems problems with staff as equal partners at the table leads to permanently solving problems rather than reprocessing them year after year. Relationship-Based Care requires that staff is free from fear of punishment since it requires staff autonomy and patient advocacy. Leaders' response to errors sets the stage for the culture to either hide errors and inspire guilt in response to them, or proactively analyze errors and near misses to seek ways to prevent future occurrences.

Institute of Medicine Standards for keeping Patients Safe used with permission.

References: Institute of Medicine. (2004). *Keeping patients safe: Transforming the work environment of nurses.* Washington, DC: The National Academies Press.

Koloroutis, M. (Ed.). (2004). *Relationship-based care: A model for transforming practice.* Minneapolis, MN: Creative Health Care Management.

PART

V

Evidence

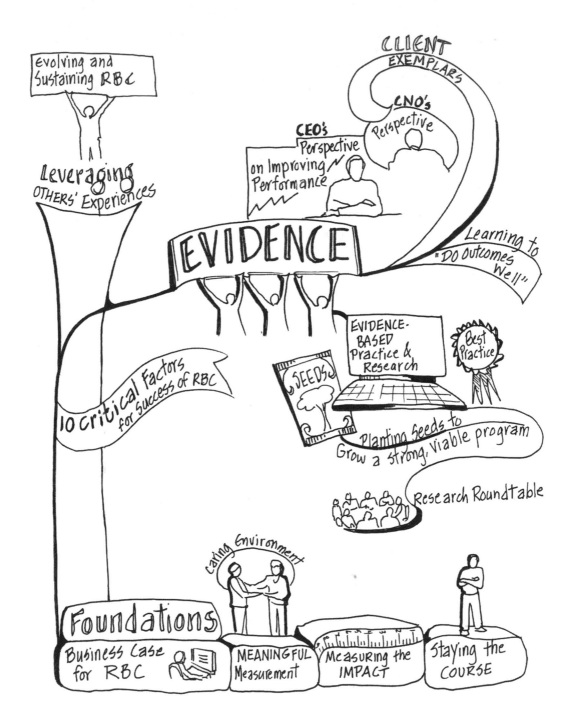

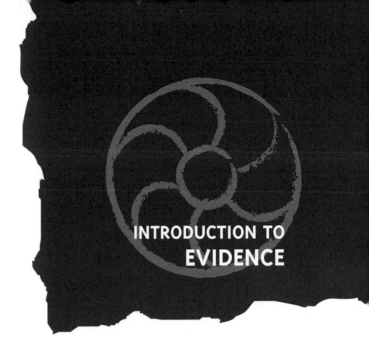

INTRODUCTION TO EVIDENCE

Evidence shows us the degree to which we have achieved what we've set out to achieve.

We always set out to measure the things that matter to us, but it is very easy to slip into the habit of measuring what we've always measured or measuring what is easily measured. It is essential, however, that we measure the aspects of the organization that demonstrate the extent to which we have achieved our vision for successfully transforming to Relationship-Based Care (RBC).

Since a primary aim of Relationship-Based Care is the quality and continuity of the patient-caregiver relationship, the most meaningful evidence we can collect is that which reveals:

- *the impact of the intentional focus on all relationships;*

- *the degree to which our every system, practice and process supports the continuity of the patient-caregiver relationship; and*

- *the level to which the benefit of this relationship is experienced by patients and their families.*

Once RBC is implemented, the challenge of collecting evidence about its success lies in the fact that some of its biggest benefits are not quantifiable. For this reason, collecting evidence that verifies the extent to which RBC is alive and well in an organization requires some departure from traditional forms of measurement and evaluation. While we might use traditional quantitative measures to determine the average number of times patient/care giver relationships are disrupted per patient stay, we may use narratives or observation to determine the exact kind of impact care givers are having on the lives of patients and their families. Collecting data on these "intangibles" and then really using that data is still fairly uncommon in most health care organizations. But in RBC, this is some of the most meaningful and useful data we collect.

In RBC we are measuring three key areas:

1. *Impact of our efforts on patients, their families and our colleagues,*

2. *Process effectiveness and process indicators, and*

3. *Persistence and focus on our commitment.*

Each organization decides in its early planning stages what outcomes will provide the clearest evidence that RBC is alive and well in the organization. Deciding what kinds of measurement will best reveal this evidence requires reaching beyond traditional outcomes evaluation. This section provides information to help organizations streamline their data collection by redefining what is really worth measuring, while providing information on the most efficient, effective ways to measure it.

In order for any measurement to be valuable, it must act to clarify "where we are now." And the greatest value of knowing "where we are now" is that we can then mine that data for evidence of our successes. When the time comes to launch ourselves into subsequent phases of our vision for change, it will be our successes that provide the foundation on which to build. Ultimately the evidence we collect becomes a new source of inspiration.

Part V: Evidence addresses the ways in which we can identify useful data, then collect and use it to inspire our workforce, to address any knowledge or skill gaps that surface, and to refine our infrastructures to provide the most potent advancement possible of Relationship-Based Care in our organizations.

CHAPTER SEVENTEEN

Foundations of Evidence

Focusing on Evidence That Helps You Stay the Course

—Jayne A. Felgen

There are only 86,400 seconds in a day, so we have important choices to make... on how we spend our time ... and to what effect.

Dr. Mae Jemison

Measuring the true impact of our efforts—the degree to which we have done what we intend to do—is far more vital than putting endless hours into collecting data that never even becomes information, much less knowledge. We must make clear decisions about what really matters and put our focus squarely on it. In Relationship-Based Care (RBC), relationships matter most, so it's the collection of evidence on the effectiveness of relationships that will do most for helping us stay on course.

We must make clear decisions about what really matters and put our focus squarely on it.

The vision statement for RBC—with all of its specific intentions for what form relationships within the organization will take—must determine, at least in part, the outcomes measures we select for our organizations. In essence, anything that the organization identifies as important to achieve through the implementation of RBC must be evaluated by quantitative or qualitative measures. The most meaningful measurements you will take are those that verify most closely your statements of intention for bringing the RBC principles into daily practice in your organization.

When implementation of RBC is based on action plans created using I_2E_2 (see page 25), each plan will begin with a clearly articulated vision and end with a section enumerating what "Evidence" the organization intends to collect in order to verify the extent to which it has brought its vision of RBC to life. When creating the Evidence section of the plan, start with your vision and decide what you can measure that will verify most directly the vital elements of the vision statement.

For example, one of your RBC vision statement's elements may be:

> *The patient and family are satisfied because they believe that their number one expressed concern regarding this episode of care is also the number one priority for their RN and the health care team.*

There are then a number of measurements you can take to verify this element. It is obvious that you can survey patients and their families to gauge their satisfaction, but if this element is important to your organization, you may also want to:

- *create a unit indicator to measure progress over time*

- *ask nurses and other members of the health care team about their patients and their number one priority for this episode of care*

- *verify that the number one expressed priority is visible in the plan of care and the medical record*

- *integrate this priority into change of shift report and monitor*

Some nurse leaders are frustrated with the difficulty in determining a cause and effect relationship between the implementation of RBC and selected quality outcomes. We need to be realistic about the many simultaneous changes occurring in any organization. It's unrealistic for most of us to design a strict research protocol that controls for every intervening variable. It is both realistic and important to look for trends and to realize that implementation of RBC is likely a significant contributor to improvements in various patient and staff outcome measures.

Quantitative and Qualitative Measures

It is important to note that evidence of some of our progress can be measured with great precision using quantitative measurement instruments. However, other evidence of our progress will be evaluated through qualitative means, such as narrative and descriptive (behavioral) information collected less formally through leadership rounds, everyday observations and interactions with staff or patients and families. When leaders can ask staff questions which are shaped to elicit responses specific to RBC, the answers can provide meaningful evidence of the degree to which we are practicing RBC in alignment with our vision (see page 270).

It is important not to limit ourselves to measuring our progress with traditional quantifiable hard-data instruments to the detriment of evaluating what is happening on the unit, in practice, every day. It is equally important to know where the baseline is for quantifiable measures of significance (i.e., patient satisfaction/loyalty measures, staff and physician satisfaction/loyalty, turnover trends; financial/productivity indicators) and then to identify targets for improvement, knowing that when we do the right thing for patients and families, we can expect improvement in all indicators reflecting the health of the organization.

When leaders can ask staff questions which are shaped to elicit responses specific to RBC, the answers can provide meaningful evidence of the degree to which we are practicing RBC in alignment with our vision.

Making a Business Case for Relationship-Based Care

—Susan Wessel

It is typically the Chief Nurse Officer (CNO) who explains the vision and benefits of Relationship-Based Care (RBC) to senior leaders and beyond. Those who have worked in RBC organizations are eager to talk about its benefits to patients, families and employees, but quantifiable data describing its more tangible benefits have been more difficult to come by. Though RBC makes great business sense, translating that into a solid business case can be a challenging task. But in reality, hospital leaders should ask, "How can we afford not to do this? Patient care delivery is our core business." Relationship-Based Care is not a project. Relationship-Based Care is a proven model of patient care delivery which drives the organization's culture and priorities.

Building a Case

Those who wish to bring RBC to their organizations can create a compelling case through four areas of focus:

- *Link the principles of RBC with the organization's established mission and strategic goals.*

- *Position RBC as a well-timed solution to current issues the organization is facing.*

- *Present RBC as way to help maintain the organization's financial health.*

- *Link RBC to measurable improvements in quality and patient safety and to patient, staff, and physician satisfaction.*

The following checklist will help the CNO build a case for RBC.

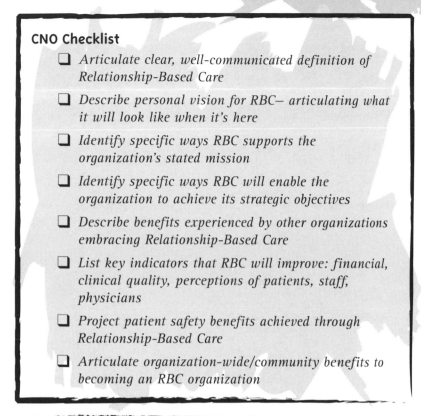

CNO Checklist

❑ *Articulate clear, well-communicated definition of Relationship-Based Care*

❑ *Describe personal vision for RBC– articulating what it will look like when it's here*

❑ *Identify specific ways RBC supports the organization's stated mission*

❑ *Identify specific ways RBC will enable the organization to achieve its strategic objectives*

❑ *Describe benefits experienced by other organizations embracing Relationship-Based Care*

❑ *List key indicators that RBC will improve: financial, clinical quality, perceptions of patients, staff, physicians*

❑ *Project patient safety benefits achieved through Relationship-Based Care*

❑ *Articulate organization-wide/community benefits to becoming an RBC organization*

Linking Relationship-Based Care to Your Organization's Mission and Strategic Goals

A model showing the powerful linkage of RBC with an organization's mission and its operational issues was created by three RBC Project Leaders from Faxton–St. Luke's Healthcare in Utica, New York. These three leaders, charged with leading the implementation of RBC in their organization, created this model which links the already established "Five Pillars" of their health system—Service, People, Quality, Growth and Finance—with the expected outcomes of Relationship-Based Care. The five pillars are based on the work of Quint Studer (www.studergroup.com), who worked with Faxton St. Luke's Health System.

This model provides a compelling picture of 24 specific ways that RBC is expected to positively affect the bottom line in this organization. Linking RBC to the already established mission of the organization meets people right where they are. It is a way of conveying, "We're on the right track and we have been all along—now let's build on our strengths and successes

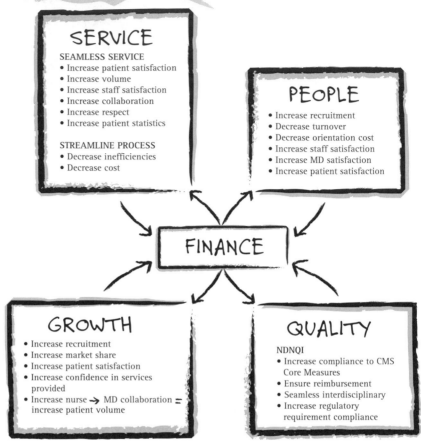

(Model for Creating the Business Case for RBC, developed at RBC Project Leader Practicum, October, 2005 by Matt Marchbanks and Tracy Hilderbran. Used with permission.)

and integrate RBC to help us carry out our mission at an even higher level of excellence!" *Note: Placing finance in the center of this model does not mean the patient/family are not central ... it was the team's way of directly demonstrating how all of these indicators interrelate to achieving financial health.*

When crafting a message to senior leaders and board members, a combination of stories and hard facts is effective. Stories of excellent patient care and outstanding teamwork can be captured through Appreciative Inquiry (see page 96) assessments. Every organization—even before RBC is formalized within it—has stories of care that illustrate the principles of RBC in action. Implementing RBC as the formal model of care creates the environment for these caring moments to occur every day in every interaction. The article by Mary Koloroutis on "Engaging the CEO and Executive Team through Patient and Family Stories" (see page 110) shows how senior leaders can come to understand the real spirit of RBC through face-to-face interactions with patients, their families and members of the care team. It is simple to tie these powerful accounts of caring and healing to the organization's stated mission, and doing so creates a more comprehensive picture of the positive effect of RBC for the framers of that mission—the CEO, the Board and the executive team.

Offering RBC as a Well-Timed Solution

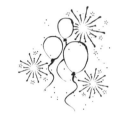

Building the case for RBC may require assessing the tough issues facing your organization. While nearly all of the assessment we do in bringing RBC to an organization is based on Appreciative Inquiry (we nearly always go looking for what is working well in order to build on it), it is also true that RBC brings with it solutions to many organizational problems. You might get at what your organization's problems are by asking yourself, "What keeps the CEO up at night?" Common issues may be lagging market share and volume, poor or plateaued patient satisfaction, safety and quality problems, poor financial performance, medical staff unrest, or employee dissatisfaction and turnover. In the always complex world of health care, these issues are difficult challenges for most organizations.

Relationship-Based Care has been found to improve relationships in the work environment, increase nursing staff satisfaction, decrease turnover, and significantly increase patient satisfaction (Nelson, 2005; Nelson, 2006).

Knowing the areas of greatest opportunity in your organization will help you identify where RBC can have the greatest impact and to communicate these opportunities to colleagues. It also will help you determine what quality data to collect before and after implementation.

No matter what issues you can identify within your organization, however, the time is not always right for change. If problems exist, but the majority of individuals within the organization are satisfied with things as they are, it may not be the optimal time for strategic change. One should never expect others to willingly accept change unless the change can be shown to help them achieve their goals. If individuals do not perceive any major obstacles in achieving their goals, they will not be primed for change.

Although there's never a perfect time for major change, it's important to trust your judgment.

In one situation, a CNO was convinced that RBC was the right strategy for her organization, but it took a year and a half for the timing to be right to begin this transformation. Although there's never a perfect time for major change, it's important to trust your judgment. As you await the time for implementation of RBC, you lay the groundwork by raising awareness, stimulating creative tension, collecting data, and linking the benefits of RBC with your organization's mission and strategic objectives.

Presenting Relationship-Based Care as a Financial Strategy

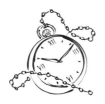

A common myth associated with RBC, if it includes a Primary Nursing role, is that it requires a larger nursing staff. This is untrue. As RBC has proven effective within a variety of staffing and skill mix situations, increasing an organization's labor cost is not a prerequisite for transformation to Relationship-Based Care. However, there are other compelling reasons for changing staffing and skill mix. We recommend, however, that these changes be kept separate from the decision to implement Relationship-Based Care. Mounting research has demonstrated that adequate staffing is linked to better patient outcomes. (Aiken, 2005). This is the most appropriate driver for senior leadership decisions about staffing.

Linda Aiken reviews the growing body of evidence linking staffing and patient outcomes from a variety of researchers in her 2005 article "Improving Quality through Nursing." This resource may help CNOs justify appropriate staffing. With appropriate resources devoted to staffing, additional financial, staff and patient benefits can be gained by implementing Relationship-Based Care.

Evidence is accumulating that adequate numbers of nursing staff, though necessary, may not be the only factor in achieving positive patient outcomes. Preliminary data from California hospitals following implementation of state-mandated minimum staffing was published in August 2005. Researchers affiliated with the California Nursing Outcomes Coalition (CalNOC) found that when the mean total RN hours of care per patient day increased by 20.8% in medical-surgical units, the units experienced no significant changes in the incidence of patient falls or the prevalence of pressure ulcers

(American Organization of Nurse Executives, 2005). Linda Aiken's recent findings (2005), which linked "better work environments" and a 19% reduction in odds on dying, further support that there are variables over and above staffing that are important to patient safety and quality.

The principles of RBC create a healthy work environment and greater RN accountability for care. The central concept is that an identified RN (Primary Nurse) manages the care of the patient for the patient's entire length of stay, and works with a consistent team of support staff (LPNs, CNAs, etc.), delegating and communicating effectively with those co-workers, physicians, and other disciplines. The patient's goals and individual needs drive care decisions. This system has been found to enhance staff satisfaction and retention, increase patient satisfaction, and improve coordination of care. An interdisciplinary implementation of RBC strengthens the relationships of all clinical professionals, improves coordination of patient care and reduces the inefficient duplication and fragmentation.

When building the case for RBC, linking the results to financial outcomes will assist you in communicating its potential benefits. Recruitment, retention and turnover may be some of the most immediate outcomes to track. Financial return should be individualized to each organization, but you may wish to consider measuring the impact of some or all of the following:

> **Elimination of Agency Staffing.** *Reduction in agency staffing can be calculated by multiplying the difference in the average hourly rate for agency and the average hourly rate of permanent staff. This dollar premium per hour is multiplied by the number of agency hours being used. Subtract from this amount the estimated cost of hiring the targeted number of permanent staff. This represents the potential savings to the organization through eliminating agency staff.*

> **The Cost of Turnover.** *The VHA Research Series on The Business Case for Work Force Stability estimates that the cost of turnover is 100% of an RN salary per individual lost— $50,000 in 2002 (Kosel & Olivio, 2002).*

Impact of Staff Turnover on Length of Stay. *Additional research sponsored by the VHA involving 235 hospitals indicates a reduction in average length of stay (ALOS) from 5.02 days in a "high staff turnover" hospital to 4.81 in a "medium staff turnover" hospital, and further decline to 3.81 days in a "low staff turnover" hospital. Low turnover organizations were defined as having turnover rates from 4 percent to 12 percent, and high turnover was 21.6 to 43.8 percent (Gelinas, Bohlen, & DeJoy, 2002).*

Impact of Staff Turnover on Cost Per Discharge. *In the same VHA study Gelinas and Bohlen concluded that organizations with high turnover rates had 36 percent higher costs per discharge than hospitals with turnover rates of 12 percent or less (Gelinas & Bohlen, 2002).*

Linking Relationship-Based Care to Improved Quality and Patient Safety

Patient safety is an additional consideration when making the case for Relationship-Based Care. The 2006 Hospital National Patient Safety Goals of Joint Commission include "Improving the effectiveness of communication among care givers" (Joint Commission on Accreditation of Health Care Organizations, 2005). In fact, failures in communication have been the leading cause of sentinel events from 1995 to 2004 as reported by the Joint Commission. Relationship-Based Care principles improve communication in a number of ways. The Primary Nurse takes ownership for communicating with other nursing staff, with other disciplines, and for facilitating a joint conversation between the patient, physician, therapist and nurse on a daily basis. There is an emphasis on communication during transitions and handoffs. Further, RBC advocates for staff assignments that ensure continuity.

Having a solid set of nationally accepted quality measures is an essential component to implementing and sustaining Relationship-Based Care. "Measuring the Impact of Relationship-Based Care" (see page 588) provides recommended nurse-sensitive outcome measures that should be compiled as baseline data and monitored throughout the transition to Relationship-Based Care. This kind of data will be important to share with senior leaders and the board throughout the transition.

Making the case for RBC can be approached in four distinct ways. It is up to you to determine which factors your organization's senior leaders will respond to most positively. Remember also to gauge carefully whether the timing is right in your organization and to be ready to spend some time laying the groundwork rather than making your case if the organization is not ready to change. And above all, spend adequate time visualizing for yourself how the formalization of Relationship-Based Care would look and feel in your organization. In the end, no matter what sort of case you choose to make, it is the clarity and steadfastness of your own vision that will allow you to make a truly compelling case for Relationship-Based Care.

References: Aiken, L. H. (2005). Improving quality through nursing. In Mechanic, D., Rogut, L., & Colby, D. (Eds.), *Policy challenges in modern health care* (pp. 177-188). Piscataway, NJ: Rutgers University Press.

American Organization of Nurse Executives. (2005). New study examines impact of nurse-patient ratios law in California. *E News Update.* Retrieved February 4, 2006.from http://www.aone.org/aone/pubs/enews/Aug%2005/081205.html.

Gelinas, L., & Bohlen, C. (2002). The business case for retention. *Journal of Clinical Systems Management,* 4(78), 14-16, 22.

Gelinas, L., Bohlen, C., & DeJoy, S. (2002). *Tomorrow's work force: A strategic approach.* VHA's 2002 Research Series. Irving, TX: VHA Inc.

Joint Commission on Accreditation of Health Care Organizations. (2005). 2006 *Critical access hospital and hospital national patient safety goals.* Retrieved December 1, 2005, from http://www.jcaho.org

Kosel, K., & Olivio, T. (2002). *The business case for work force stability.* VHA's 2002 Research Series. Irving, TX: VHA Inc.

Nelson, J. W. (2005). *Leadership at the point of care: Measuring the impact.* Northeast Health Care System, U.S.A.: 1-21.

Nelson, J. W. (2006). *Results of the Healthcare Environment Survey.* Northeast Health Care System, U.S.A.: 1-26.

Measuring the Impact of Relationship-Based Care

—Susan Wessel and Jayne A. Felgen

Measuring the impact of Relationship-Based Care (RBC) is essential to inspiring the effort and sustaining results. There is truth in the adage, "You get what you measure." When staff see that elements of RBC are being tracked, it serves to reinforce their progress and lets them know that the results are important.

An effective example from the field is to use simple graphs that can be posted in a shift report room during the initial weeks of implementation. Two examples are provided below,

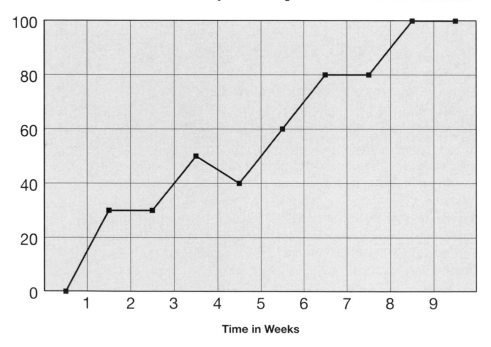

Percent of Patients with Primary Nurse Assigned within 12 Hours of Admission

Time in Weeks

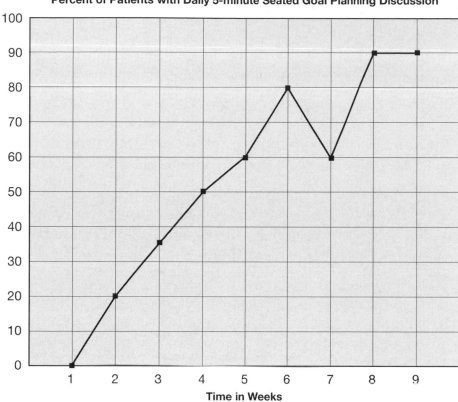

Percent of Patients with Daily 5-minute Seated Goal Planning Discussion

but the specific elements should be decided by each Unit Practice Council. When progress is made it's important to celebrate even small steps toward the ultimate goal.

A quality report card with two levels of data is recommended: hospital-wide and unit level. Hospital-wide indicators should represent macro measures including: human resources, financial, clinical quality, quality perception and Relationship-Based Care. Many of these measures will be recognized as nurse-sensitive indicators as endorsed by the National Quality Forum and the American Nurses Association (ANA) (National Quality Forum, 2004). We have found all of these measures to be impacted favorably by Relationship-Based Care.

Hospital-Wide Indicators

Before RBC is implemented the Results Council should select and adopt indicators from the following table or similar measures that are currently being tracked. Most often this information will already exist in the organization. Pulling it together in one place will allow those leading RBC to compile baseline data and to track ongoing results. The Results Council, working in conjunction with the Quality Improvement Department, has responsibility for establishing and maintaining these measures over time to monitor the status of implementation.

An important element for both RBC and attaining Magnet designation status is measuring the health of the work environment. Organizations should select a practice environment scale for use at least annually during implementation of Relationship-Based Care. John Nelson, a nurse researcher specializing in this field, has developed nurse environment surveys that have been helpful in measuring the impact of Relationship-Based Care (www.hcenvironment.com).

Unit-Specific Indicators

A second level of indicators is presented for individual patient care units. Members of each Unit Practice Council, working in conjunction with their manager, should be asked to select a set of measures appropriate for their unit. One of the universal challenges with quality measures is finding the time and reliable systems for data collection. It's better to have a smaller number of measures at the unit level that are meaningful and realistic to track rather than a large number that are overly burdensome. It can be very rewarding to staff to compare their patient satisfaction results with the progress toward various elements of RBC that they have selected.

It's better to have a smaller number of measures at the unit level that are meaningful and realistic to track rather than a large number that are overly burdensome.

The following table includes the hospital-wide and unit-specific measures to track the status of Relationship-Based Care. The table offers a rich collection of process and outcome measures, both organization-wide and unit-specific. You may choose those that best measure your desired impact.

A chart defining indicators and giving references for each can be found on pages 594 to 596.

RBC Quality Indicators

Hospital: _____

Change Implementation Date: _____

Note: Collect data before and during implementation.

INDICATORS		Date:	Date:	Date:	Date:
Human Resources Voluntary turnover rate	RN Other				
Vacancy rate	RN Other				
Nursing job satisfaction (annual)					
Skill mix	RN Contract				
Financial Dollars per adjusted patient day					
Average hourly salary rate					
Total nursing care hours per patient day					
Average patient length of stay					
Clinical Quality Nosocomial infection rate (UTIs)					
Ventilator-associated pneumonia for ICU & high risk nursery patients					
Falls prevalence					
Patient falls with injury					
Mortality*					
Pressure ulcer prevalence					
Quality Perception Patient satisfaction overall					
Patient satisfaction with nursing care					
Patient willingness to return or recommend					
Relationship-Based Care Percent of discharged patients with RBC					
Practice environment scale (annual)					

RBC Quality Indicators

Hospital: _____

Change Implementation Date: _____

Note: Collect data before and during implementation.

INDICATORS	Date:	Date:	Date:	Date:
Responsibility for Relationship & Decision Making:				
Percent of patients at discharge with a Primary Nurse assigned from admission to discharge				
Percent of patients whose relationship with their primary nurse began on admission (or within 12 hours of admission)				
Percent of patients whose answer to "what is the most important issue/concern for this episode of care" drove care plan				
Percent of patients who experienced a 5-minute conversation about their goals with their nurse seated at the bedside				
Work Allocation and Assignments:				
Percent of shifts worked that Primary Nurse cared for primary patient				
Percent of primary patients/shift whose nurse was "pulled" off assignment or unit				
Communication with Health Care Team:				
Percent of patients whose Primary Nurse, physician, & AHP met jointly with patient about care every day				
Percent of physician calls or rounds about patient made by Primary or associate nurse (vs. charge nurse, others)				
Practice Environment--Patients:				
Percent of patients asked to describe at admission how they prefer to experience caring				
Percent of patients with at least 5 hours of uninterrupted sleep per night				
Percent of patients whose call bells are answered in less than one minute				

INDICATORS	Date:	Date:	Date:	Date:
Patient satisfaction with pain management				
Patient satisfaction with educational information				
Patient satisfaction with noise/quiet				
Practice Environment--Staff: Percent of staff taking lunch breaks off the unit or in a peaceful place without interruption				
Percent of staff involved in communication network				
Percent of staff saying they practice good self-care				
Percent of staff saying they receive good care from colleagues				
Process Improvement: Minutes spent waiting for care (such as meds, transportation, discharge...any process at issue)				

Measurement Instructions for Quality Indicators

INDICATORS	NUMERATOR	DENOMINATOR	REFERENCE
Voluntary Turnover Rate	Number of voluntary uncontrolled separations during the period for RNs and APNs Number of voluntary uncontrolled separations during the period for LPNs and nursing assistants/aides	Number of employees (full-time plus part-time) on the last day of the period for RNs and APNs (exclude per diem and agency nurses) Number of employees (full-time plus part-time) on the last day of the period for LPNs and NAs	NQF—National Quality Forum (VHA)
Vacancy Rate	Number of budgeted unfilled positions (full-time plus part-time) on the last day of the period (exclude perdiem)	Total number of budgeted positions (full-time plus part-time) for the period (exclude perdiem)	
Nursing Job Satisfaction	Job satisfaction expressed by nurses working in the hospital setting as determined by scaled responses to a uniform series of questions designed to elicit nursing staff attitudes toward specific aspects of their employment situation		ANA
Skill Mix % of RNs % of contract	Number of productive hours worked by RN nursing staff (employee and contract) with patient care responsibilities Number of productive hours worked by contract staff (RN, LPN and UAP) with patient care responsibilities	Total number of productive hours worked by nursing staff (RN, LPN, UAP) with direct patient care responsibilities (employees and contract)	NQF (ANA-NDQI)
Dollars per Adjusted Patient Day	Total expense dollars for all patient care departments	Adjusted patient days	
Average Hourly Salary Rate	Total salary dollars for all patient care departments (include contract staff)	Total hours worked in patient care departments (include contract hours)	
Total Nursing Hours per Patient Day	Total number of productive hours worked by nursing staff with direct patient care responsibilities on acute care units during the period	Patient days for the period	ANA
Average Length of Stay	Number of patient days	Number of discharges	Aiken
Nosocomial Infection Rate (UTIs)	Number of urinary tract infections developed after 3 days of hospitalization X 1000	Total patient days	ANA
Ventilator-associated pneumonia, ICU and High Risk Nursery (HRN)	Number of ventilator-associated pneumonias in ICU X 1000 Number of ventilator associated pneumonias in HRN X 1000	Number of ventilator days for ICU patients Number of ventilator days for HRN patients	NQF (CDC)

INDICATORS	NUMERATOR	DENOMINATOR	REFERENCE
Falls Prevalence	Number of inpatient falls X 1000	Total number of inpatient days	ANA, NQF
Patient Falls with Injury	Number of inpatient falls with injuries X 1000	Total number of inpatient days	ANA, NQF
Mortality Rate	Inpatient deaths	Total number of discharged patients	Aiken
Pressure Ulcer Prevalence	Inpatients with National Pressure Ulcer Advisory Panel (NPUAP)-Stage II or greater hospital-acquired pressure ulcers	Inpatients in the prevalence study (Exclude <16 years of age and skin breakdown due to arterial or venous insufficiency, diabetes neuropathy or incontinence)	NQF, CalNOC
Patient Satisfaction with Care Overall	Patient opinion of care overall received during service as determined by scaled responses to a uniform series of questions designed to elicit patient views regarding global aspects of care		ANA
Patient Satisfaction with Nursing Care	Patient opinion of care received from nursing staff during the hospital stay as determined by scaled responses to a standardized patient survey		ANA
Patient Satisfaction with Educational Information	Patient opinion of nursing staff efforts to educate them regarding their condition and care requirements as determined by scaled responses to a standardized patient survey		ANA
Patient Satisfaction with Pain Management	Patient opinion of how well nursing staff managed their pain as determined by scaled responses to a standardized patient survey		ANA
Admissions Receiving RBC	Number of patients admitted who receive Relationship-Based Care (Primary Nurse from admission to discharge)	Total number of patients admitted to the facility	

INDICATORS	NUMERATOR	DENOMINATOR	REFERENCE
Practice Environment Scale—Nursing Work Index (composite and five subscales)	Composite score is the mean of all subscales Subscales = mean of all items comprising each subscale: • Nurse participation in hospital affairs • Nursing foundations for quality of care • Nurse manager ability, leadership and support of nurses • Staffing and resource adequacy • Collegial nurse-physician relations	Staff RNs Note: Random sample with a minimum response of 30 completed surveys (all 31 items completed) is consistent with the NQF-endorsed consensus standard	NQF (Kramer, Aiken, Lake) Lake, E. (2002). Development of the practice environment scale of the Nursing Work Index. *Research Nurse Health* 25:176-188.

Measurement Instruments for a Caring Environment

—John W. Nelson

This article will review the use of three different instruments that can be used for measuring impact and outcomes in the dynamic environment of health care. Each of the instruments was designed by people who have experience in health care, working to improve patient care either at the bedside or at the organizational level. These scientifically tested instruments have been designed to measure the core factors of a caring environment from the perspective of all participating parties including the patient, the employee and the organization.

Instrument I: The Caring Factor Survey (CFS)

This measure is founded on the work of Dr. Jean Watson and was created to measure caring as perceived by the patient. Caring, according to Dr. Watson, is premised on ten caring processes (also known as Carative Factors and/or Caritas Processes) which make up this construct of caring for patients. Twenty questions were created, with two questions for each process, and all questions were validated by other experts in the Caritas Processes. Authors of the original twenty questions were Dr. Jean Watson, Dr. Karen Drenkard, Gene Rigotti, and the author of this article, John Nelson. The CFS uses a 1-7 Likert scale with higher scores indicating a greater sense of caring from the patient's perspective. Various methods of validity testing were employed (face, content and criterion), along with reliability testing.

The 10 caring processes, based on Dr. Watson's work (www. uchsc.edu/nursing/caring) include:

- *Formation of a humanistic-altruistic system of values*

- *Instillation of faith-hope*

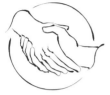

- *Cultivation of sensitivity to one's self and to others*
- *Development of a helping-trusting, human caring relationship*
- *Promotion and acceptance of the expression of positive and negative feelings*
- *Systematic use of a creative problem-solving caring process*
- *Promotion of transpersonal teaching-learning*
- *Provision for a supportive, protective, and/or corrective mental, physical, societal and spiritual environment*
- *Assistance with gratification of human needs*
- *Allowance for existential-phenomenological-spiritual forces*

The Caring Factor Survey can be used to examine the impact of various caring interventions. If you use this instrument, please contact any of the authors of the CFS to inform them of its use so ongoing testing can be conducted. Contact information for the authors is included with the CFS.

Instrument II: The Health Environment Survey (HES)

A contemporary instrument that measures the work environment of patient care, including the effectiveness of patient care itself, as perceived by all disciplines and employees within health care, has not existed before the recent development of the Healthcare Environment Survey (HES). Prior instruments did not measure operational issues related to patient care, were not tested scientifically, or were limited in that they were specific to only certain disciplines. Both archival and contemporary literature were used to understand the evolution of measuring job satisfaction in health care. *Quantitative methods* are used to gather data that can be examined statistically, and are meaningful alongside other indicators like financial and patient outcomes. *Qualitative methods*, however, are used to capture unique aspects of the work environment and are also collected for the purpose of conducting ongoing validity assessment—for example, asking, "Does the quantitative portion really measure what is important for job satisfaction?" These aspects of the HES make it a one-of-a-kind tool, applicable to anyone who works in health care. What follows is a general overview of the HES and how it can be used in your organization for process improvement, various sorts of certifications, and in pursuit of quality awards like the Malcolm Baldrige National Quality Award.

Measuring the work environment is important in order to create the most efficient and satisfying work places. The work environment has historically been examined within each discipline, using different instruments for each discipline, thus prohibiting meaningful comparisons of the state of affairs among disciplines and departments. We also found that job satisfaction data for those in many disciplines and departments were scarce. For example, while there is a vast amount of literature on nurse and physician satisfaction with the workplace, the number of studies on job satisfaction for other disciplines declined in the following order: pharmacists, physical therapists, respiratory therapists, occupational therapists, managers, care and technical assistants, support staff and volunteers. To rectify this deficiency, the author of this article conducted an extensive examination of the work environment as experienced by all workers in health care. (Readers of this paper who would like a list of references for each discipline should contact the author of this paper.)

Upon examination of the literature, it appears that the more distant the care provider is from the patient, the less literature about job satisfaction was available. For example, no studies were found for housekeepers and cooks working in health care settings. Despite the distance of some of these workers from the patients, however, a qualitative study (Nelson, 2005) found that many of the workers considered peripheral to patient care brought their talents to health care in a deliberate effort to contribute to the well-being of patients. For example, cooks stated, "The aspect of my job that I enjoy the most is cooking for patients." Housekeepers similarly stated, "The aspect of my job that I enjoy the most is making sure the patient's room is clean." This instrument was designed to capture what makes work meaningful for all employees within health care, and it correlates meaningfully with other organizational indicators

> Connecting patient and employee outcomes to human resources outcomes can and should influence decision-making and report writing for quality improvement and return on investment.

> Despite the distance of some of these workers from the patients, a qualitative study found that many of the workers considered peripheral to patient care brought their talents to health care in a deliberate effort to contribute to the well-being of patients.

like financial and patient outcomes. Connecting patient and employee outcomes to human resources outcomes, for example, can and should influence decision making and report writing for quality improvement and return on investment.

The HES uses all of the common variables identified in the literature by all of the disciplines and employees within health care. These variables include:

- *job satisfaction*
- *promotional opportunities*
- *staffing and scheduling*
- *work relationships*
- *autonomy*
- *participative management (unit management)*
- *pride in the organization*
- *intent to stay with the organization*
- *distributive justice*
- *workload*
- *staffing and scheduling*

When we do ask staff what they value most, we can give them what they really want—rather than what occurs to them to ask for.

While the intent of the Health Environment Survey is to allow us to compare the experience of individuals in all disciplines and departments, it also includes questions specific to:

- *direct care providers (relationship with the patient)*
- *those who work directly with physicians (relationship with the physician)*
- *those who work directly with nurses (relationship with nurses)*
- *nursing staff only (perception of nursing administration)*

Having the same questions asked of all disciplines allows staff and administration to see what is happening in each department or discipline within the same area, using the same questions. However, rather than including questions that would not have relevance to certain survey takers (for example, asking someone in housekeeping who has no physician contact about his or her experience with physicians), we tailored the mix of questions to suit the work scope of those surveyed.

Below is an example how various employment groups responded to a question on "perception of workload" (See Figure 1).

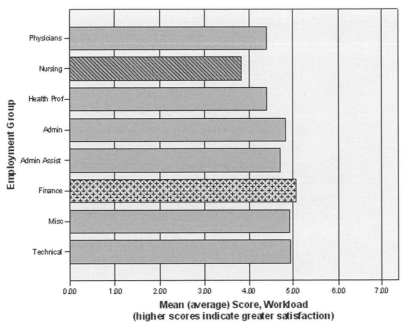

Figure 1 Perception of Workload, All Employment Groups

As you can see, the greatest discrepancy in how individuals in this organization perceive their workload is between those in finance and those in nursing. This sort of data is useful because it facilitates conversations about efficient allocation of resources. An organization that has only limited resources to address the issue of workload can begin with the most distressed by evaluating the work process for possible work redistribution or purchase of updated equipment.

Utilizing graphs like Figure 1 above to examine quantitative data helps facilitate understanding of what is occurring within each department of the organization. Combining these data with qualitative data provides for a deeper understanding of what is working to motivate employees and is captured no other way. It's important to know what people enjoy in their work so you can give them the support and resources to do more of it. If you're unaware, for example, that cooks and housekeepers are significantly emotive about being in service to patients and their families, there can be a great disconnect between those who are peripheral to the patient and those who provide resources for them. We may perceive that they desire newer and better equipment and fail to identify that it is the patient's well-being that makes cooks and cleaners show up for work. Having data that reveal that cooks and housekeepers value most knowing that they're having an impact on patients, you may find that their satisfaction is not increased as much by new equipment as it is by receiving regular reports on patient satisfaction and outcomes. This may not only be less expensive to do, but may also create more motivated employees who are happy to do more with less, just knowing they make a difference for patients. These peripheral "care givers" are so distant from the patient that it doesn't occur to either staff or management that things like patient reports may be what creates a deep feeling of reward for these care givers. When we do this qualitative study to find what they value most, we can give them what they really want—rather than what occurs to them to ask for.

The HES uses questions that ask people to report the quality of their experiences in order to understand some of the work environment's more emotive aspects. Responses to the following qualitative questions are acquired from all employees, and examined by various demographics (i.e., by hospital, discipline, shift worked, etc.):

> *You may find that cooks' and housekeepers' satisfaction is not increased as much by new equipment as it is by receiving regular reports on patient satisfaction and outcomes.*

- *The one aspect of my current job or work environment that really makes me want to LEAVE my current job is:*

- *The one aspect of my current job or work environment that makes me feel the most STRESS is:*

- *The one aspect of my current job or work environment that really makes me want to STAY is:*

- *The one aspect of my current job that I ENJOY the most is:*

Qualitative data are examined by researchers trained in qualitative research, and it is then themed and graphed. Figure 2, noted below, is from a study of nursing staff from 17 different facilities. These data not only provide ongoing validation of the aspects being measured in the quantitative section of the HES©, but help leaders of the organization understand the emotive responses to the aspects of the organization on the employees' minds the most. These data can be broken up by unit and department to evaluate where relationships are found to be stressful, and where successful relationships are being enjoyed. Comments can be examined to understand the specific aspects of the relationships that are found stressful or enjoyable in the respects areas of the organization. (See

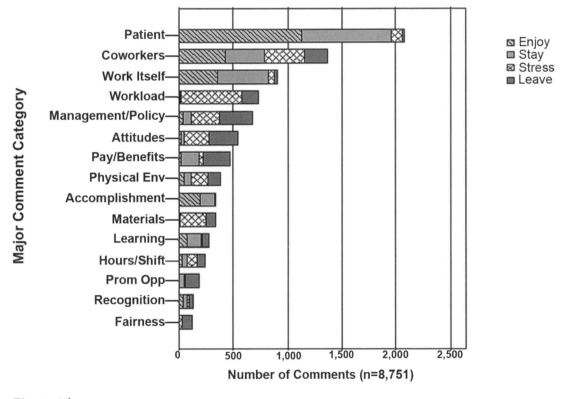

Figure 2.)

Figure 2. Qualitative Data by Themes

This graph is showing us which aspects of the job give the most satisfaction and least stress and which aspects are causing people to have the highest stress and thoughts of leaving their jobs. It reveals that in this organization, "patient care" is an aspect delivering relatively high satisfaction and low stress, while "workload" is causing tremendous stress and even causing people to want to leave the organization.

Instrument III: The Health Care Organization (HCO) Report Card

The HCO Report Card[1] was developed to connect labor, financial and patient indicator data in order to establish a better understanding of organizational effectiveness. It can be used manually, or it can be automated using interface technology to connect the existing databases within the organization. Users of the automated data can then select data they want examined, and on what frequency—daily, monthly, quarterly or annually. Access codes can be used to provide security. This article will provide a brief example of how this process can be used to facilitate understanding of how very different aspects of the organization relate to one another.

Example:

An organization contacted me desiring to know how to conduct a staffing effectiveness report as required by Centers for Medicare and Medicaid Services (CMS). Organizations are required to select and measure two human resource indicators, and two clinical indicators. This particular organization wanted to examine how its current staffing levels related to patient falls. Data were collected and then examined in a correlation table, and it was found that the "nurse-to-patient ratio" factor was most sensitive to increased falls. In other words, the more patients the night nurses took on, the higher the occurrence of falls. Such understanding facilitated discussions of process improvement and the possibility for ongoing analysis of the impact of the interventions implemented. This example offers only a small window into the possibilities of what might be examined in this very user-friendly format.

It is noted in Figure 3 that the number of patient falls has a range on the vertical axis from zero to 20. The higher the unit is in the graph, the more falls occurred on that unit. It is also noted that the horizontal axis has the number of patients each nurse, on average, is responsible for on the night shift. Patient load ranges from 1.70 patients, on average, to 7.30 patients. The number of patients increases on the horizontal axis from left to right. It is noted that there is a general trend for patient

---

falls to increase as the number of patients per nurse increases. This relationship (also referred to as a correlation) was found to be statistically significant at the .05 level. (See Figure 3.)

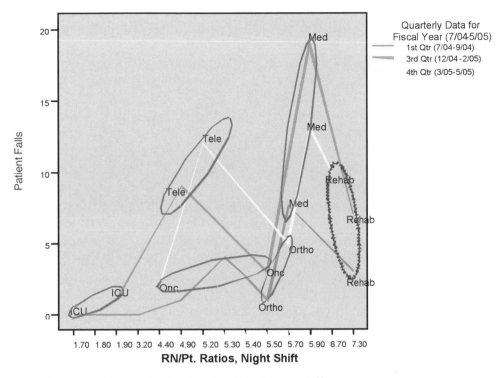

Figure 3. Relationship of Staffing on Night Shift With Patient Falls

It is the intent of this brief article to illustrate how measuring in a caring environment and showing the impact of interventions is possible if the appropriate instruments and methods are used and that the methods were created by people who have experience in health care and understand the most important variables.

For more information on these measurement tools, visit www.hcenvironments.com.

Research in the Dynamic Environment

—John W. Nelson

The following document is a very basic guide to conducting organizational research within the dynamic environment of health care. The first section identifies essentials for research; the second section is an algorithm to follow.

Use of both quantitative and qualitative methods. This approach is sometimes referred to as "triangulation." Some purist researchers will argue against using both methods; however, in a dynamic environment using both is essential to properly understand the current state of affairs.

Use of several types of data. If the data collected represent a minority percentage of the population of interest, several types of data should be used. For example, if you have job satisfaction data from only 45% of the staff, the data cannot be used alone to assert the degree of job satisfaction among the staff as a whole. Rather, supplemental data (i.e., notes from staff meetings, focus groups outcomes, etc.) should be utilized in conjunction with the job satisfaction data for proper decision making. If, however, the data represent 80% of the population of interest, the data alone can be used for discussion.

Validity. Do the data capture the primary content of interest? For example, if primary care is being implemented for all direct-care disciplines, is the perception of primary care being measured from both the patient and care giver perspectives? (Primary care includes measuring perception of the patient/care giver relationship, care planning, interdisciplinary collaboration and continuity of care.)

Reliability. Quantitative (numerical) data that are used should be gathered by instruments that have a reliability of at least .80 (technically this is called a Chronbach's Alpha). This number indicates that, of those who responded, 80% had a common understanding of the questions being asked. For example, if the survey asks the question "I am respected by the organization," and one half of those surveyed understand this to mean respected professionally, while the other half understands this to mean respected personally, the reliability (Chronbach's Alpha) would be .50 because only one half of those surveyed shared an understanding of the meaning of the question. An instrument with a reliability of less than .70 is considered risky to use. The reliability of an instrument can be found by contacting the author of the instrument, or in literature about development of the instrument under the "methods" section.

Feedback loop. The feedback loop should always be connected to some evaluation of return on investment (ROI). The ROI may be turnover rate, number of sick calls, productivity, patient outcomes or any other indicator that can be related to cost and quantified.

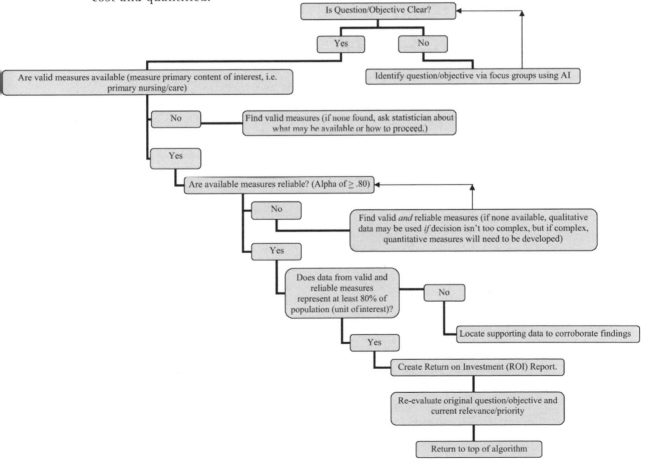

CHAPTER EIGHTEEN
Impact: Client Exemplars

A CNO's Perspective on an Organization-Wide Relationship-Based Care Implementation

—Patricia A. Roach (Interviewed by Susan Wessel)

Background: *Pat Roach is the Chief Nursing Officer at Faxton-St. Luke's Health Care, a 370- bed hospital in Utica, NY. She was interviewed by Susan Wessel.*

Could you talk about how you got your senior leadership colleagues so excited about Relationship-Based Care?

I think it was really sharing the vision for Relationship-Based Care and linking it to what we are trying to achieve. We had just developed a 2010 Vision, which was behind our goal of reaching the 95th percentile for patient and physician satisfaction using our established satisfaction tools. When we talked about it at the senior level, I said that I really thought that Relationship-Based Care could help us—it can be the vehicle to get to the patient and the staff and the physician satisfaction targets. So I used the existing vision and said, "This is going to be the vehicle." I think that was probably the best thing to do—to tie it into corporate strategy and that way there was buy-in right out of the gate.

It sounds like you had a very strong desire from the beginning to make RBC interdisciplinary in your organization. Talk about why that was so important and how you achieved it.

I think the interdisciplinary piece was a "natural" for us because of what we are trying to accomplish. We are working with the VHA "Tomorrow's Work Force" initiative, and that's really about employee engagement—getting staff involved in decision making. This fit in nicely with Relationship-Based Care as well. Relationship-Based Care isn't a replacement of Tomorrow's Work Force, but rather enhances the work we are already doing. Nursing cannot run the hospital by itself. If every nurse reported to work tomorrow morning we still couldn't run it by ourselves—we need the other disciplines. So having all the key people—individuals from literally every discipline in the organization—at the table sends an excellent message as we move forward. I think if the nursing department alone attempted to bring in RBC, it might've been viewed as something just the nurses are doing, rather than having everybody in the organization focus on the patient and come together as a team.

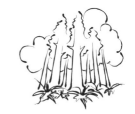

I know from the very beginning you invited all the disciplines to participate in the educational programs for Relationship-Based Care. Explain your structure for the Results Council and how that helped get everyone involved.

The Results Council leadership is multidisciplinary with two enthusiastic co-chairs. Matt Marchbanks is an Executive Chef as well as the Director of Nutrition and Environmental Services, and Tracy Hildebran, the nurse manager on the oncology unit. Additionally, Donna DeFrank, our Assistant Vice President for Nursing Operations, is the project coordinator. She makes sure that details are facilitated and she coordinates the overall project. As the executive sponsor, I see my job as creating the patient care vision and securing the resources and/or removing barriers for implementing Relationship-Based Care. The leadership structure also includes key leaders serving as functional subgroup leaders. Every member of the Results Council shares the passion for RBC and serves as a champion.

We have the interdisciplinary team well represented at the table. We have an occupational therapist, two pharmacists, the director from Facilities Management, a representative from Materials Management, our union president, and Human Resource professionals just to name a few. We've also included a board member who is a nurse educator and is interested in participating in helping us move the vision forward. An internal medicine physician and a surgeon also are members. Nursing is prominently at the table with the five nursing administrators, the nurse managers who are involved in "Wave 1" implementation, nurse clinicians, charge nurses and a Staff Nurse. It really helps having some staff members from the point of care at the table who can see the vision and help create the roadmap to achieve it.

So tell me one of the things you're most proud of in getting RBC off the ground. Give me an example of something you feel really good about.

I would probably say that I feel really good about the interdisciplinary approach and getting the entire team focused on seeing the importance of all of us working together toward a common goal—understanding that our shared purpose is to take care of the patient. That was probably our greatest achievement. You know there is always "whitewater" in health care, and we're trying to channel the resources we need to make RBC happen. Again, we were able to do that by linking it back to the corporate strategy and focusing on what we're all trying to achieve—the vision of trying to be a GREAT place to work and a GREAT place to receive care.

I know your organization has chosen to use Reigniting the Spirit of Caring (RSC) as a very specific intervention. Tell me about how you're using that program and what you hope to achieve.

During the first months after the merger, I brought all the nursing leadership together—nurse managers, nurse administrators, nurse clinicians, and we went off site and spent three days in *Reigniting the Spirit of Caring*. There were still a lot of people in the room who didn't know each other as colleagues, and didn't even know each other as people because they were on two separate campuses. I think the greatest benefit of that 3-day experiential workshop was really to get to know each other and to respect each other.

> I feel really good about the interdisciplinary approach and getting the entire team focused on seeing the importance of all of us working together toward a common goal.

We decided that it was such a wonderful coming together of the nursing leadership team that it was really something that we wanted to roll out to our charge nurse group. They were faced with a lot of the same issues; they didn't know each other, there was a lot of interdepartmental conflict, and units were moved over from one hospital to the other hospital. So staff were working with people they hadn't necessarily worked with before. There were also union/nonunion issues for nursing—nurses having to leave the union when they went to the other campus due to aspects of certain labor agreements, and nurses having to join a union when they didn't necessarily want to. There was a lot of conflict and anger—all the things that you would expect with such a dramatic change.

We decided that our *RSC* work had been so powerful that we got a commitment all the way through the board level to support *Reigniting the Spirit of Caring*. It is in our strategic plan for the next five years—that every member of the organization will participate in *Reigniting the Spirit of Caring*. We've had several of our vice presidents already go through this program and have a commitment from our chief executive and chief operating officer that they will also go through the program.

RSC has been a great sort of building block, if you will, toward our mission and vision. It's been a great starting place and now we are building on this with Relationship-Based Care. We are committed to giving our leaders the tools they need to make this happen and this is where *LEO* (*Leading an Empowered Organization*) fits in so that we can be sure that managers can facilitate this enormous change. Many of our senior leaders refer to this change as "Turning the Titanic." It is a slow process that must be done with skill. We were an organization with patient satisfaction scores in the 20th percentile and employee satisfaction scores close to the 14th percentile. We're proud to say that after just one year, we've been able to, for the first time, get our patient satisfaction scores up to the 47th percentile and employee satisfaction scores up to the 48th percentile. So we know that the investment is definitely worth it. We know that it's a huge commitment in terms of time, money and training staff (getting people off-site for a 3-day workshop), but we can see the power of it, and it's really making a difference.

Many of our senior leaders refer to this change as "Turning the Titanic." It is a slow process that must be done with skill.

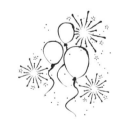

Finally, I'd like you to describe how your CEO, Keith Fenstemacher, envisions meshing Relationship-Based Care with the organization's mission and pillars and how he has articulated that so that it can be spread through the whole organization.

Getting to Great—Vision 2010

Vision

RBC in Concert with TWF as
Means & Method to Express Excellence and Achieve 2010

G R O W T H	P E O P L E	Q U A L I T Y	S E R V I C E	F I N A N C E

VALUES

Honesty, Respect, & Integrity *Quality of Service*	*Teamwork & Pride* *Communication*

Mission

Keith talks about our organization's mission and vision in terms of building a house. The foundation of the house is our mission—our common shared purpose, why are we doing this, who we are, and what are we trying to do for our community. Then he puts on the next layer of the house, which are the values of the organization in terms of how Relationship-Based Care's conceptual framework fits into our organizational values. He talks about respect and dignity and teamwork and communication, which makes perfect sense—it's really linked into the Relationship-Based Care domain and its principles—so it really goes hand in hand with the whole framework.

Then he talks about our pillars; we have five strategic pillars: quality, finance, growth, people and service. Again, he sees Relationship-Based Care as driving us towards the vision, which is to have the highest possible patient, staff and employee satisfaction. With the pillars we feel that Relationship-Based Care fits into all of them. If you give the best service, your employees are going to be happier and service is handled through the caring of patients. This is sitting down at the bedside, knowing a particular patient's story, taking the 5 minutes to understand what the patient wants for the day and to maybe allay their fears, or just get to know them as a person. Nurses can and want to spend much of their time at the bedside, so the people pillar automatically falls into place—with a focus on patient care, we increase employee satisfaction. The quality pillar, with the outcome measures, will set us apart. Relationship-Based Care fits nicely into all the quality and satisfaction outcomes we are trying to achieve. It also helps us in our journey to become a Magnet designated facility.

Going back to the people pillar, the staff involved in the Unit Practice Councils have told us repeatedly that our early success in moving those employee satisfaction scores was due to employee engagement, and getting them involved in decision making and the process of deciding what's the best practice. We did that for our Tomorrow's Work Force initiative, setting up teams where employees were engaged as part of the process. Well, Relationship-Based Care takes that one step further because each unit (and we've decided to make each department part of the practice council so they'll also have their own multidisciplinary approach) has their own say in what they can do to contribute to Relationship-Based Care. This is a new development that the entire Results Council is excited about, which also helps fulfill the people pillar.

As for the quality pillar, one of the things we're doing now is making the linkage of Relationship-Based Care to the quality program in the organization. We're not only looking at outcome measures, but we're also looking to, as the book says, "measure what our vision is," and that is very easy for us because our vision has always been around these satisfaction initiatives. I think when we link it into the quality program

Our CEO sees Relationship-Based Care as driving us towards the vision, which is to have the highest possible patient, staff and employee satisfaction.

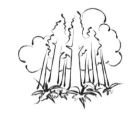

(staff involvement, understanding processes from their level) that's really going to be an added benefit.

As you look at the house drawing, the finance and growth pillars are on the outside of the house encasing the people, service and quality pillars. If they fall we would be fine because we have strong service, people and quality. With strong service, people and quality, financial stability and growth are going to follow.

Then, of course, the top of the house, or the roof, is our vision, which I've said many times is to have high satisfaction scores in all groups. One of the important messages we're trying to get to our staff is that Relationship-Based Care doesn't replace our initiative of employee engagement through Tomorrow's Work Force, but rather enhances it, and this is a method or vehicle to get us there. So that's the house that Keith built.

Relating Outcomes to Excellence in Nursing Practice

—Diane E. Allen

Nurses often say that what makes their work satisfying is the ability to make a difference in patients' lives. When asked how they know when they have made a difference, nurses are usually able to provide anecdotal descriptions of their positive influence, yet they hardly ever have any hard data to support their success. Even though clinical nurses have extraordinary access to and influence over patient care data, they often underestimate their roles as data managers and innovators of change, and relinquish control of data to others. In order to motivate clinical nurses to make evidence-based changes in practice, data must be presented to clinical nurses in a manner that makes sense and readily relates to the work that nurses do.

At New Hampshire Hospital (NHH), a publicly funded acute psychiatric hospital in Concord, NH, clinical nurses not only collect and report data; they use data to demonstrate their impact on patient care. Nurses at NHH have taken deliberate steps to incorporate evidence-based practice into everyday clinical interventions and decision making. They have selected the dynamic nursing process described by Ida Jean Orlando (1961) as the foundation for practice and implemented a Relationship-Based Nursing model (RBN) for patient care delivery. A Nursing Practice Outcomes Committee (NPOC) was created to measure the impact of the RBN delivery model.

The committee's goals were to identify outcomes measures that reflect nursing practice at NHH and to plan an outcomes measurement process that would be realistic and relevant for

Clinical nurses not only collect and report data; they use data to demonstrate their impact on patient care.

psychiatric nurses giving direct patient care. The committee is composed of assistant directors for clinical nursing practice and nursing education, managers for clinical units, nursing education coordinators, educational resource nurses and clinical Staff Nurses.

New Hampshire Hospital is a data-rich environment, with measurement processes already in place for falls, nosocomial infections, assaults to staff, seclusion and restraint, adverse medication events, patient satisfaction and a myriad of other indicators. Committee members were interested in identifying indicators that reflect the quality of relationship-based patient care provided by professional psychiatric nurses and that can be tracked long term. *Nurse Job Satisfaction* and the *Development and Implementation of a Patient Care Delivery Model* (American Nurses Credentialing Center, 2002) was used as a resource. The process for identifying indicators began by asking two simple questions: "What do we always want to see?" and "What do we never want to see?" Three indicators were selected as relevant to relationship-based psychiatric nursing:

- *use of seclusion and restraint as emergency interventions,*

- *patient's familiarity with the name of his/her Primary Nurse, and*

- *nurse job satisfaction.*

Seclusion and Restraint

Seclusion and restraint are inherently dangerous interventions used during psychiatric emergencies that can have a negative impact for both staff and patients. NHH nurses celebrate their ability to avoid the use of restrictive interventions as a reflection of empowered nursing in action. RBN promotes trusting relationships between nurses and patients that are invaluable during times of psychiatric crisis. The Primary Nurse who is familiar with the patient's needs, strengths and coping methods is able to help the patient during times of crisis without the need for restrictive interventions. As committee members sought to find a way to quantify and validate the role of the empowered nurse, they recognized the value of connecting nursing interventions to seclusion and restraint data already being collected.

Patient Satisfaction

Kinnaird and Dingman (2004) found that both the nurse and the patient are mutually responsible for determining the desired outcomes of each episode of care. Patient care is driven by the needs of the patient and the patient's significant others. It is expected that nurses identify themselves to the patient as the responsible agent for the patient's nursing care—his/her Primary Nurse. Therefore, the outcomes committee determined that the patient's ability to identify the name of his/her Primary Nurse would be a simple process indicator to measure. Three nursing theory-based questions were added to the hospital's patient satisfaction survey. These questions were formulated with the intent to capture the essence of both Primary Nursing and Orlando's Nursing Process. In addition, nurses designed their own parallel data collection process. Unit managers conduct a "blitz" survey once every 3 months, asking all patients on their units that day if they knew the name of their Primary Nurse, if the nurse talked with them and if the nurse helped them.

Nurse Job Satisfaction

The project to design a patient care delivery model gave nurses a voice in designing their own jobs and in deciding how they could best contribute to patient care and make a difference in people's lives. RBN promotes the autonomy, professional status and collaborative relationships that are important components of nurse job satisfaction. Therefore, a study was planned, using the Index of Work Satisfaction (IWS) (Stamps, 1997) as a survey tool, to explore the relationship between nurse job satisfaction and the development and implementation of a patient care delivery model unique to NHH (Allen, 2005).

RBN promotes the autonomy, professional status and collaborative relationships that are important components of nurse job satisfaction.

Increasing Investment of Clinical Staff

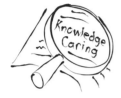

Once indicators had been selected and data collection methods identified, the committee discussed ways to increase the investment of clinical nursing staff in collecting and managing the data. The Staff Nurse committee members played a pivotal role in making data understandable and usable at the unit level. As they came to understand the meaning of the data, they became more aware of the impact of seemingly mundane decisions, as they were translated into measured data. They quickly recognized data as a source of power (American Psychiatric Nurses Association, 2005), and were eager to look at data that clearly related to the interaction between nurse and patient.

The Nurse Practice Outcomes Committee (NPOC) took deliberate steps to close the communication gap that existed between collecting, reporting and using data, with seclusion and restraint as the initial example. Nurses had been the long-standing and primary source for data collection regarding the use of seclusion and restraint, but they found the presentation of aggregated data to be confusing and less than meaningful at the unit level. The Staff Nurse committee members provided the feedback that shaped the form of the data distribution. They wanted to see unit-specific, actual data—not usage rates that were adjusted by average daily census—and they wanted to see it in a timely manner—not months later.

Data collection forms were simplified, and a simple auditing process was implemented to assure validity. (Night nurses verify the data during 24-hour chart checks.) Nurse leaders were engaged in discussions about the importance of presenting the data in a constructive manner. The Staff Nurses sought to use the data to inform and contribute to knowledge to improve practice, without shame or blame for practitioners. Their recommendations were incorporated into the reporting method that has communicated—and perhaps contributed to—the continued downward trend in the use of restrictive interventions.

Actual, unit-specific data about seclusion and restraint use are now reported to units in colorful graphic format, every week and in monthly trend graphs. "Talking points" were added to the graphs to facilitate discussions among interdisciplinary treatment team members. The information is easy

Actual, unit-specific data about seclusion and restraint use are now reported to units in colorful graphic format, every week and in monthly trend graphs.

to read and interpret, and nurses can see what they need to change, as well as the impact of their efforts to change. Nurse managers have taken on the role of champions for the reduction of the use of seclusion and restraint and have established daily and weekly forums to use the data in discussions with physicians and other members of interdisciplinary teams about issues surrounding the use of all restrictive interventions.

Actual Outcomes

The data collected by NHH nurses show that the use of seclusion and restraint is steadily (see Figure 1 below) declining at NHH, in spite of a more than 50% increase in the rate of admissions over the past 2 years. There has been a steady increase in the percentage of patients who know the name of their Primary Nurse (see Figure 2 on the following page)—one indicator that implementation of relationship-based nursing has been a success. Nurse job satisfaction as measured by the Index of Work Satisfaction increased 14% 6 months after implementing the Relationship-Based Care.

Unit Seclusion/Restraint
December 10 - 16, 2006

	12/10	12/11	12/12	12/13	12/14	12/15	12/16
Seclusion (Hours)	0.25	0	1.5	0	0.5	0	0
Restraint (Hours)	2.5	1.5	0	0	0	0	0
Episodes	1	1	1	0	1	0	0

Figure 1

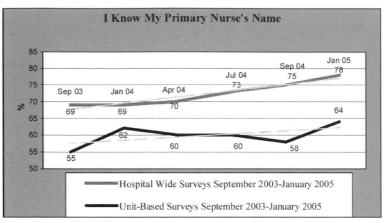

I Know My Primary Nurse's Name

Figure 2

Conclusion

Nurses must find effective ways to promote the diffusion of new knowledge in order to keep pace with changes in the future. They must clearly articulate their knowledge to others in order to help patients and improve the professional status of nurses. This knowledge will be more readily accepted if it is presented in ways that are understandable, meaningful and usable for those who deliver patient care. NHH nurses have demonstrated that nurses have the ability to lead change at all organizational levels through the use of outcomes data. Effectively packaging and disseminating nursing-sensitive outcomes data will help nurses to understand that they are the experts in their profession, with the power and responsibility to share their unique knowledge of patient care.

References: Allen, D. (2005). *Nurse job satisfaction and the development and implementation of a patient care delivery model.* Academic Dissertation, Master of Nursing, University of Dundee, Scotland.

American Nurses Credentialing Center. (2002). *Health care organization instructions and application process manual.* Washington, DC: American Nurses Publishing.

American Psychiatric Nurses Association. (2005). *Position statement: Psychiatric-mental health nurse roles in outcomes evaluation and management.* Washington, DC. Retreived August 31, 2005 from http://www.apna.org.

Kinnaird, L., & Dingman, S. (2004). Outcome measurement. In M. Koloroutis (Ed.), *Relationship-based care: A model for transforming practice* (pp. 215 - 248). Minneapolis, MN: Creative Health Care Management.

Orlando, I. (1961). *The dynamic nursing-patient relationship.* New York: National League for Nursing.

Stamps, P. (1997). *Nurses and work satisfaction: An index of measurement.* Annapolis Junction, MD: Health Administration Press.

Measuring Organizational Effectiveness: Learning to "Do Outcomes Well"

—Paula Ellis

I love hot fudge sundaes. I could easily eat three a week, but I only allow myself one sundae a month. When I go to Dairy Queen, I know I'll get exactly the same sundae each month, same size, same amount of hot fudge, same delicious ice cream.

If I received a different quality hot fudge sundae on one of my visits, that visit would be my last. Dairy Queen knows that my consistent return—and the return of millions of others—depends upon a consistent product. Every Dairy Queen manager wants a predictable hot fudge sundae, a consistent, nonvarying *outcome.*

I offer the example of the hot fudge sundae as a way to understand the value of consistent, predictable outcomes in health care. Leah Kinnaird (consultant with Creative Health Care Management) got my attention the first time I met her when she stated: "Most organizations don't do outcomes well. This is a chance for your organization to do outcomes well." At first I was irritated; I wanted to let her know I'd worked in nursing for more than 25 years. I knew nursing process. I knew nursing theory. Unfortunately, she proved right: I held little understanding of how the care experiences of my patients varied as a result of my not-always-completely-consistent nursing practices—that is, I didn't have a clear picture of the outcomes of my efforts. To add to my discomfort, my assignment as chair of the Outcomes Subcommittee for Kindness Connects—St. Francis Health Center's organizational intervention aimed at improving relationships between all employees and customers house wide—our vision for Relationship-Based Care initiative now haunted me. I hate feeling incompetent. After recognizing a new learning opportunity, the subcommittee started the journey toward identifying what we needed

What measurement would capture "our existing excellence?"

to accomplish, toward setting measurable goals, and toward using the information we would obtain to improve our efforts. Clearly this was a chance for our organization to learn to "do outcomes well."

The Beginning

Dr. Kinnaird met with the outcomes subcommittee. Our initial task loomed large. We needed to develop a process by which we could help others in the organization (not just those in nursing services) figure out what they wanted to accomplish and to understand that changes in their behavior based on the principles outlined in St. Francis Health Center's Kindness Connects initiative could improve their work on patients' behalf. Our overarching goals were to be health care provider of choice; to be employer of choice; to build on the excellence already existing.

keep the process simple and strive to make the organization culture "all about outcomes."

This group needed to develop a process for determining outcomes at both the organizational (*macro*) and departmental (*micro*) levels for our health center. We heard Dr. Kinnaird's reminder frequently as we worked. She said that health care organizations that jump on the benchmarking bandwagon consistently face two problems: First, if the data they collect look good, leadership feels no compunction to do anything, and second, if data look bad, leaders defend it. She also challenged us to keep the process simple and strive to make the organization culture "all about outcomes." I wondered if our organization would ever be "all about outcomes?"

The Middle

The questions we ask drive the changes we desire.

I'd already learned from Colleen Person of CHCM that the questions we ask drive the changes we desire. By asking questions, we collect data specific to those questions. The questions we ask around what we want to accomplish—our intended outcomes—ultimately determine what practices, processes and behaviors within the organization will be eliminated, improved or replaced. I knew our health center was already drowning in data, but suddenly I could ask some new questions: What were we doing with it? Did the data compiled on Kindness Connects make any difference? I decided to find out.

The overarching goals for the Kindness Connects initiative are:

- *to be the provider of choice for health care in northeast Kansas*

- *to be the employer of choice for health care workers in northeast Kansas*

- *to build upon our existing excellence*

The first task for our subcommittee involved translating these goals into organizational (macro) outcomes. Starting with our first goal, to become the provider of choice, any data we found that measured how satisfied our patients reported feeling with their care seemed a natural fit. Now we needed to determine which data related to patients' satisfaction with care might correlate directly to the Kindness Connect initiative. Since Kindness Connects focused on enhancing relationships between and among patients, staff, physicians, co-workers and/or other customers, we looked at every question on our current patient satisfaction survey, eventually zeroing in on three items thought indicative of improved relationships:

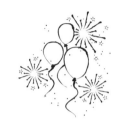

- *I consistently received respect and compassion while at St. Francis Health Center (SFHC),*

- *Compared to other local or regional hospitals, SFHC provides the best care, and*

- *I would recommend SFHC without hesitation to others.*

We determined that an increase of two (2) points for both the "Agree" and "Strongly Agree" categories would indicate that the Kindness Connects initiative was having a measurable, positive effect on practice.

For our second goal, to become the employer of choice, we turned to our biannual employee survey to choose questions corresponding to improved relationships among and between employees. We looked at four general areas: supervisor relationships, work role compatibility, personal growth and development, and the employee's opinion of the organization. Specific items targeted were:

- *I am proud to work for this organization.*

- *I am satisfied with the career development*

opportunities available to me at SFHC.

- *I would recommend SFHC as a good place to work.*

- *I receive the training necessary for me to be successful at my current job.*

- *My job makes good use of my skills and abilities.*

- *My supervisor provides constructive feedback and coaching to help me improve my performance.*

- *I am confident in the ability of my supervisor.*

We targeted an increase in this indicator of three (3) percentage points in the combined "Agree" and "Strongly Agree" categories as evidence of positive growth in these areas.

The final goal, to build upon our existing excellence, provided the greatest challenge. Our health center enjoyed a positive reputation and solid financial success. But what measurement would capture "our existing excellence?" After much discussion, we concluded we would look at physician satisfaction as the best indicator of this goal. Historically, an outside firm performed a medical staff survey for us biannually. We targeted three questions from the survey we thought captured the impact of Kindness Connects as it related to this final goal:

- *Overall, how would you rate SFHC as a place to practice?*

- *How would you rate the quality of care at SFHC? and*

- *How would you rate the nurses' knowledge of patient status and needs?*

We set the target at 80% satisfaction in the combined "Very Good" and "Excellent" categories. Having finished the macro indicators for the three organizational goals, I found myself feeling more competent.

After we as a subcommittee selected the macro indicators for the organization as a whole, we turned to helping department directors develop their own unit-based micro indicators. Dr. Kinnaird clearly stated that leaders must set the outcomes for their own work areas. We'd piloted the micro indicator development for the Kindness Connect initiative on the work

> Departments experiencing the greatest successes related to Kindness Connects, without exception, were led by Directors who spent the time investing in and learning about the outcomes measurement process.

areas represented by the outcomes subcommittee members. Using the project goals and macro indicators as guides, Dr. Kinnaird worked the subcommittee members through the process of determining micro indicators for use at their own departmental levels. She asked the following questions:

- *What helps your work group know your vision?*

- *What would you always want to see in your work area?*

- *What would you never want to see?*

Subcommittee members reported seeing the value of articulating the expectations for their work areas through this process. This created recognition that we subcommittee members needed to tell our staff what our expectations were so they could better focus their efforts. Our mantra became: "We have the power to improve from outcomes; data does drive change."

Now just for a moment, in order to review what we've learned about goals, indicators and outcomes, let's go back to the hot fudge sundaes. Dairy Queen's success rests on producing a consistent product. Thus, Dairy Queen's overarching goal might be something like "In the midst of life's ups and downs, Dairy Queen consistently provides a superior ice cream product to the customer." Next, a possible organization-wide (macro) indicator for such a goal might be a measurable increase in ice cream product sales. This takes us then to the level of individual stores where they may develop their own micro indicator in support of the overarching goal of the organization. Each store manager would determine "what they always wanted to see" and/or "what they never wanted to see" and translate that vision into an indicator of a quality outcome. For example, a micro indicator for Franchise X could target a 5% increase in its own hot fudge sundae sales.

Generic Outcomes Grid

What to collect		Source of data and who will collect			How to evaluate and trend/track			Celebration
Indicator	Definition	Method	Source	Report Format	Numerator Denominator	Validity Reliability	Target	
Patient Satisfaction with Overall Care. (This is a macro indicator related to the organization's vision to be the Provider of Choice.)	Indicator is defined as patient opinion of care during a health center encounter as determined by specific questions asked on a vendor-supplied survey as a set of scaled responses (from 1–5).	Vendor survey sent to randomly-selected patients four weeks post discharge.	Patient relations department coordinates survey process internally. Data summarized by vendor.	Data collected monthly; reported quarterly; reports sent to executives and department directors and managers simultaneously.	Numerator is the number of patients who reported at the level of "strongly agree" on the set of scaled responses (level 4 on a scale of 1–5) over the denominator of the total number of patients responding to the survey questions.	Vendor provides validity and reliability data in background information describing the instrument.	An improvement in the responses from the "agree" (level 3) to "strongly agree" (level 4) by 2% on the identified questions. Track the data until the target is stable and sustained. Trend line kept in common area for staff to discuss ways to continue to improve.	Reward and recognition for improving is determined by staff and managers who are accountable for the change.

The Outcomes Grid (above) brought this whole process to the point where something useful resulted. First, working with the grid itself offered a learning experience; that is, completing the grid taught us more about outcomes as well as reinforcing much of what we'd already learned. The grid allowed us to put key principles Dr. Kinnaird taught us into practice. These principles include:

- *valuing the importance of accurate data to ensure data reliability over time,*

- *reporting the data directly to the people who can do something about it, and*

- *defining your indicator and determining a good measure of it.*

Second, adherence to the grid decreases the variability of the process itself, and we know from best practice research that decreasing *the variability in any process provides the most consistent outcomes.* Third, we worked with each subcommittee member so that each left the session with at least one micro indicator specific to his or her work area.

After successfully piloting the process on our subcommittee, we moved house-wide to all department directors and supervisors, requesting that they attend a 2-hour educational session. With background provided in the educational session, the participants then utilized the outcomes grid for micro indicator development for their work areas. Department directors were expected to report quarterly on progress relative to their micro indicator to both their Vice President and to me.

The Finale

Our first wave of the Kindness Connects initiative rolled out in January of 2003. Now, 3 years into the project, we are still using the project goals and macro indicators we selected initially. Many departments altered their micro indicators two or more times as circumstances evolved. The increasing comfort of leaders with the process has led to more sophisticated micro indicators than those used in the early stages of the project.

Mixed results followed. On one hand, not every department director discusses micro indicators with the Vice President quarterly and not every department director provides me with quarterly data. On the other hand, measurable progress was noted in several areas including patient satisfaction. For instance, the laboratory wanted to impact patient satisfaction, and by looking at the emergency department (ED) as a laboratory customer, they realized that if they could decrease the turnaround time (time from specimen receipt into the lab until verification of results) for key tests, patients could be treated faster, decreasing time in ED and improving patient satisfaction with the ED experience. The laboratory's goal was for a 30-minute turnaround time on nine tests. In the early months, they attained the goal 80+% of the time. For the last six months, the laboratory averaged meeting the goal 95.65% of the time.

A busy medical nursing floor, also looking at patient satisfaction, focused on noise levels on the units that disturbed patients' rest. Patient response to the question "My room was restful and quiet" improved from a score of 78 to a score of 85 over a 30-month period. Patient response to the question "My sleeping hours were disturbed only when necessary" improved from a score of 84.7 to a score of 88.2 over a 30-month period.

Most organizations don't do outcomes well. This is a chance for your organization to do outcomes well.

Another department focused on employee satisfaction—specifically on two questions from the biannual employee survey:

- *My supervisor respects the unique background, skills and viewpoints of every employee, and*

- *I am confident in the ability of my supervisor.*

The target involved raising the "Agree" and "Strongly Agree" categories (cumulatively known as favorable) for each of these questions by three (3) percentage points between March 2003 and March 2005. In this particular department, for the first question, the "Agree" and "Strongly Agree" categories increased 25 percentage points, from 50% favorable to 75% favorable. The second question saw a 42 percentage-point increase, from 50% favorable to 92% favorable.

Departments experiencing the greatest successes related to Kindness Connects, without exception, were led by directors who spent the time investing in and learning about the outcomes measurement process. Leadership interest and enthusiasm definitely translated into staff interest and enthusiasm.

Learning about the outcomes measurement process meant adopting the language of the process. Those leaders in the organization who spoke in terms of macro and micro indicators, who asked about outcomes, and who recognized and addressed key behaviors were the leaders whose staffs blossomed the most in conjunction with this process. Those staff members generated great ideas in meetings, looked at different ways of tackling problems, and provided enthusiastic support of change within the organization.

Once a leader has invested staff with authority to not just "see a problem and fix it," but rather to see a problem, identify causes, look at alternatives, and choose the best course of action (knowing that the present course can be changed at any time), then staff will not experience the feeling of helplessness rampant in so many organizations. Allowing staff to experience the power of meaningful data requires the leader to continue providing more data to satisfy staff needs. We have put a good deal of focus on our outcomes measurement process over the last several years and have improved measurably because of it. We at St. Francis Health Center now "do outcomes well."

Leadership interest and enthusiasm definitely translated into staff interest and enthusiasm.

A CEO's Perspective on Improving Performance and Achieving a Vision of Excellence Through Use of the Balanced Scorecard

—Ron Bachman (Interviewed by Mary Koloroutis)

Background: *Marion General was built in the early 1920s and has been viewed since that time as the community hospital in Marion, OH. MedCenter Hospital was built in 1962 and was acquired by Marion General in 1998. Marion has a population of 35,000 with a county population of over 70,000 and Marion General is the central point of a seven-county area. Marion General and MedCenter were competitors for many years. During that time MedCenter had one third of the total market share and Marion General had two thirds. Marion General has been affiliated with Ohio Health System since 1986 and MedCenter was independent until the merger. The merger of the two organizations was announced in 1996 and MedCenter was officially closed in 1998. Marion General became the inpatient facility with an emergency department and all outpatient services went into the MedCenter Building. A for-profit joint venture was created to run ambulatory surgery and all other out-patient diagnostic services such as lab, radiology, physical therapy and occupational therapy.*

Combining staff and managers from the formerly competitive facilities into one inpatient facility was a devastating time. The community didn't like it because MedCenter was taken out of service. The medical staff who admitted to MedCenter Hospital had a building attached to the old facility so that 98% of patients came from their clinic. Suddenly, two medical staff—formerly archrivals—were forced to partner with each other. Prior to the merger, medical practices had been exclusive to one hospital or the other. Most physicians and surgeons never "crossed the street!"

There was a crisis of confidence even within the hospital management team regarding whether one emergency department and one hospital could serve the needs of the community. Medical staff members were reluctant to come together; hospital staff members had been in a friendly rivalry, and suddenly there was an effort to combine management teams and relocate, moving hospital staff from one facility to another. A lot of construction was required in the Marion Hospital building to accommodate the influx of an increased volume of inpatients from 1998 to 2001. Twenty-eight million dollars was invested in capital improvement to accommodate the merger—the planners built a new ICU, renovated the medical units, gutted a unit and built a new unit, and all of the operating rooms had to be made larger to accommodate inpatient surgeries (outpatient was to the MedCenter building across the street)—including orthopedic, total joints, and open heart. This was a huge period of change and turmoil.

Patients didn't like the merger initially. The very first winter after the MedCenter's emergency department was closed there was a tremendous flu outbreak. This happened while one half of the emergency department was under construction and more than two times the number of patients were being seen—it felt like patients were hanging from the rafters! Patient satisfaction was at the 4th percentile for inpatient initially and at the 9th percentile in late 1999 to 2000. It was pretty ugly! We had a vision of creating a different model, nothing that we could point to, and we had a lot of Doubting Thomases in the community—including our management team!

Ron Bachman, was interviwed by Mary Koloroutis.

Congratulations on being awarded the "Performance Improvement Leaders Award" for 2005 from Solucient Top 100 Hospitals. We'd like to understand how you have used the balanced scorecard as a tool for successfully using evidence to chart progress and inspire action and change in your organization.

We have a balanced scorecard approach to our business planning and incentive compensation programs. As we write goals and measure progress, it is all driven by the balanced scorecard. We have four quadrants to the balanced scorecard:

- *Clinical quality*
- *Customer service*

- *Quality of work life*

- *Financial performance*

I know a lot of organizations say they have a balanced scorecard, but unless they reach their financial numbers nothing else seems to matter. At both Marion General and in our system, we have kept all four areas religiously in balance. As we evaluate our hospital performance, there are times that we can have a great quality year and not such a great financial year, and if we do well in three of the four quadrants, that still means we had a pretty darn good year. And our incentive compensation systems reflect that balance.

I think it's helpful, too, that we don't dwell on a quadrant that we come up short in; if everything else is a success, but we don't meet our bottom line, it doesn't mean we're a failure. We say, "Well, 75% of our balanced scorecard was great and we'd like to do better, and we will strive to do better, but we are still going to celebrate the success we had in three quadrants." I think being zealous about the balanced scorecard—making sure people understand that it's a good representation of what we stand for, that it's how we measure our performance and it is here to stay—has about as big an impact as anything.

For example, in the quadrant that measures clinical quality, we measure performance not on anecdotal comments from patients and physicians, but on industry-wide benchmarks. Within the clinical quadrant we track about 25 clinical quality indicators that are common to all the hospitals within OhioHealth—in diseases that all of us take care of whether we are a 1,000-bed hospital or a 50-bed hospital. Once people in the organization saw that we are using that information and that we are standardizing our goals and measures, they eventually accepted that those things were here to stay.

Initially it was a challenge to get people past critiquing the tool, or the collection mechanism, or the validity of the tool. I remember that CHCM [Creative Health Care Management] used a term I liked; you said that people have to learn to have "functional trust." We had to get our staff and medical staff to accept the science behind these tools instead of trying to invalidate the results because they had determined that the tools weren't scientific, or significantly valid, or that only

I think being zealous about the balanced scorecard—making sure people understand that it's a good representation of what we stand for, that it's how we measure our performance and it is here to stay—has about as big an impact as anything.

negative people fill out Press Ganey, or whatever other reasons they could come up with to resist the change.

You recently experienced a big jump in physician satisfaction scores. What was the "tipping point" for improving physician satisfaction?

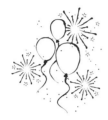

We had to communicate to the physicians on a regular basis those things that we do all the time that are geared to make this a satisfying place for them to practice. It's similar to how we improve our patients' perception by communicating in a way that lets them know what we are doing for them—"I am going to close this curtain to ensure your privacy"; "Is there anything else I can do for you? I have time." We know what is needed to improve satisfaction, so we remind physicians of the things that actually happen that we've put into place to satisfy them.

The very first question on our physician satisfaction survey is the only question that Ohio Health uses to compare us from hospital to hospital, and it is the only one that is counted in the balanced scorecard. That question is: "When you think of Marion General Hospital, how do you rate it as a place to practice medicine?" The only answer that counts is "excellent," so we are evaluated on the percentile responses of "excellent" that we receive from our medical staff. "Very good" doesn't count; we only get credit for "excellent." In spring of 2005, 64 physicians took the survey and only 16 answered that question with "excellent." In spring of 2006, 74 physicians took the survey and 34 have rated us as an "excellent" place to practice medicine. The 16 out of 64 last year put us at approximately the 36th percentile of "excellent" responses compared to the Professional Research Consultants (PRC) database. This year's 34 out of 74 puts us in the 83rd percentile. That is how sensitive the measure is. Even though less than 50% rated us as excellent, when compared to the national PRC database, it puts us up there in the 83rd percentile!

What has happened to your patient satisfaction scores over time?

Five or six years ago when we started to consolidate the two hospitals here in Marion we were in single digits on both inpatient and emergency department patient satisfaction. The community didn't like us because we were taking away one of the hospitals, we had construction going on here, and our staff was in an uproar because we were consolidating staffs. We were changing the physicians' world drastically, trying to combine two medical staffs that used to be rivals. Slowly but surely over the past 6 years we have brought our scores up. Our inpatient satisfaction year-to-date (as of June 30, 2006) is in the 94th percentile, including the fourth quarter where we finished in the 99th percentile, which placed us as number one in the country—first time we have ever been there for inpatient satisfaction. The emergency department finished at the 89th percentile for the full year and the fourth quarter was in the 93rd percentile. We are going to have a major celebration over these results. Our inpatient satisfaction over the last ten quarters averages above the 85th percentile, so we have reached a plateau of consistency. The emergency department is still on the rise, but even there we probably have six quarters in a row where we are above the 85th percentile.

Inpatient Overall Percentile Rankings

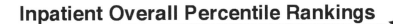

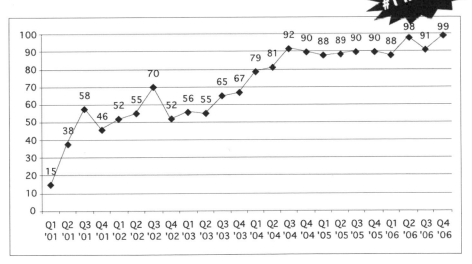

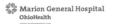

Amazing Consistency!

Marion General Hospital
OhioHealth

How do you measure employee/work-life satisfaction?

We use an employee opinion survey that is system wide. The survey has 84 questions; there is a subset of 13 core questions that make up the "employer of choice index" (EOC Index) and that's what we use system wide to compare scores hospital-to-hospital. All 84 questions are of interest to us, but the 13 core questions are what we use to compare ourselves to other organizations and to trend progress, and that is what we use on the balanced scorecard. For each of the last 3 fiscal years, Marion General earned the best EOC scores among the OhioHealth system hospitals

Marion General Hospital

EMPLOYER OF CHOICE RESULTS				
Question	2006	National Norm	Best Practice	OhioHealth Norm
Good Job Communicating Organization Objectives	5.3	4.3	5.1	4.7
Quality/Service Improvements a High Priority	5.3	4.9	5.2	4.9
Taking Steps to Keep Competitive Edge	5.1	4.8	5.1	4.7
We Will Use Survey Info to Make Improvements	4.9	4.4	4.9	4.3
I Would Recommend Employment to Friends	5.3	4.5	5.6	5.0
I am Proud to Work for This Organization	5.5	5.1	5.9	5.3
My Manager Communicates Performance Expectations	4.7	4.9	5.3	4.6
My Manager Seems Interested in Employee Motivation/Satisfaction	4.6	4.7	5.4	4.6

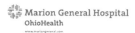
Marion General Hospital
OhioHealth

How have you been doing in the financial quadrant?

This year we are doing better than we have in the last 7 years—it has been our lagging quadrant. We have been at or near budget, but this year we are far in excess of our operating margin target and should score very high. We track two indicators as a system: one is "operating margin as compared to budget" and the other is "cost per adjusted discharge," which looks at our overall cost per case in relation to our prior year's results. We are doing very well in both of them.

Obviously something we are curious about is whether you see any of the work with Relationship-Based Care (RBC) as having an effect over these last five or six years.

Oh, it absolutely did. Particularly in customer service and patient satisfaction. Relationship-Based Care helped all our staff understand that it is "all about the relationship" and that the one-to-one relationship with the staff is critical. I think RBC is one of the things that has contributed to our success.

It sounds like one of the key factors for you and your team was gaining alignment around the use of the balanced scorecard as a source of shared purpose and inspiration.

We got the team aligned in a very practical way—through our Teamwork Incentive Plan (TIP Program). We started using the balanced scorecard almost 6 years ago after we established board-approved hospital goals for each quadrant of the scorecard. Then we picked out the most significant goal out of each of the four quadrants and we developed a Teamwork Incentive Plan (TIP program), through which we put money at stake for all of our staff. We then designed a program where individuals earned bonuses if we as an organization achieve any of the "stretch targets" for these goals in a given year.

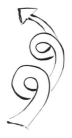

Here's how it works: our scoring guidelines are zero to 5, with 3 being the expected level of performance—i.e., for the financial quadrant, meeting budget would be a 3, beating budget by a significant portion would be a 4, and really hitting a financial "home run" would score a 5. Scores of 4 and 5 are reserved for stretch performance; they represent "going beyond the call," where we would have had to intentionally do something that would drive a different result. For these TIP goals we set the "stretch" at a score of 4 on our hospital scoring guidelines. So in our financial performance goal for this year our budgeted operating margin is 1.6%, but our stretch goal is a 2.1% operating margin. If we reach 2.1% or greater, full-time staff members earn an additional $150.00, and we prorate that amount for part-timers.

> At the end of the day being evaluated on these objective measures was a tough transition for some people.

Was this "TIP" incentive part of your strategy as you began as CEO almost 6 years ago?

Absolutely. It was a way to get people aligned and show them we were serious enough about this that we were willing to put money behind it. We are also careful to choose goals that we believe most people in the organization have an opportunity to impact. We know that not every housekeeper or person working in nutrition has a direct impact on quality indicators, but we picked indicators that have the broadest audience possible.

For the first 5 years this program was in place, we achieved three out of the four TIP goals. The mix was different over each of the 3 years—some years we hit financial, some not; some the quality, some not; we weren't consistently weak in any one quadrant—but we hit three out of four for the first 5 years. This year, it looks like for the first time we will hit four out of four!

That means $150 per goal achieved for every full-time employee. Last year we spent $345,000 in TIP bonuses, and this is just for front-line staff—management receives bonuses through a different incentive program. People know what it takes to reach the goals. We have town hall meetings every 4 months or so and part of the agenda is to give an update on how we are performing in relation to our hospital goals on the balanced scorecard. Within that presentation we also highlight how are we doing on the TIP goal within each quadrant on the balanced scorecard so people know how we are doing.

What have you done to bring your leadership team along?

We had a few casualties earlier on—people who didn't buy into the balanced scorecard, or may have not bought into one particular quadrant of the scorecard. It wasn't that difficult to get people to rally around the balanced scorecard. The scorecard itself is really "common sense"; where people struggled was with the accountability piece. At the end of the day being evaluated on these objective measures was a tough transition for some people.

We had some people who were used to sitting down with their boss at the end of the year and saying, "I think I had a pretty good year ... this happened, and that happened ... it all felt pretty good; we accomplished a lot." We had to transition them to a process whereby you set your goals in the springtime for the year that begins July 1. Not only do you set your goals; you set your scoring guidelines, so that when it comes to your evaluation, or at any given time throughout the year or at the end of the year you can measure exactly how you are doing. It's set up so that that score is meaningful, because that score is going to be how your bonus will be determined and how your individual merit increases will be determined.

We also put significant money into a risk pool for the top 25 people in the organization—directors on up. Most of our directors have the ability to earn 12% of their base pay in bonuses, and those bonuses are split evenly into two components—how well the hospital does as a whole in relation to its goals and how well individuals perform in relation to their goals for the units they lead.

You referenced "celebrating your successes" earlier. What does that look like in your organization?

When we do the TIP bonus checks in August, we have two big parties, one for the day shift and one in the evening. We decorate, we eat well, and the leadership team is there to pass out checks to their respective staff and to congratulate them personally. We have a great time.

Awards are given for quality and customer service each month. In the course of a full year, we give out 52 customer service awards and 26 quality awards as we give out two per category per month. We do customer service recognition every other week and quality each month. We present the awards at the end of an administrative council meeting. We also do customer service banners and trophies for departments that have objectively received a particular result based on Press Ganey data or the internal report card measurement that we use. We present them with a banner and a box of candy. We also have a customer service trophy that we use in the same way.

The administrative council does the presentation on the unit. We gather people around, read from the printed chart that we will leave with them (if there are physicians on the floor we make sure to have them join us and be a part of the team picture), and in the very next newsletter the picture

Awards are given for quality and customer service each month.

is published so the world can see. Each person is identified and there is a story about what they achieved to receive the banner!

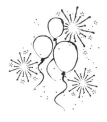

Just a postscript that I want to share because we are really excited about it. We had our Joint Commission survey last week (summer 2006) and it was a huge success. Our overall results were the best since we consolidated the two hospitals. Our overall performance was 4.5 on a 5-point scale. In fiscal year 2006 we added two expanded cardiac services to include angiography and open heart and we have grown our inpatient admissions to 6% greater than year-end 2005. We are feeling incredible about our movement and growth and plan to continue with a focus on excellence in all four quadrants.

The Impact of *Reigniting the Spirit of Caring* on the Work Environment of the Nurse

—John W. Nelson

Data from three rigorous CHCM client studies will clearly show the positive impact that the *Reigniting the Spirit of Caring* (*RSC*) workshop has on the work environment of Staff Nurses, as reported by Staff Nurses. Findings revealed an improvement in all of the most important variables in a nurse's work environment for nurses who participated in the *RSC* workshop. This brief paper will review the results of these three studies. Power analysis, instrument psychometrics, and confounding variables were all included in analysis, but are beyond the scope of this brief paper. Readers who would like a more extensive review of the methods and limitation of any of the studies are invited to contact the author of this paper, or of this Field Guide.

The Intervention, *RSC*

In brief, *RSC* is designed to explore challenging aspects of the nurse's job through reflection, dialogue, journaling and storytelling. It is built on the premise that by sanctioning time for reflection and conversation and by gathering colleagues together, nurses will be able to tap into and benefit from the wisdom, collective intelligence, and support and appreciation of each other. Nurses gain personal insights and develop new ideas and skills and strategies that will help them thrive in their daily work and lives.

This program was developed on the belief that through reflection and learning, through intentional thought and action, through leadership and collegial support, and through enhancing awareness and refocusing on what matters most—people have the power to transform work cultures. Organizational environments can be transformed into cultures in which personal responsibility prevails, healthy relationships thrive,

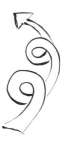

appreciation is openly expressed and caring and healing are the constant and core reason for existence. It was the hypothesis of all of these studies that such training would benefit nurses by helping them to gain insight into their working world and how they might respond to it.

Study Number One, Tertiary Care Center

The Healthcare Environment Survey (HES) was used to measure the work environment as perceived by the Staff Nurse. It was sent out to 182 randomly selected nurses at an East Coast tertiary care center. Eighty-three of the nurses had participated in *RSC* and 99 had not. Sixty-three nurses from the *RSC* group returned the surveys (a 76% response rate) and 63 nurses from the control group returned the survey (a 64% response rate) for an overall response rate of 70%. Results revealed nurses who attended *RSC* reported greater overall job satisfaction on every variable measured than those who did not attend. It is important to evaluate both trend and statistical significance (see Figure 1).

Figure 1. Comparing Nurses Who Attended and Nurses Who Did Not Attend *RSC*, 2003 Study

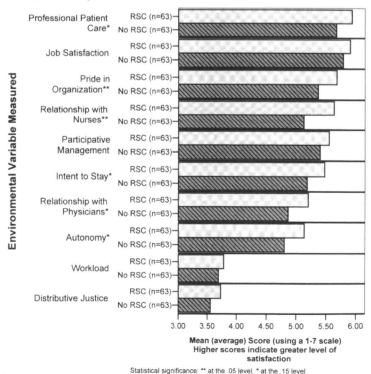

Statistical significance: ** at the .05 level, * at the .15 level

Certain demographic groups had an additional positive impact by RSC, including (using a two-way ANOVA):

- *certain units,*
- *more advanced age groups, and*
- *nurses with higher levels of education in nursing.*

The qualitative portions of the data revealed:

- *a greater number of perceived stressors relating to workload and work relations.*

- *65 of the 123 nurses who participated in this study reported the patient relationship to be the aspect of their job they enjoyed the most. If employees are able to engage in what they enjoy the most (the relationship with the patient in this case), they will be productive and go the second and third mile, not because they are asked to or required to, but because they want to.*

Additional Findings from Study Number One

ANOVA: analysis of variance

The Healthcare Environment Survey (HES) was used to measure the work environment as perceived by the Staff Nurse. Surveys were made available to 859 staff members on 79 units/departments/clinics through an online process. There were 347 responses, which represents a 40.4% response rate. When comparing the staff who attended *RSC* (n=73) to those who did not attend (n=258), it was found those who attended *RSC* were more satisfied with 12 of the 14 variables, including nurse leadership, job satisfaction, professional patient care, participative management, intent to stay, promotional opportunities, pride in the organization, autonomy, relationship with nurse, relationship with co-workers and distributive justice. It is important to evaluate both trend and statistical significance (see Figure 2).

Study Number Two, Pediatric Hospital

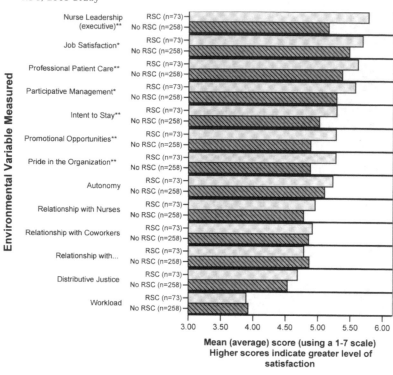

Figure 2. Comparing Nurses Who Attended and Nurses Who Did Not Attend *RSC*, 2005 Study

Statistical significance: ** at the .05 level, * at the .15 level

| Additional findings from Study Number Two | Certain demographic groups had an additional positive impact by RSC, including (using a two-way ANOVA): |

Additional findings from Study Number Two

Certain demographic groups had an additional positive impact by RSC, including (using a two-way ANOVA):

- *certain units,*
- *staff who worked the 8-hour shift (versus 12-hour shift),*
- *nurses in administrative/managerial roles, and*
- *nurses with higher levels of education in nursing.*

Of the 199 comments regarding what they enjoy most within their role

- *139 nurses reported patients' families (70%),*
- *48 nurses reported coworkers (24%), and*
- *23 nurses reported professional growth (12%).*

Opportunities for advancement and taking care of the patient were the two variables that explained 51% of what makes people feel pride in their work (using regression analysis). Feeling pride in one's work has implications for not only being glad to show up for work, but wanting to go the second and third mile to ensure the organization is a success.

The purpose of this 3-year study was to examine whether the level of job satisfaction improved during implementation of various organizational initiatives, including *Reigniting the Spirit of Caring.* Multiple initiatives limited this study to being descriptive in nature. However, the consistency of the results of the improved environment when interventions like *RSC* are utilized adds to the understanding of the impact of *Reigniting the Spirit of Caring.*

Six of the nine variables of job satisfaction improved sequentially over the 3-year period, including the nurses' perception of workload, autonomy, professional patient care, pride in the organization, intent to stay with the organization and job satisfaction. Three of the variables had the highest level of satisfaction in the second measurement period, but did end up with higher scores in the final measurement when compared to the baseline in 2002. These three variables included relationship with nurses, relationship with physicians and perception of distributive justice (rewards). Only one variable declined every year, perception of participative management. Figure 3 shows the findings for all the environmental variables that were measured all 3 years.

Study Number Three, Time Series Study in a Community Hospital

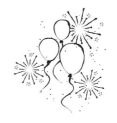

Figure 3. Scores for All Environmental Variables During the 3-Year Project, which Included *RSC*, 2002-2004 Study

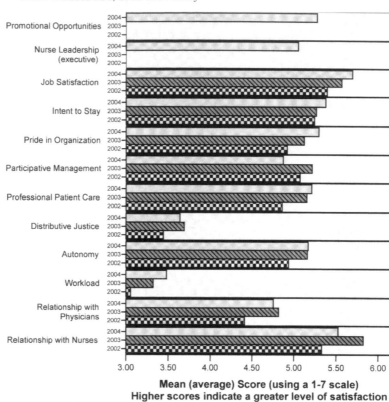

Mean (average) Score (using a 1-7 scale)
Higher scores indicate a greater level of satisfaction

Summary

All three studies show the impact that *Reigniting the Spirit of Caring* has on the environment that nurses work within. The collaborative work of *RBC*, creating new insight and strategies through reflection and conversation, does appear to help nurses thrive in their daily work and lives. Implications for such improvement include happier and healthier staff, which ultimately spills over into patient care, the reason for the existence of nursing.

The Impact of *Leadership at the Point of Care* on the Work Environment of the Nurse

—John W. Nelson

In 2005, a client requested Creative Health Care Management's help in improving the work environment for registered nurses on 65 units in 17 facilities on the East Coast of the United States. It was determined in consultation that their specific goals would be to improve staff morale, strengthen leadership at all levels, and reduce RN turnover. As CHCM's *Leadership at the Point of Care* (*LPC*) workshop facilitates leadership development by exploring the interchange of leadership, communication and Human Dynamics (see page 396), we offered it as one of the primary interventions for this client.

What follows is a review of the intervention and the positive changes found in all 13 aspects of the work environment that were measured after implementation, when compared to the baseline data. A noteworthy finding within this study was that the successful execution of unit-specific action plans was a key determinant for staff who reported an improved work environment, including increased satisfaction with unit and executive nurse leadership. In addition, *LPC* was found to raise scores relative to healthier work relationships which have a positive correlation to lower rates of nurse turnover. Using *LPC* to create action plans that utilize leadership at every level of care delivery has implications for not only an improved work environment, but also lower turnover created by healthier working relationships.

The Intervention

Leadership at the Point of Care is based on the belief that everyone has the capacity to be both a leader and a follower. We have found that bringing out the leader within every individual at every level of the organization is possible when

• *645*

one understands the interplay of leadership skills, communication, and Human Dynamics. Participants in *LPC* examine this interplay and work with facilitators and other colleagues attending *LPC* to create action plans for personal and professional change. (Refer to page 424 for additional information on the *LPC* workshop.)

The *LPC* workshop is divided into two sessions: *Leadership at the Point of Care* (also referred to as *LPC*), a 3-day learning session, and World Café (WC), a one-day debriefing of successes following the first session, anywhere from a few days to, ideally, several months later.

In the first session, participants explore leadership theory and concepts as they apply to individuals in roles at all levels of an organization. On the final day of *LPC*, participants are guided in the development of personal, collegial and professional action plans. They develop personal action plans (for their use only) which focus on their own individual development. They develop collegial plans focused on improving relationships in the work environment, the customization and execution of which are to be completed later with their unit members. They develop professional action plans focused on improving individual care and service to patients, also to be completed with their unit members.

In the follow-up World Café session, which takes place after individuals have had time to begin collaborating with their colleagues to execute their action plans, participants share with other units their stories of implementing their action plans on their own units, and in turn listen to what other units have experienced with their action plans. The shared successes and challenges of the action plan execution from the variety of units and facilities provide a venue for learning from each other for the purpose of refining all action plans.

In the case from which this study emerged, *Leadership at the Point of Care* was offered to 1,010 participants within the client's 17 organizations as the centerpiece of what the client called the "Nursing Leadership Project." The 3-day *LPC* session was attended by 79% of the allocated RNs, nurse managers, supervisors and CNOs. The one-day World Cafe' session was attended by 69% of the same allocated staff.

Nurses surveyed after taking both sessions of Leadership at the Point of Care expressed increased satisfaction with all 13 variables relative to the work environment.

The primary aims of this study were to discover the impact of the entire *LPC* workshop on morale, leadership and turnover. The analysis would begin by examining the impact of *LPC* on the 13 variables of the work environment, using a pre-post comparative design, including a paired t-test, to examine the difference in satisfaction scores in the environment before and after the *LPC* program. The Healthcare Environment Survey (HES) was used to measure changes in perception of the work environment. The HES used a 1-7 Likert scale, with higher scores indicating greater satisfaction with each respective aspect of the work environment. This is an 86-item instrument that has been extensively tested for validity and reliability, and designed specifically for the health care setting. Aspects of the work environment that were measured included:

- *Professional patient care*
- *Job satisfaction*
- *Promotional opportunities*
- *Work relationships*
- *Autonomy*
- *Physician relationships*
- *Participative management (unit management)*
- *Nurse relationships*
- *Nurse leadership (executive nurse leadership)*
- *Pride in the organization*
- *Intent to stay with the organization*
- *Distributive justice*
- *Workload*

The focal outcome of the *LPC* workshop is for participants to begin writing their own colleague and professional action plans on day three of the *LPC* session. After the action plans begin to take shape, the nurse participants went back to their units and worked with their colleagues to execute the plans. In this study, participants from *LPC* had anywhere from 6 to 256 days to execute their action plans before they were assessed in World Café (WC). We decided to examine whether having more time to execute action plans, as measured by the number of days between *LPC* and WC, would improve scores related to nurses' perceptions of the work environment. The date each participant attended the *Leadership at the Point of Care (LPC)* workshop was used as the time for measurement of the preintervention. The second date recorded for each participant was the date each attended the World Café (WC). We expected to find that nurses who had more days between sessions, and therefore more time to execute their actions plans and observe related successes, would be more satisfied than nurses who had fewer days between sessions.

Next, we wanted to examine the nurses' intentionality, which refers to the degree to which the nurses were committed to their action plans and felt equipped to be successful in executing them. In order to measure intentionality, a tool was created that asked participants about the positive energy they'd put into creating and executing their action plans, their perception of the success of their plans to date, and their levels of satisfaction with the contributions of their colleagues and the subsequent professional action plans generated and executed in professional collaborations on their units. Again, we used a 1-7 Likert scale. Higher scores would indicate greater positive energy and satisfaction with their respective action plans. This instrument was assessed for content validity by four consultants involved in the program. We expected to find a lower level of satisfaction among nurses who did not voice commitment to their plans. In contrast, we expected to find higher scores for those who felt committed and supported in the execution of their plans.

The above data were also evaluated relative to turnover data collected in phone interviews with 14 unit managers. The intent of examining these data was to see whether we could show a correlation between improved work environment and decreased turnover.

Findings Directly Related to the Study

As to the efficacy of the workshop in general, nurses surveyed after taking both sessions of *Leadership at the Point of Care* expressed increased satisfaction with all 13 variables relative to the work environment, as is shown in the following graphic (See Figure 1)

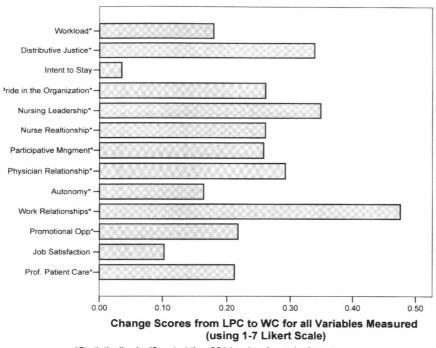

Figure 1. Difference Scores of All Variables Measured

We found that as the perceived success of the execution of unit-specific action plans improves, satisfaction with the work environment also improves. In contrast, nurses who were not satisfied with the execution of their action plans did not show an improved score or showed a decline in the variables measured.

We found that an increase in time for nurses to execute their action plans (to then be farther along, and presumably witness more evidence of the changes they intend to bring to their units) was not a predictor of increased nurse satisfaction with the work environment. Nurses who had only 6 days to execute their plans did not report a statistically significant difference in satisfaction with the execution of their plans from those who had several months to execute their plans. If there was an improvement noted in the work environment it was based on their intentionality, not time.

While "time spent executing action plans" did not prove to be significant to the nurses' perception of success, inten-

Additional Findings

As the perceived success of the execution of unit-specific action plans improves, satisfaction with the work environment also improves.

tion—the degree to which the nurses were committed to their action plans and felt equipped to be successful in executing them—proved notably significant. We found that those who were committed and confident stayed committed and confident and expressed satisfaction with the execution of their action plans whether they had a few days or several months to execute them, and we found that those who were not inclined to put energy into executing their plans were no more or less inclined after several months than they were after a few days.

After *LPC* we found that nurses reported a greater satisfaction with their work environments and subsequently reported lower turnover rates.

Recommendations Based on Findings

We found that 66% of the participants who expressed satisfaction with the execution of their action plans said that what made their plans successful was creating those plans in collaboration with consultants and colleagues on the last day of the *LPC* workshop. These findings have operational implications, including how to follow up with individual participants after an organizational intervention like *Leadership at the Point of Care.* Because we found that strong intention was such a significant predictor of nurses' satisfaction with the execution of their action plans—and by implication, with their work environments in general—we recommend that follow-up to *LPC* within the organizations to which *LPC* participants are returning consist of 6 days of concentrated focus on helping *LPC* participants to bring their action plans to life within their units, rather than months of periodic reviews and check-ins on how the action plans are going.

As intention was found to be such a powerful predictor of nurse satisfaction, efforts within the organization to help sustain the participants' positive energy make good sense. If participants come out of *LPC* ready to make things happen, the best way to sustain their enthusiasm is to "go with the energy" of the emerging participants. It is vital that participants receive the appropriate instruction, materials and support to ensure success of collaborative action plans.

The outcome of this study has implications for increased productivity and lower turnover derived from enhanced teamwork and happier workers. Subsequently, the new environment that results from the successful execution of action plans created in *LPC* should decrease cost by the increased productivity, decreased turnover and greater marketability of the organization.

For more information on the Healthcare Environment Survey, visit www.hcenvironment.com.

CHAPTER NINETEEN

Evidence-Based Practice and Research

We Make Evidence-Based Practice Much More Complicated Than It Needs to Be

—Donna Wright

Many health care professionals talk about the importance of evidence-based practice. But when I ask them about what evidence-based measurement is, they give me answers like:

- *"It's research done by clinical specialists and nursing scientists."*

- *"That is data collected by our quality coordinator."*

- *"The health center has several quality improvement and performance improvement monitors that collect that kind of information."*

When I ask them what kind of evidence-based data they collect, they look confused and I hear:

- *"I don't do that."*

- *"I do not have access to that."*

- *"I am not the one in charge of that."*

Oh, they are so sadly mistaken. We have access to so much data every day, but we don't recognize it.

Evidence-based data can be research and Quality Improvement/Performance Improvement (QI/PI) monitors, but it can also be much more than that.

Let's say you start three IVs today. One or two days later, check if those IVs are still in place. With a quick look at the chart you can see if the IV was discontinued or not. After a few days of looking at the IVs you started, you can begin to see evidence of what taping jobs best secure the IVs you start and any other techniques that help contribute to a healthy, long-life IV site. This is the beginning of evidence-based practice.

Here's another example: Let's say at the end of each day you discuss, as a team, for 3 minutes, how report went for the day. After just 3 or 4 days of 3-minute discussions, you will start to see trends in your discussion: what is working and what is not. This becomes an evidence-based measurement that will help you create a better reporting process.

Evidence-based data is NOT your "gut feeling." It is always grounded in data collection. Even if data collection is informal, it is still data collection. Basing decisions and practice on a gut feeling is not evidence-based practice. I am not saying that following your gut is wrong, but it reflects Intuitive decision making, not evidence-based decision making.

For example: You hear a nurse state, "The night shift never does a good job collecting I and O information." Is this statement accurate? Is this statement evidence-based, or is it based on the speaker's gut instinct?

For further inquiry, you ask the nurse to collect data on this judgment. You (and she) may find something very different.

Here is the dialogue to investigate further:

"So the night shift NEVER collects good I and O data?"

"No. Most nights it is pretty good. But this week we had some areas that fell short."

"So did everyone this week on the night shift not collect I and O data?"

"No. Marcia forgot to do totals and collect data, two nights in a row."

So now we discover through actual evidence-based data collection that it is not true that the night shift never does a good job with data collection, but instead that Marcia really bugged you two nights in a row and you need to address this problem with her. But you can see how your gut may lead you to say, "We have a problem with the whole night shift."

Evidence-based practice is in our daily reach. It is our obligation to our patients, our practice and our profession.

Evidence-based measurement is very important to making good decisions and choosing appropriate interventions and actions. We cannot just rely on our gut feelings, but we cannot also become paralyzed in thinking that evidence-based measurement is out of our reach. It is not that complicated. Start collecting your data today, and every day. It is the best way to work and motivate yourself and your practice in the right direction. Evidence-based practice is in our daily reach. It is our obligation to our patients, our practice and our profession.

Evidence-Based Practice and Best Practice: What's the Difference?

—Kathryn Ewers

The term *evidence-based practice* was first popularized by a group of physicians from McMaster University in the early 1990s, in an attempt to shift physicians' practice decisions from opinion-based to evidence-based practice. Sackett, Straus, Richardson, Rosenberg, and Haynes (2000) defined evidence-based medicine as the "integration of best research evidence with clinical expertise and patient values." Since that time, the evidence-based practice movement has spread to include many disciplines other than medicine. In the nursing world many international nursing organizations have included the principles of evidence-based care into nursing practice standards. For American nurses, evidence-based practice is a key component for receiving designation as a Magnet organization by the American Nurses Credentialing Center.

The term *best evidence* means that the evidence is of the highest level currently available. In the research world there are evidence hierarchies that provide levels of evidence. For example, evidence that comes from systematic reviews or a meta-analysis or randomized clinical trials would be considered to be more valid than lower-ranking opinion-based evidence. Studies have shown that even when higher levels of evidence exist, both physicians and nurses still prefer to rely on other forms of evidence, like experience or opinions of colleagues. The evidence-based practice movement is helping health care professionals move from more traditional opinion-based care to more evidence-based care. Given that the research to health care practice gap is still between 12 and 17 years, this has proven to be a very critical but complicated undertaking.

For academics, especially those of us who hail from the United Kingdom or Canada, the term *best practice* is synony-

> Studies have shown that even when higher levels of evidence exist, both physicians and nurses still prefer to rely on other forms of evidence, like experience or opinions of colleagues.

mous with the term *evidence-based*. Evidence-based practice guidelines are good examples of this. If you are in Canada, Britain, Ireland, Scotland or Australia, these guidelines may be referred to as Best Practice Guidelines. In the United States, evidence-based practice guidelines are usually referred to as clinical practice guidelines.

The term can cause confusion. In common American usage, however, a best practice is a process or method that has been refined over time and is still subject to further improvement. Under this common definition, a best practice is based on experience and opinion, not on research. In some instances, *best practice* simply means *most common*.

Another source of confusion is that the term *best practice* is sometimes inappropriately substituted for the term *standard*. A practice standard defines what is acceptable or unacceptable behavior, as well as the process for making decisions (Registered Nurses Association of Ontario [RNAO], 2000). Not all standards are evidence based. Sometimes, like best practices, standards are simply based on common industry practices. These practices may or may not be up to date and research or evidence based.

In summary, when you hear the term *best practice*, you should find out the source and level of the evidence being used to describe the practice. Initially this may seem uncomfortable and burdensome. However, skills can be rapidly built with help from clinical nurse specialists, nurse researchers, or a hospital librarian. It is crucial that nurses begin to increase their comfort with research terms if we are going to embrace the concept that nursing is an intellectual discipline as well as a caring profession.

To see firsthand how guidelines provide levels of evidence for practice decisions, visit the Registered Nurses Association of Ontario at www.rnao.org and click on the Best Practice Guideline Project. You will be able to download 29 nursing clinical practice guidelines as well as a variety of implementation and teaching resources without cost. You can also access guidelines via the Web from the National Guideline Clearinghouse at www.guideline.gov.

Best Practice A practice that may be based on evidence of varying levels, from observation and opinion to best evidence.

Best Evidence is evidence of the highest level currently available, for example, evidence that comes from systematic reviews or a meta-analysis or randomized clinical trials.

Clinical Practice Guideline "Systematically developed statements (based on the best available evidence) to assist practitioners with patient decisions about appropriate health care for specific clinical (practice) circumstances" (Field & Lohr, 1990, p. 38).

Evidence-Based Practice Practice that integrates the best research evidence with clinical expertise and patient values.

Levels of Evidence "A hierarchy of evidence, usually ranging from strongest to weakest" (RNAO, 2002, p. 86).

Meta-Analysis "A technique for quantitatively combining and thus integrating the results of multiple studies on a given topic" (Polit & Beck, 2004, p. 723).

Systematic Review "A rigorous scientific approach to consolidate the research evidence on a specific topic" (RNAO, 2002, p. 88).

References: Field, M. J., & Lohr, K. N. (Eds). (1990). *Guidelines for clinical practice: Directions for a new program.* Washington, DC: Institute of Medicine, National Academy Press.

Polit, D. F., & Beck, C. T. (2004). *Nursing research: Principles and methods.* (7th ed.). Philadelphia: Lippincott Williams & Wilkins.

Registered Nurses Association of Ontario. (2000). *Introduction to RNAO best practice guidelines PowerPoint.* Available from Registered Nurses Association of Ontario Web site, www.rnao.org

Registered Nurses Association of Ontario. (2002). *Toolkit: Implementation of clinical practice guidelines.* Toronto, Canada: Registered Nurses Association of Ontario.

Sackett, D., Straus, S. E., Richardson, S. W., Rosenberg, W., & Haynes, B. R. (2000). *Evidence-based medicine: How to practice and teach EBM.* New York: Churchill Livingstone.

The Development of a Nursing Research Program: From Planting the Seeds to Growing a Strong Viable Program in a Small Community Hospital

—Marlene Dufault and Dorothy Anne Garman

History: Planting the Seeds

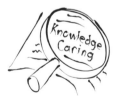

Our research program developed out of the desire of the nursing division to attain Magnet designation from American Nurses Credentialing Center (ANCC). Prior to completing a Magnet gap analysis in June 2002, the nursing division was very much aware that the most challenging task in the journey toward Magnet designation would be to show compliance with the research standard. We attained Magnet designation in November 2004. This article describes how we began from "scratch" to build a research infrastructure, and how over a 2-year period, we were able to obtain extraordinary outcomes and successes, some of which extend not only beyond the immediate work environment but internationally. Outcomes include:

- *the development of a formal research committee;*

- *the development and implementation of research roundtables as mechanisms to translate research into practice;*

- *the review, implementation and evaluation of several research proposals;*

- *the presentation of a symposium at an international research conference in Denmark in August 2004;*

- *the publication of an article entitled "Translating Fall Prevention Best Practices in the Hospital Setting: Reflecting on McInnes and Askie's (2004)*

658 •

Evidence Review" in the June, 2005, issue of Worldviews on Evidenced-Based Nursing; and

- *the presentation of both a symposium and a research study at the annual spring research conference of Sigma Theta Tau Delta Upsilon Chapter in April 2004.*

Nursing leadership identified several steps that needed to be completed in order to build an infrastructure and culture to support nursing research. The steps included:

Creating a Culture and Structure to Support Research

1. Contracting with a research consultant

The hospital's close affiliation with the School of Nursing at the University of Rhode Island was key to gaining access to credentialed nurse researchers. An experienced consultant was hired with a program of translation research spanning 20 years and who also had considerable experience in research development.

2. Gaining access to an Institutional Review Board (IRB)

Newport Hospital is part of the Lifespan Health Care System, which consists of four hospitals in Rhode Island. Active IRB support was available in two of the four hospitals. The vice president of nursing and patient care services at Newport Hospital gained membership of the IRB, at The Miriam Hospital, the 10th Hospital to achieve Magnet designation, and one of the two academic Lifespan hospitals.

3. Articulation of research as an integral component of nursing practice

Several initiatives were implemented to ensure that we all would be able to articulate and operationalize the philosophy and goals of our nursing research program.

Our research consultant met with all nursing directors, nursing professional development and the director of performance evaluation and improvement to assess individual degrees of readiness, goals and expectations related to research development. Meetings were held with unit-specific nursing professional practice councils. This provided opportunity for members of the nursing staff to discuss and identify nursing problems and specific practice issues that they deemed important and critical to review. We revised our nursing philosophy to emphasize our beliefs that empirical knowledge is essential to support nursing practice, change, and innovation and that we embrace evidence-based practice as integral to quality care. The care delivery principles, which operationalize the nursing process and therefore drive our professional practice model, were revised to incorporate the concepts of best practice and nursing research as fundamental to nursing and to quality care.

4. Creating a nursing research committee

Our research consultant paved the way and was highly instrumental in ensuring that we got off to the right start with regard to the development of a nursing research committee. The first meeting was held in 2002. Membership included four external nurse researchers from affiliating colleges, the vice president of nursing and patient care services, nursing directors, Staff Nurses representing each patient care unit, the director of performance evaluation and improvement, the coordinator of nursing professional development and the coordinator of staff and community education.

Bylaws, policies, procedures and guidelines were developed for reviewing research proposals. Our principal research mission was defined as providing the ongoing development and utilization of clinical and organizational outcomes with research as an integral component of nursing care. Functions of this committee include:

- *assisting in ensuring that standards of care, policies and procedures are evidence based and reflect best practice,*

- *fostering a climate of inquiry,*

- *providing nursing staff access to nursing research,*

- *disseminating research findings, and*

- *promoting clinical investigation among nurses.*

The committee meets monthly and the research consultant serves as chair.

5. Providing education to promote the development of research competencies

Formalized programs on nursing research were developed and implemented for the nursing staff as a means to develop competency in nursing research and a working knowledge of the research process. These programs were also incorporated into the graduate nurse internship program. Programs focused on the ethics of research, how to read and critique research, methodologies in evidenced-based practice, and the link of research to continual quality improvement. It was extremely important to emphasize this quality improvement link because many research proposals and roundtable agendas would be generated from quality and nursing data and results i.e., changes in a standard of care would be monitored in our database system.

Education programs have also served to foster positive attitudes among nursing administration and staff toward research and have been instrumental in developing competency in research skills. This is evident by the increased participation of nursing staff in roundtable discussion and in various research activities.

6. Providing opportunities for nurses who provide direct care to participate in research activities

Research roundtables were implemented and conducted on an ongoing basis as an approach to increase Staff Nurses' awareness of the relevancy of research to their day-to-day care giving activities. These roundtables are co-led by nursing staff and affiliating nursing students and facilitate a collaborative effort to increase knowledge of the research process and the translation and application of research to actual clinical problems. The roundtables are also an approach to help us measure our success with meeting our research mission and goals (see page 664).

7. Incorporating research expectations into each step of the clinical ladder

The final step in the development of the formal research program was incorporating research expectations into our clinical ladder advancement program. This program recog-

Programs focused on the ethics of research, how to read and critique research, methodologies in evidenced-based practice, and the link of research to continual quality improvement.

nizes and rewards the clinical excellence of Staff Nurses. Participation in research is necessary for a nurse to advance in the program. For example, one of the key behaviors that must be met for advancement is that he/she cites examples of how they have incorporated evidence-based practices to validate nursing policy, procedures and standards of care.

8. Extending beyond the work environment

Presentations on our research activities have been presented by nurses internally (Newport Hospital's Health Fair), externally at research conferences (such as local chapters of Sigma Theta Tau, March 10, 2004, and the Eastern Nursing Research Society Conference, April 1-3, 2004) and internationally (International Research Conference, Aahrus, Denmark, August 2004). One of the most significant outcomes of our research activities is the extent to which bedside nurses have participated in research dissemination and translation beyond the work environment. Staff Nurses have joined the ranks of nurses publishing works in renowned international research journals, including *Worldviews on Evidence-Based Practice and Nursing Research*.

Our research consultant provided the impetus for us to participate in an international research conference in Denmark, where members of the research committee presented a symposium entitled "Using a Collaborative Research Utilization Model to Translate Best Nursing Practices." The major theme of this presentation was planting, growing and sustaining the seeds of research. Presenters of this program included our research consultant, the vice president of nursing and patient care services, the director of surgical nursing, and most significantly, a Staff Nurse. They discussed the model's application to Newport Hospital's quest for research-based practice and practice-based research. Major themes included the importance of a culture that merges research and continuous quality improvement, the role of nursing management as mentors in the research utilization process for nursing staff, and outcomes in the nursing staff such as increased competency in research utilization with more positive attitudes towards research, becoming integral members of the nursing research team, enhanced professional image, and increased

> One of the most significant outcomes of our research activities is the extent to which bedside nurses have participated in research dissemination and translation beyond the work environment.

motivation to provide evidence-based, highest quality of care to patients. This conference has been recently published in the journal *Nursing Research* (Tracey, Dufault, Kogut, Martin, Rossi, & Willey-Temkin, 2006).

Conclusion

We are enjoying the fruits of our labors and are committed to ensuring that our research garden continues to flourish. As previously stated and supported by the research literature, benefits to nursing resulting from the development and implementation of our research infrastructure include the following: 1) increased competency in research utilization, 2) more positive attitudes towards research, 3) the opportunity to become integral members of the nursing research team, 4) enhanced professional image, and 5) increased motivation and ability to use innovations of evidence-based research to provide the highest quality of care to patients. Each year we would like to see continued growth that provides evidence that we are meeting our research mission.

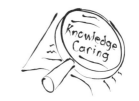

Reference: Tracey, S., Dufault, M., Kogut, S., Martin, V., Rossi, S., & Willey-Temkin, C. (2006). Translating best practices in nondrug postoperative pain management. *Nursing Research* 55(Suppl 2), 57-67.

The Research Roundtable: A Strategy to Build Ongoing Nursing Staff Competency in Translating Research into Practice

—Marlene Dufault and Dorothy Anne Garman

The implementation of research roundtables has been instrumental in providing a means to increase staff and student nurse awareness of the relevancy of research to everyday clinical practice. The roundtables have also facilitated collaboration and dialogue between nursing staff and affiliating nursing students by jointly participating in research activities that focus on clinical problems identified in the practice setting. Topics for the research roundtable are generated from different resources such as the Nursing and Patient Care Performance and Evaluation Committee (nursing quality committee), nursing professional practice councils, and nursing policy and procedure committee.

Once a topic has been identified, literature searches are conducted in cooperation with the affiliating nursing faculty, students and health reference librarians and forwarded to all roundtable participants. Discussion guidelines are used to help Staff Nurses and students arrive at a decision regarding the usefulness and readiness of a study for translation into a "best practice" standard of care, policy or protocol. In the roundtables, students present two or three studies relevant to the topic for translation into a standard of care. Students also lead the discussion about the study's methodology. The role of the Staff Nurse is to examine the studies for feasibility and applicability for practice changes on his or her unit.

For example, some members of the nursing staff on a surgical unit were puzzled as to how to put in practice the "foot paddling" exercises as required in the nursing policy related to postoperative care in the prevention of deep vein thrombosis (DVT). Staff noted that the policy lacked instructions as to how to perform this intervention and that this intervention lacked supporting empirical evidence to reflect its efficacy and best practice. The DVT roundtable emerged from this confusion and inconsistency among the nursing staff. The unit's professional practice committee requested a roundtable to review DVT-related empirical research. Two of the studies showed relevance to the present foot paddling exercises to prevent DVT. Participants discussed the study's findings on the effect of ankle exercises and the corresponding increase in venous flow.

As a result of the roundtable discussion, members from this professional practice committee revised the standard of care for DVT prevention based on the empirical evidence presented in the roundtable discussion. The standard includes that the patient will perform 12 repetitions of ankle exercises every one hour while awake until the patient returns to a pre-admission level of activity. The findings were presented to the Nursing Quality Committee where the recommendation to adopt the new standard of care was approved. In addition, nursing staff members developed a patient education video on post-operative care that provides information for patients on how to perform the technique of ankle exercises.

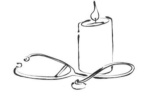

A roundtable on the "Efficacy of Texted Messages in Changing Nursing Practice" had its roots in a nursing and patient care leadership council meeting in which data were shared reflecting a problem related to the documentation of patient teaching. The roundtable discussion focused on three studies supporting the use of texted messages as an effective way to cue nurses to action. As a result, a texted message which read "What have you taught your patient today?" was integrated into the computer screen savers on the computerized documentation system. The effects of this intervention have been most positive and the data reflect much improvement in this area.

"What have you taught your patient today?"

As a result of a roundtable on falls prevention strategies from the perspective of the patient, an article for *Worldviews on Evidence-Based Nursing* was published in June 2005.

Authors include the coordinator of nursing professional development, the director of performance evaluation and improvement, the director of nursing clinical systems and two Staff Nurses from the Vanderbilt Rehabilitation Center. Objectives for the roundtable participants were to:

- *determine the strength, usefulness and feasibility of findings evaluated in the evidence,*

- *review the summary titled "Evidence Review on Older People's Views and Experiences of Falls Prevention Strategies" published in Worldviews on Evidence-Based Nursing in 2004,*

- *examine current policies and practices on a subacute and acute hospital unit in view of the strength of this evidence,*

- *suggest strategies for translating these findings into practice, and*

- *identify implications for research.*

Nursing staff members found the summary particularly valuable in comparing their current practices and standards of care to the most current research.

Through a roundtable discussion, the best practice for the use of music, massage and guided imagery as comfort enhancements resulted in the director of the volunteer department initiating a comfort care team in which volunteers provide proven alternative therapies to alleviate pain and enhance well-being with massage, music and guided imagery. Volunteers are trained to offer patients techniques that reduce stress and aid relaxation. This has been a highly successful source of satisfaction for patients.

We are presently testing a best protocol for shift handoffs, which was generated from a roundtable discussion. We will be testing on the variables of feasibility, usefulness and nurse-patient satisfaction.

Other priority topics coming up for roundtable research discussion for 2006 include:

- *Developing an evidence-based procedure for maintenance of central venous catheters, and*

- *Assessing the efficacy and technique for capillary refill, developing evidence-based guidelines.*

> Through a roundtable discussion, the best practice for the use of music, massage and guided imagery as comfort enhancements resulted in the director of the volunteer department initiating a comfort care team in which volunteers provide proven alternative therapies.

Conclusion

In conclusion, the implementation of research roundtables continues to confirm that this is an excellent approach to preserve a culture of research by fostering a climate of inquiry, ensuring that standards of care policies and procedures and protocols are evidence based and reflect best practice, providing clinicians access to nursing research and promoting clinical investigation among nurses.

Reference: Hollander Feldman, P., & McDonald, M. (2004). Conducting translation research in the home care setting: Lessons learned from a just-in-time reminder study. *Worldviews on Evidence-Based Nursing*, 1(1), 49-59.

Focused Evidence as Inspiration

—Jayne A. Felgen

In order to understand what it means to use "evidence as inspiration" you must first understand I_2E_2 (see page 25), the formula for leading sustainable change.

When an organization finds itself ready to commit to a whole new way of being, I_2E_2 provides a formula to ensure that all planning and implementation activities for that change are both comprehensive and inclusive. I_2E_2 takes its name from the first letters of the four elements of sustainable change:

Inspiration (I_1)

Infrastructure (I_2)

Education (E_1)

Evidence (E_2)

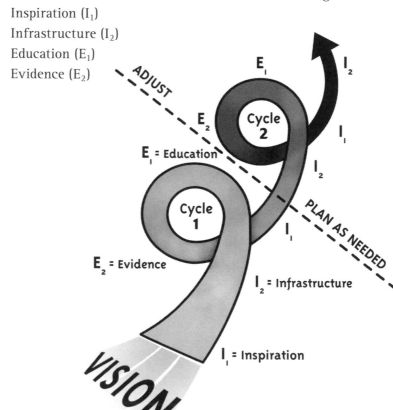

It's important to note, however, that the formula for change that these elements comprise is not linear. The I_2E_2 formula for change is cyclical, and therefore continual.

As you can see, the I_2E_2 model cycles continually so that once change has begun, after every cycle of refinement to the Inspiration, Infrastructure, Education and Evidence pertaining to the change, a new cycle begins again with Inspiration. In practice, the simplest, most effective place to go for more Inspiration is right to the Evidence of our success.

When we use I_2E_2 in the implementation of Relationship-Based Care (RBC), the Evidence we seek to collect is that which will show us most directly the degree to which RBC is up and running in the organization. For this reason, the decision about what Evidence to collect is based largely on the intentions we set in our RBC vision statement. If we said we intend to create it, we commit to collecting Evidence of our progress toward it.

In organizations implementing RBC, units develop and display posters that reflect the impact of their changes on patient satisfaction and safety.

If we say, for example, that we intend for each patient to be assigned a Primary Nurse within 12 hours of admission, we'll collect evidence as to the consistency with which patients are being assigned and a Primary Nurse accepts this responsibility within 12 hours of admission. And if when we collect that evidence, we see that we have moved to any degree at all toward our goal, we then have information that is easily used to inspire further forward movement in those who have already begun to succeed, as well as a real-life success story to inspire those on other units about to take on the same challenges.

In a health care organization undergoing integrated cultural change, Evidence helps us monitor the impact the new changes are making on our primary areas of concern—patient and family satisfaction and clinical quality. Furthermore, Evidence helps us to monitor the impact of related variables like staff retention scores, nurse and physician satisfaction scores, and other staffing-sensitive patient quality indicators—all of which ultimately affect patient loyalty, clinical quality and robust fiscal positioning. It is typical that most if not all of what we monitor will show measurable improvement, and every bit of that improvement can be used to further inspire everyone in the organization.

In organizations implementing RBC, units develop and display posters that reflect the impact of their changes on patient satisfaction and safety. With their visual impact, posters like the one below provide a clear and compelling picture of both intention and impact.

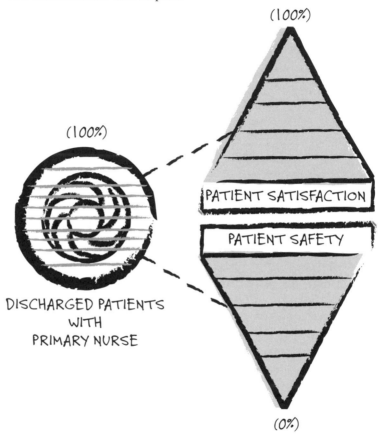

The assessment of Evidence is one of the most obvious opportunities we have to practice Appreciative Inquiry (see page 96). It is a core value of ours that we always build upon the strengths we find in an organization (rather than looking for what's "broken" in order to fix it), and using Evidence of the organization's own successes as Inspiration is one of the more overt ways we express this value. Using Evidence as Inspiration helps us to recognize and celebrate any and all forward movement in the most meaningful way possible.

CHAPTER TWENTY

Evidence From the Field: Critical Success Factors

Ten Critical Factors for the Successful Implementation of Relationship-Based Care

—Colleen Person

In more than 13 years of experience in bringing Relationship-Based Care (RBC) to health care organizations, I've been both an active participant and an invested witness. I've witnessed what works, and I have identified 10 factors that all but guarantee the successful implementation of Relationship-Based Care. The 10 critical factors for the successful implementation of RBC are listed below and explained in detail throughout this piece.

Success Factors:

- *Appreciative Inquiry becomes the standard way of thinking, working and interacting within the organization.*

- *Commitment and excitement for RBC are built at the executive level from the beginning.*

- *Relationship-Based Care is integrated into all of the organization's strategic, operational, tactical, and individual behaviors and actions.*

Editors' note: *Colleen Person and Jayne Felgen have worked side by side with hundreds of individuals implementing Relationship-Based Care in facilities across the country. Throughout these experiences, Colleen and Jayne each developed her own unique set of "critical factors" for successful implementation. Together they show the power of two different voices delivering a consistant message.*

- *Leaders exhibit constancy of purpose in implementing and sustaining RBC in the organization.*

- *Middle managers align with executive management in understanding the depth, breadth and tactical realities of Relationship-Based Care.*

- *Managers become leaders.*

- *Staff members are inspired to deliver professional and compassionate care.*

- *Unit Practice Councils are recognized as the essential component for real change in daily practice and are supported and empowered to own and change their practice to meet the RBC principles.*

- *Individuals in the organization own their personal responsibility, authority and accountability for living RBC in their daily work.*

- *Successes are acknowledged and celebrated.*

Success Factor One:
Appreciative Inquiry becomes the standard way of working and interacting within the organization.

Appreciative Inquiry (AI) invites us to discover our past and current strengths and successes so that we can build on them. (See page 96.) We have found that discovering and discussing successes increases our positive energy, and that the positive energy AI generates is highly contagious. Appreciative Inquiry creates a deep appreciation for our own strengths, which translates into the realization that we can replicate our past successes and build on them to meet the goals of Relationship-Based Care. An AI assessment of current practice, for example, can give us a touchstone in our quest for RBC, because it leads us to conclude, "I know I can practice RBC consistently because I've already been practicing it in the very best moments of my individual practice."

An AI assessment of current practice leads us to conclude, "I know I can practice RBC consistently because I've already been practicing it in the very best moments of my individual practice."

Success Factor Two:
Commitment and excitement for RBC are built at the executive level from the beginning.

Both the vision and strategy for Relationship-Based Care begin at the executive level. When the executive team is excited about its commitment to RBC and embraces it as a key organizational strategy for achieving the mission, vision and values of the organization, the likelihood of a highly successful transformation that proves sustainable over time is greatly enhanced.

This is how it usually works:

- *An "executive champion" (often the vice president of Patient Care) introduces RBC to the team.*

- *This champion links RBC with the mission, vision, values and business goals of the organization.*

- *The champion then articulates the hopes and possibilities for RBC in the future of the organization—including why it makes good business and quality sense.*

- *The executive team integrates RBC as the means to achieving desired outcomes such as service to the community, patient satisfaction, quality indicators, financial indicators, and staff and physician satisfaction.*

It is important for the executive champion to embody the possibility and hope of Relationship-Based Care and to engage the others at the executive level in creating a shared vision and strategy to support a structured implementation of RBC over time. A key to executive commitment is the understanding that RBC will positively impact the fiscal health of the organization—in essence, that RBC is a wise investment.

The *Relationship-Based Care Leader Practicum*—a workshop offered early in the process to members of the executive team, the executive champion (CNO), and RBC Project Leader—has been a successful forum for building shared knowledge, understanding, and commitment to Relationship-Based Care. As a result of attending the workshop, participants have consistently reported a greater ability to move RBC forward as they have greater clarity about what it will mean in their orga-

A key to executive commitment is the understanding that RBC is a wise investment.

nization and a common understanding of what RBC means to them individually and collectively. This translates into greater ease and confidence in leading the design, implementation and integration of Relationship-Based Care (see page 468).

Success Factor Three:

Relationship-Based Care is integrated into all of the organization's strategic, operational, tactical and individual behaviors and actions.

The third critical success factor is for:

- *Relationship-Based Care to become the umbrella under which the primary strategic initiatives of the organization fit, and*

- *Relationship-Based Care and Creative Health Care Management's I₂E₂ framework for transformation become the structure and change process that bring the mission, vision and values to life at all points of service.*

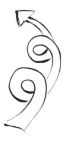

All of us have experience with initiatives and programs that are generated and "rolled out" at the executive level but don't actually have any measurable impact at the point of care delivery. We may hear our staff members refer to these as the "flavor of the month." Integrating RBC into all of the organization's strategic, operational, tactical and individual behaviors and/or actions means that it gets fully integrated into the organization's infrastructure. This means that policies, procedures, position descriptions, competency assessments, hiring practices and educational offerings are assessed and adapted to assure that they are congruent with RBC principles. It means that individuals identify specific changes in their practice and ways of relating to patients and families that move them from task-based to Relationship-Based Care. When RBC is implemented systematically and thoughtfully, it brings the desired vision into alignment with day-to-day care, service and relationships. I see RBC as a methodology to promote integration and alignment between the strategic mission of the organization and daily practice.

Success Factor Four:
Leaders exhibit constancy of purpose in implementing and sustaining RBC in the organization.

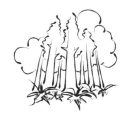

When the decision is made to implement Relationship-Based Care, a commitment is made to transform the organization's culture. But since such deep transformation takes hold in phases over a period of many months, there are instances in which crises and other issues will interrupt the executive team's focus on Relationship-Based Care. It could be a fiscal crisis, or issues with electronic medical records, or something going on with the physician group, or a Joint Commission review. Granted, these are all things that the executive level and middle managers need to attend to, but it is important that they not significantly disrupt the continuous development of Relationship-Based Care. Executive level leaders must be attentive to what modifications need to be made in order to address issues not directly related to RBC so that while something may briefly interrupt the implementation of one phase or another, *nothing* interrupts the overall flow of RBC implementation for long. When RBC is brought to a complete halt (it has happened), managers and staff members become disheartened and cynically conclude that the commitment to doing business differently was simply a passing phase. When this happens, it is very difficult to regroup and reinspire energy and to refocus on the vision.

Part of what helps leaders stay on course is recognizing that RBC puts an infrastructure in place that actually helps us move out of cycles of continuous crises. In an RBC culture, the question becomes "How can RBC principles guide how we move through this crisis and what will it take to fortify us for next time?" Relationship-Based Care becomes the framework through which the organization addresses crises, not because the organization has committed itself to RBC, but because looking at a crisis with RBC as the lens guides us to devise excellent, inventive solutions with patients and their families front-of-mind.

Success Factor Five:

Middle managers align with executive management in understanding the depth, breadth and tactical realities of Relationship-Based Care.

The biggest challenge I see for middle managers in implementing RBC is to understand, right along with those at the executive level, how RBC isn't "just another initiative." In organizations where RBC takes a firm hold, middle managers are helped to see how it makes a positive, measurable difference in the experience of patients and their families, as well as for care givers themselves. It is critical that managers see RBC as a practical source of hope in the midst of all of the challenges they are dealing with.

I've seen RBC implementations really take hold when middle managers begin to form their own visions about how RBC can help them in developing staff in providing exceptional care and service on a day-to-day basis. Once they understand how RBC provides a clearer and more systematic way to manage their clinical units, they will do everything in their power to make RBC operational wherever they have influence.

Success Factor Six:

Managers become leaders.

Because of the empowerment that is part of RBC, all individuals in the organization are called to lead, so it's essential that managers are equipped to model and teach effective leadership qualities and practices. Every conversation a manager has becomes a conversation in which RBC can be either actively practiced (and therefore more solidly embedded into the organization's culture) or ignored.

Managers need to feel cared for in the organization in order to care for staff.

The leadership that makes the biggest difference is not in what managers do, but in what managers adopt as a *way of being.* Managers do the most good by modeling the attitudes and behaviors they want from others. If managers slip into a task-based approach for their work and are so involved in daily operations, problem solving, decision making, and putting out fires themselves, it is very difficult for them to see the bigger picture and to lead staff in an inspirational, facilitative way. Furthermore, managers need to feel cared for in the organization in order to care for staff.

A key dimension of an RBC organization's infrastructure is a shift to decentralization and empowerment—particularly for RNs at the point of care. For this reason, the changes in expectations for clinical managers are significant, and whether or not they are able to make that shift determines the success of implementation. They have to make a shift to the work of empowering the staff, which in practical terms means:

- *articulating expectations,*

- *helping their team understand the full scope of each individual's responsibility, accountability and authority,*

- *teaching and modeling both the fundamentals and nuances of healthy interpersonal relationships, and*

- *continuously focusing on developing people.*

Leadership for RBC requires that managers' practice be aligned with the principles. They must hold the RBC vision as their own, see themselves as front-line developers of staff, and—like leaders at the executive level—see to it that no crisis has the power to derail their commitment to the goals of Relationship-Based Care.

Success Factor Seven:
Staff are inspired to deliver professional and compassionate care.

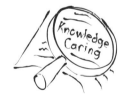

Inspiration, both individually and collectively, is a critical success factor for those at the staff level. It's important to acknowledge, right from the start, that in many organizations, staff members need inspiration on a continuous basis. In the organizations in which we've seen the most successful transformations, there is a methodology in place to inspire and reconnect staff with their core values, initially through an inspirational workshop focused on professional practice and caring and on an ongoing basis through leadership support for professional practice and caring for patients and families. To this end, the *Reigniting the Spirit of Caring* (*RSC*) workshops have been a key intervention in many organizations. *Reigniting the Spirit of Caring* helps individuals feel reconnected and reinspired. It helps people get out of some of the pain they've been in with the whitewater and chaos of health care and to really celebrate the caring aspect of what they do.

It brings participants back to the most basic human aspects of health care—seeing others as people and being seen as people themselves. Furthermore, the renewed commitment and energy engages staff in proactively and creatively addressing process issues and solving problems.

It has delighted me to facilitate the *Reigniting the Spirit of Caring* workshops where leaders and staff from all disciplines and departments from the Board of Directors to housekeeping have participated. It's wonderful to see all the new energy around the importance of their relationships with patients and families (whether it be direct or indirect) and the recognition that they share a common purpose and mission regardless of the specific work they do.

Success Factor Eight:
Unit Practice Councils are recognized as the essential component for real change in daily practice and are supported and empowered to own and change their practice to meet the RBC principles.

The most successful RBC implementations I've seen have been those in which Unit Practice Councils (UPCs) are resourced, supported and empowered to truly design, implement and own the practice changes on their units. Unit Practice Councils lead the design and implementation of RBC for their unit. Through their planning and implementation, they turn vision and principles into behavior and action. The members of these councils have been selected by their peers to lead the change and are diligent about communicating with their colleagues and assuring that they have integrated the input of their colleagues into the unit design.

It's important to acknowledge, right from the start, that in many organizations, staff members need inspiration on a continuous basis.

The most successful Unit Practice Councils are those that have an experienced facilitator who participates in their meetings and helps them stay on course. This facilitator may be someone from human resources or a clinical specialist or other individual who has had education and experience in the art of facilitation. This facilitator coaches the council members on effective communication, consensus decision making, how to manage meetings, and other council functions. The clinical manager serves as a sponsor to the council. This manager opens pathways and provides guidance for getting new processes implemented. The UPC itself needs to develop a vision that is in alignment with the executive and middle management vision and then focus on achieving it on the unit level.

We have found also that UPCs always need help with communication—particularly what I call "effective dialogue." We tend to think we are good communicators because we talk all the time! However, when we learn to listen to each other, amazing things can happen. This is an important point of awareness and may require "unlearning" the way we have traditionally communicated. We all have to understand that we don't always listen; we don't always listen to patients, and we don't always listen to each other. Our challenge is to listen in order to hear.

One of the expectations for Unit Practice Council members is that each one is assigned a group of staff with whom they are expected to have two-way communication. This is one of the biggest success factors within the council infrastructure. When members know how to communicate effectively—not just send out a questionnaire and consider communication "accomplished"—the system can work exceptionally well. If they don't have a two-way conversation with folks—"What's important to you about this work? What are your ideas related to the principles? What suggestions do you have?"—things break down pretty quickly. Effective UPC members will take the answers to questions like these back to the Unit Practice Council so that they have everybody's suggestions and then create the best plan for that unit using everyone's input. It's not just about polite conversations and giving everybody a chance to feel like they've been heard; it's about co-creating.

When UPCs are carefully formed and fully supported, we find that they can change mindsets. UPCs are key in influencing their staff colleagues to own their own work and to make decisions about the ways they will accomplish it. Empowered, inspired staff members become decision makers and reactive problem solvers.

Success Factor Nine:
Individuals in the organization own their personal responsibility, accountability and authority for living RBC in their daily work.

This success factor goes beyond individuals merely knowing their jobs and doing them efficiently. The really critical success factor here is the ownership of practice by each individual. Since true transformation to RBC happens one relationship at a time, it's essential for each individual to internalize what that means to his or her own practice or work responsibilities.

In successful transformations, individuals ask themselves:

- *What am I being called to do?*

- *What am I being called to transform?*

- *In what ways can I make RBC live in my practice or on my unit, or my work area?*

- *In what ways can I "live" RBC in my relationships with patients and their families?*

- *In what ways can I "live" RBC in my relationships with my colleagues?*

Practitioners at all levels get very inspired when we get into Jean Watson's and Kristen Swanson's work on the caring and healing relationship. However, though deep integration of RBC at the individual level can be taught, encouraged and coached, unless it is also modeled by those in leadership positions, it will not take hold in the organization. When leaders "model the way," there's no end to how deeply the RBC principles can become embodied in the work of individuals.

Success Factor Ten:

Successes are acknowledged and celebrated

Celebrating Caring Relationships is another workshop to help leaders and staff get reconnected with their values. It is a way to come together with positive energy and possibility. Celebrating successes includes everything from formal gatherings with public acknowledgement of progress, to inspirational seminars, to recognition programs in which individuals or teams are formally recognized for extraordinary care and service, to less formal celebration and appreciation on a daily basis. This less formal culture of celebration and appreciation is one in which thank-yous are extended for a job well done, people are supported when they navigate complex situations, kindnesses are acknowledged and returned, and people are conscious of the privilege and power of caring.

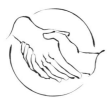

Celebrating successes includes everything from formal gatherings with public acknowledgement of progress to less formal celebration and appreciation on a daily basis

Critical Success Factors for Implementing, Evolving and Sustaining Relationship-Based Care

—Jayne A. Felgen

Every implementation of Relationship-Based Care (RBC) is different because every organization is unique. While each implementation is therefore customized to harness the unique strengths found in each individual organization, those facilitating the implementation must be aware of a number of factors that we know to be critical to the success of Relationship-Based Care. In more than ten years of bringing RBC to health care organizations, the critical success factors for implementing, evolving and sustaining RBC that I have identified are as follows:

- *The Chief Nurse Officer in each organization has a deep understanding of Relationship-Based Care and is willing to be its "champion," when called upon, throughout the organization.*

- *The vision for RBC in the organization is so widely inclusive that it touches the practice of everyone in the organization—from those at the bedside, all the way to those who have no one-to-one patient contact at all.*

- *There is unwavering and widely articulated buy-in from the executive team.*

- *The oversight team or Results Council has Level 3 authority and a shared leadership model—meaning there are four leaders of the project, not one.*

Editors' note: *Jayne Felgen has served as the client manager for a large number of organizations implementing Relationship-Based Care across all disciplines and departments. This piece is the result of an interview with Jayne to tap into her wisdom and experience on what has made organizations successful in implementing and integrating Relationship-Based Care.*

- *A subgroup of the Results Council called the "Integration" functional group (generally consisting of the CNO and VP of Human Resources) integrates the output of all Results Council functional groups and Unit Practice Council (UPC) innovations into the fabric of the organization.*

- *There is visible leadership and buy-in across the multidisciplinary executive teams—particularly from the allied health or service support departments.*

- *Trustees and medical staff are involved from the outset and over time.*

- *Education is offered in which team immersion helps individuals to rediscover a collective shared purpose in their work.*

- *The workshop Leading an Empowered Organization (LEO) is presented to line leaders, project managers and the executive team.*

- *Baseline documentation of the organization's current status using a report card format is collected so that it can be used to support and build the mechanisms to capture and disseminate reports of periodic progress over time.*

While there is no one way to implement RBC, the combination of strong internal leadership and experienced consultants has proven especially effective.

Another item that bears mentioning—a sort of overarching critical success factor—is one that is hard to articulate without sounding self-serving. We have found that the organizations that have experienced the most successful implementations are those that have had a combination of strong leadership from within and a solid functional partnership with Creative Health Care Management (CHCM). Because of our experience we are able to save organizations time and help them maximize their productivity from the earliest stages of implementation. While there is no one way to implement RBC, the combination of strong internal leadership and experienced consultants has proven especially effective.

As an organization's vision of RBC is implemented using I_2E_2 as the formula for sustainable change (see page 25), I have used the elements of Inspiration (I_1), Infrastructure (I_2), Education (E_1) and Evidence (E_2) to create a practical framework through which each critical success factor can be understood.

Inspiration is not a luxury in this work.

I have found that in order to make any implementation of RBC complete and sustainable, it is essential to kindle a deep inspiration in everyone involved. Since RBC is brought into an organization by someone at the executive level, that's where inspiration starts. While inspiring others is some of the most important work I do in implementing RBC, it's also the easiest. Relationship-Based Care reminds all of us in health care why we came to this work in the first place. "Selling" the idea that patients and families should come first is never necessary. Inspiring individuals to the idea that it is both possible and pleasurable to improve the relationship between every care giver in the organization and our patients and their families takes little effort and meets no resistance.

The fire of inspiration that circles RBC must be kindled and fanned in the Chief Nursing Officer, the entire executive team, and throughout the entire staff—from those at the point of care to those who have no direct patient contact. I am addressing the first two of these success factors together as they are intrinsically related.

Inspiration is not a luxury in this work.

Success Factor One:
Each organization has a Chief Nurse Officer who has a deep understanding of Relationship-Based Care and is willing to be its "champion" when called upon, throughout the organization.

Success Factor Two:
The vision for RBC in the organization is so widely inclusive that it touches the practice of everyone in the organization—from those at the bedside, all the way to those who have no one-to-one patient contact at all.

First there is a champion (usually the CNO) who is the one who really understands that RBC is not just good for business—Relationship-Based Care is the business. He or she is willing to persevere and work out the details and innovations as RBC moves into the organization.

A CNO who has experience with or knowledge of RBC will contact us because he or she knows that his or her role is to support nurses to provide the best possible care. The CNO who champions RBC has both passion and purpose, is emotionally and intellectually resilient and consistently demonstrates a working knowledge of what we call "the 5 Cs."

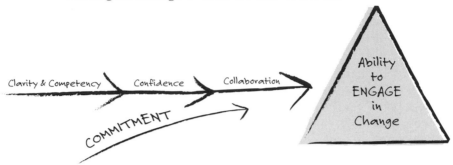

Those organizations that are successful are those in which at least the CNO, and perhaps others, have clarity about who they are and a sense of purpose and meaning that their leadership role makes a difference. They're also clear that everyone has a gift to bring in the patient care arena, and nurses have a unique gift that needs to be lifted up and made more visible. They have clarity that there is only one care delivery model that supports Professional Nursing Practice and that is Primary Nursing. Relationship-Based Care is broad enough to encompass Primary Nursing and a role for other professionals and service support staff to play as well.

In skillful RBC implementations, the leader (the champion) of this transformation is one who is very savvy in the executive role. He or she is profoundly competent—having the tools, the financial know-how, the operational skills, the interpersonal tools, the visionary leadership and the technical skills to make such a deeply integrated cultural change possible. When clarity meets competence, it inspires the confidence of all those who experience it and further inspires them to collaborate in order to create the kind of environment that everyone in the organization wants. The whole model is underscored by the 5th C: commitment. It is easy to see how when clarity and competency meet confidence and inspires both confidence and collaboration, everyone involved would feel very committed to the outcome along with whatever process will bring that outcome to life.

They have clarity that there is only one care delivery model that supports Professional Nursing Practice and that is Primary Nursing. Relationship-Based Care is broad enough to encompass Primary Nursing and a role for other professionals and service support staff to play as well.

Success Factor Three:
There is unwavering and widely articulated buy-in from the executive team.

The buy-in from the executive team is clearly also a factor in the entire organization's ability to stay inspired throughout implementation. It is the CEO who holds others accountable, so the support from the top leader becomes visible and tangible as he or she coaches others. Each member of the executive team must buy into the notion that RBC will really help them to reach their organizational (and personal) vision for excellent patient and family care. And then each member must embody that vision every day. In every bit of communication (even in one-to-one conversations) members of the executive team will either embody or undermine the organization's implementation of Relationship-Based Care. There is no middle ground.

When executive buy-in is strong (and in our experience, it always is), embodiment of RBC becomes natural for the executive team. Once they have reconnected with the reason they went into health care in the first place—to create the best experience possible for patients and their families—they are inspired to embody whatever it is that will bring that about. And when they understand the full scope of what RBC offers, they become willing to do whatever it takes to sustain their own inspiration and that of those around them over the long haul.

There is, of course, an intangible element in this part of the work—the work that keeps the not-at-all-literal flame of inspiration burning. But there's also a very tangible role that this inspired executive team ends up playing. An executive expresses support and provides inspiration for the rest of the organization in part by holding others accountable to the implementation plan and to the integration and application of innovations within the organization. When others in the organization see that this is being done, they know on an even deeper level that they can trust that what's going on in the organization is important.

An executive expresses support and provides inspiration for the rest of the organization in part by holding others accountable to the implementation plan and to the integration and application of innovations within the organization.

Infrastructure (I_2)

An organization's infrastructure comprises its physical structure along with every process, practice, procedure and behavior found in it. In order to bring about a fully integrated cultural change, every process, practice, procedure and behavior that happens in the organization must be configured to support that change. In all successful implementations of RBC, certain well-chosen individuals must be given the authority to refine all aspects of the organization's infrastructure.

Success Factor Four:
The oversight team or Results Council has Level 3 authority and a shared leadership model—meaning there are four leaders of the project, not one.

Level 3 authority and a shared leadership model are essential aspects of the Results Council. Level 3 authority is the right to take action after gathering and evaluating the information required for reaching sound decisions, and involving key stakeholders in the decision-making process in order to discern implications (impact) and gain their investment and support.

It is also very important that this oversight team understands the gravity of its work. I have had several CEOs who have conveyed to their entire leadership team that embracing RBC implementation would provide the single most significant impact they would make in their professional careers. These CEOs "got it." They knew to convey to those empowered to implement RBC in the organization that if they could get this right, it would be their single most significant contribution to health care and the highlight of their careers.

The members of the Results Council and the executive team must be clear that the Results Council is not just an ad hoc group. The fact that they have Level 3 authority is made abundantly clear to them as is the fact that they will become the experts on the part of the organization as far as RBC principles and practice are concerned. They will make the crucial recommendations that will allow the implementation to succeed.

Within the Results Council and throughout the organization there is a clearly understood shared leadership model that allows for each of the functional subgroups of the Results Council to have teams of two or more leaders. Each of these functional subgroups has outcomes and expectations that are critical to the overall success of the implementation, so sharing the load is very important. In every implementation I

It is very important that this oversight team understands the gravity of its work.

facilitate, there are at minimum a project leader, co-leaders of the Results Council and one executive sponsor. The executive champion CNO must be on the Results Council, as must an HR executive and a chief medical officer or another representative of the medical staff.

Inexorably linked with this success factor is the importance of selecting the RBC Project Leader. We believe this person needs to be someone who is highly regarded for having values consistent with Relationship-Based Care. It also is a plus if the person is in a position of authority and/or is given Level 3 authority (see page 486) that others will honor. It's beneficial for this person to already be in an operational role so that his or her leadership for RBC is consistent with his or her typical role responsibilities, making it very apparent that this is not an ad hoc position. Some of our best Project Leaders have come from the director level. Often the lead for organizational development is thought of highly in the organization and frequently reports directly to the CEO and is therefore also a good choice.

At McKee Medical Center in Loveland, Colorado, the Rehab Director and an Oncology Clinical Nurse Specialist are Project Leaders. The Results Council leaders are a Respiratory Therapy director and a nurse administrator, while executive sponsors are the associate administrator responsible for Operations and the CNO.

It also helps, of course, if the person selected as project leader is organized and an excellent leader. In summary the following are essential qualities for the project leader:

- *Highly regarded in the organization with recognized values consistent with RBC,*

- *Already in a position of authority,*

- *Enjoys a reputation as an effective leader, coordinator, facilitator, and*

- *Someone with a proven ability to make things happen.*

Success Factor Five:
A subgroup of the Results Council called the "Integration" functional group (generally consisting of the CNO and VP of

Even if the RBC implementation begins with nursing at first, other allied health and service departments must be invited in to support the patient care delivery model.

Human Resources) integrates the output of all Results Council functional groups and Unit Practice Council innovations into the fabric of the organization.

Integrating the output of all Results Council functional groups and UPCs into the fabric of the organization is the unique role of the functional group called the "Integration" group. This group ensures that innovations become embedded into standards, policies, procedures and roles and are linked to the mission and vision.

Success Factor Six:
There is visible leadership and buy-in across the multidisciplinary executive teams—particularly from the allied health or service support departments.

While the initial implementation may involve only nursing, I believe there must be a multidisciplinary involvement across the executive team. Even if the RBC implementation begins with nursing at first, other allied health and service departments must be invited in to support the patient care delivery model. It is up to the organization needs to determine their own timing for bringing these allied health and service departments into alignment with RBC, but it is essential that they do.

Success Factor Seven:
Trustees and medical staff are involved from the outset and over time.

It is important, of course, to get RBC integrated into every facet of the organization's infrastructure, so the board of trustees and medical staff must be explicitly included. Engaging board members and the medical staff helps integrate into the day-to-day workings of the organization the notion that RBC is the way to achieve and express its existing mission, vision and values. Relationship-Based Care is the ultimate business case.

Education (E_1)

The implementation of RBC challenges everyone in the organization to think, relate and practice in new and more fulfilling ways. While there are practical changes to make, the individuals involved in the change also have internal changes to make in order to embody the principles and practices of Relationship-Based Care.

I believe that all of us in health care are here for the same fundamental reason—to make a positive difference for patients and their families. That's why the educational offerings that have become critical success factors in successful RBC implementations are those that put individuals at literally every level in the organization back in touch with their core purpose for going into health care in the first place.

Success Factor Eight:
Education is offered in which team immersion helps individuals to rediscover a collective shared purpose in their work.

The *Relationship-Based Care Leader Practicum* or another alternative where a team immersion happens in which there is a collective shared purpose discovered must be offered at minimum to every member of the Results Council and at best, to anyone who has a major leadership role like directors or managers on the units involved in each wave of implementation. (See *RBC Practicum*, page 468.)

I've seen time and again that team immersion is key. Having a group of directors attend the practicum together, for example, helps them get off the "gerbil wheel" long enough for them to come together and become clearer about how to lead Relationship-Based Care. Then when they return to the hectic pace, they know how they can find support among themselves to stay the course and not get caught up in dysfunctional dynamics that prevent them from reaching their vision.

Success Factor Nine:
The workshop Leading an Empowered Organization (LEO) is presented to line leaders, project managers and the executive team.

Leading an Empowered Organization (*LEO*) is an essential offering for leaders in an organization that wishes to experience any real measure of empowered decision-making from individuals at any level in it.

The *LEO* workshop's greatest contributions are these:

- *it provides a common sharing of language and concepts, and*

I believe that all of us in health care are here for the same fundamental reason—to make a positive difference for patients and their families.

Having a group of directors attend the practicum together, for example, helps them get off the "gerbil wheel" long enough for them to come together and become clearer about how to lead Relationship-Based Care.

- *it provides an opportunity for individuals to learn together the real skills required to create a trusting and decentralized environment where the staff will actively engage in change.*

It is ideal for leaders to participate in *LEO* before any RBC implementation work is done with the staff (see page 483).

Evidence (E$_2$)

In order for us to know when we have achieved our vision for change, it is essential for us to be clear about where we are beginning and where we want to end up so that we can find meaningful evidence of our progress.

Success Factor Ten:

Baseline documentation of the organization's current status using a report card format is collected. This baseline documentation can then be used to support and build the mechanisms to capture and disseminate reports of periodic progress over time.

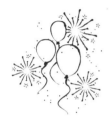

It is critical that we assist our clients in capturing and reporting where they are now, including the nurse-sensitive indicators and other indicators from the literature that we know are directly related to patient care delivery. It's also critical that it be assembled in an easy to read and use report card format. The outcomes functional group of the Results Council needs to understand that its role and responsibility are to help support the UPC in building mechanisms to capture and disseminate meaningful evidence of periodic progress over time. It means they measure what matters, and that can only be measured accurately if thorough, accurate baseline measurements are taken before implementation.

Some of the most important work I've been privileged to do is this work of bringing Relationship-Based Care to organizations throughout the world. I have seen organizations that appeared to be in deep pain find within their walls individuals who were able to step up magnificently in order to implement Relationship-Based Care. When the way is clear and success is well planned for, many who might otherwise hesitate find the courage to move confidently toward what matters most to them.

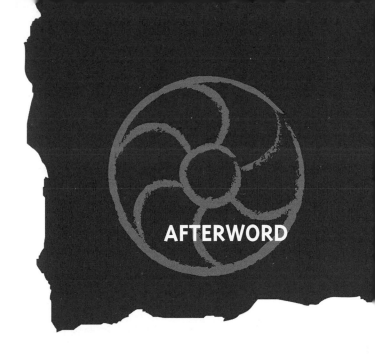

AFTERWORD

Dear Readers,

We appreciate each of you for your commitment to Relationship-Based Care and your interest in our Field Guide. Your leadership and work in the field is what makes Relationship-Based Care come to life. Through your leadership there is hope that health care will deepen and expand to become a field that is universally known as compassionate and humane. Health care will be recognized as the milieu in which technology and caring and healing are integrated and complimentary. Through your leadership individuals will thrive, teams will excel and patients and families will experience the power of human connection. Patients and families will know that they are "seen as people" and are central to our activities and interactions on their behalf. They will know that they are safe in our care—emotionally, physically and spiritually.

We have been profoundly affected by the response to our book, *Relationship-Based Care: A Model for Transforming Practice.* By putting our years of personalized consulting into a conceptual framework and publishing it, many more of you have learned about Relationship-Based Care and are moving into action! You have told us that it represents a fundamental truth about care and service and that there is a hunger and yearning for "getting back to the basics" of what our work is all about. Additionally, you have told us that leading and achieving these "basics" in our complex health care environment can be daunting and lonely.

As we come together to bring Relationship-Based Care to life, we experience the power and inspiration that results in collective wisdom and energy. Our shared vision becomes achievable, and the isolation and loneliness that comes from simply trying to survive in a system that seems too immense and depersonalized to change fades away. Relationship-Based Care is personal! We have the "power of one", we have the "power of many" and we can make Relationship-Based Care a way of life—a way of doing business.

Our mission is to help you succeed in your vision for Relationship-Based Care. We hope you will let us know how we can partner with you and support you in achieving your vision of care and service. We have clients who have invited us to enter into a full consulting partnership. In this situation, we provide consultation through each phase of design and implementation and provide a full range of educational and support services. We have clients who have established a more intermittent (prn) relationship with us and access our services and educational programs to support them at specific junctures in their implementation. We also have clients who have read the book, attended our *Relationship-Based Care Leader Practicum*, accessed resources through our company to support their design and implementation and are working quite independently. Whatever your situation, we are here to partner with you and provide consultation, coaching, and education so that your goals and outcomes are successfully achieved.

We want to express our sincere thanks to each of our contributing authors for sharing their insights, tools, and experiences. You have brought Relationship-Based Care to life in your writing and sharing with others in the field. Our vision is to keep the fire burning. To do so, we would love to publish an update to this field guide in a couple of years. We know that you are doing incredible work and we invite you to share it with us. Our next updated edition will be organized in the same five part sections: Vision, Inspiration, Infrastructure, Education and Evidence. If you have examples and insights to share in these areas, please contact us. We would also love to share specific stories about how you have "Sustained the Gains" of Relationship-Based Care. Because you are reading this, we know you understand that Relationship-Based Care is NOT another "flavor of the month." It is a commitment to leading and caring that must be nurtured and sustained over time. We hope to hear from you and include you as a contributing author in our next edition.

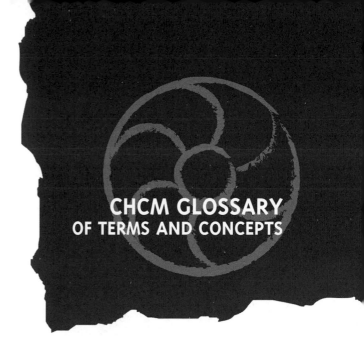

CHCM GLOSSARY
OF TERMS AND CONCEPTS

Accountability: Ownership for the consequences of one's decision and actions. The retrospective review of the work done and decisions made to determine whether or not they were appropriate. This may take the form of reflective practice, peer review, quality improvement or performance feedback.

Articulated Expectations: The clear and consistent expression by leaders of expected behaviours in three crucial relationships: 1) staff reporting to them, 2) their peers and 3) their immediate supervisors. These expectations serve to inspire, guide and direct others. They shape the culture by setting boundaries for what is acceptable and not acceptable behaviour in the work area. Effective articulated expectations serve to promote growth and learning. (*Creative Health Care Management, 2007*)

Authority: The legitimate right to act and make decisions in areas where one is given and accepts responsibility. The level of authority delegated should be commensurate with the scope of responsibility.

The four levels of authority are as follows:
Level 1: Data/Information/Idea Gathering
Authority to collect information/data and *provide to another to make the final decision and determine what action will be taken.*
Level 2: Data/Information/Idea Gathering and Recommendations
Authority to collect information, weigh the options, and *recommend actions to be taken to another who will make the final decision.*

Level 3: Data/Information/Idea
Gathering and Recommendations;
Pause to Communicate, Clarify, or
Negotiate and then Take Action
Authority to apply critical think-
ing, weigh the options, recommend
actions, negotiate the final decision.
*Includes pausing and collaborating
with others before taking action.*
Level 4: Act and Inform Others After
Taking Action
Authority to assess, decide and act.
May follow up and inform another
of the actions taken as required by
the situation.

Accountability: Ownership for the consequences of
one's decision and actions. The retrospective
review of the work done and decisions made
to determine whether or not they were appropriate. This may take the form of reflective
practice, peer review, quality improvement or
performance feedback. (*Creative Health Care
Management*, 2007)

Building relationships: Successfully forming a
connection with others as an essential skill
for leaders in achieving the common goals
of the group. Building healthy relationships
requires trust, mutual respect, open and direct
communication and consistent visible support
(*Creative Health Care Management*, 2007).

Care Delivery System: A method of organizing
nursing, allied health, professional and service
support care to meet the needs of patients and
families. Includes a set of organizing principles
for nursing and allied health departments that
define how the work will be allocated and
how the staff will function. The organizing
principles cover decision making, work allocation, communication channels and management responsibilities. Of the four prototypical
systems, Primary Nursing, total patient care,
functional nursing and team nursing, only
Primary Nursing supports professional practice.
Variations of the four prototypes are abundant.

Care Giver: A person responsible for carrying out
work activities to meet the needs of patients and
families in conjunction with the plan of care.

Care Provider: An agency or person responsible for
rendering services.

Care Team: Two or more care givers from key disciplines who accept responsibility for planning,
providing and reviewing the plan of care for a
defined group of patients and their families.

Care Team Pairs: A care delivery unit including
an RN and one or two support staff who collectively own the responsibility, authority and
accountability for carrying out the plan of care
for a defined group of patients. They work at
the direction of the RN and organize their work
at the beginning of each work shift. The membership can vary daily.

Care Team Partners: A care delivery unit including
an RN and one or two support or ancillary staff
who voluntarily work with one another, consistently over time. The team partners have shared
responsibility, authority and accountability
for carrying out the plan of care for a defined
group of patients at the direction of the RN.
Members commit to managing their relationship and to professional and personal growth.

Caring and Healing Environment: A therapeutic
milieu in which the primary purpose is to provide humane and compassionate patient care.
Practitioners attend to the whole person (body,
mind and spirit), patients and families are
actively involved in their care, and the physical
environment is designed to facilitate healing
by attending to such areas as providing for
privacy, noise management, facilitating rest,
integrating alternative therapies. Care givers'
focus on patient well-being includes assessing,
monitoring and preventing physical complications as well as safeguarding human dignity
and emotional safety (Felgen, 2004).

Caring Leader: A leader who creates an environment
in which caring relationships happen. Caring
leaders directly influence caring interactions
with patients and families by virtue of their own
caring interactions with staff members. Their
leader behaviors are built on the Five Caring
Processes by Swanson (Koloroutis, 2004).

(The) Caring Model: A customer service program
developed by Sharon Dingman that complements professional practice principles and customer service objectives of any health care
service department. It includes five behavioral
interactions (Dingman, 1999):
1. Introduce self to patient and family and
explain role,

2. Call patient/family by preferred names,
3. Use touch appropriately,
4. Sit at the bedside for at least five minutes to review care, and
5. Reinforce the mission, vision, values of organization when planning care or service.

Caring Processes: Five processes with specific behaviors that are present in an intentional caring relationship (Swanson, 1993):
1. Maintaining belief—believing in persons and their capacity to make it through events and transitions and find meaning.
2. Knowing—striving to understand an event as it has meaning in the life of the other.
3. Being with—being emotionally present to the other.
4. Doing for—doing for the other what they would do for themselves if it were possible.
5. Enabling/informing—guiding the other's passage through life transitions and unfamiliar events.

Coach: One who encourages, supports, guides and facilitates another to raise competency in areas of performance, critical thinking and interpersonal domains.

Collaboration: Occurs when people work together in a joint intellectual effort for the purpose of attaining a common goal.

Collaborative Practice: A relationship between care givers with common mission, vision and values. It is based on clearly defined goals, roles and responsibilities as well as authority and accountability and involves sharing decision making, resources, risks and rewards. Related to patient care, it references the consistent and coordinated care of a patient through a unified plan of care, information sharing and respect for the important contribution of each member.

Competency: The knowledge, skills, abilities, and behaviors needed to carry out a job (Wright, 2005).

Competency Assessment: A mechanism for directing and evaluating the competencies needed by employees to provide quality health care services to our customers (Wright, 2005).

Continuum of Care: The delivery of health care services that involves three dimensions: levels of health, intensity of services, and settings of care over time. It provides a longitudinal integration of the provision of an individual's care throughout an episode of illness or over an entire lifetime, and supports a seamless transition from responsible care givers in one setting of care to another.

Decentralization: An approach to management where responsibility is clearly allocated and accepted, where authority is defined and accountability is commensurate with the responsibility and authority. The primary aim of decentralization is to acknowledge the wisdom and appropriateness of decision making by those closest to the work.

Delegation: Assigning responsibility to another individual who has the knowledge, skill and appropriate experience to carry out a task.

Design Team: A group selected by an organization for the purposes of planning the structure and implementation process of a specific project. It may or may not provide oversight for the implementation of the project. When it does have accountability for the implementation of Relationship-Based Care, it is often called the Results Council.

Developing Capability: Enhancing the competency and confidence of followers so that they realize a potential beyond their expectations. Leaders lay the ground work for the success of others by articulating expectations, learning their needs, providing necessary resources and encouragement, and standing by them even when things don't go well. (*Creative Health Care Management*, 2007).

Differentiated Practice: Defined levels of nurse roles and responsibilities based on educational preparation and defined competencies. Differentiated Practice may have salary levels associated with it and is generally defined by clinical, education, research and leadership criteria. Is sometimes also used to describe the distinction between the scope of practice for the registered nurse and the licensed practical nurse in a way that honors both.

Discipline: A field of study or a branch of knowledge with the inherent attributes of self-regulation, practice, mentorship, order, an ethical code and reinforcement of standards.

Empowerment: Empowerment exists within individuals and groups who accept responsibility, authority, and accountability for decisions that affect their lives and work. Individual empowerment is an intrinsic quality. Leaders and mentors can create an empowered environment where others gain greater ownership and control over their work. In an empowered environment:

• healthy relationships thrive,
• teams are interdependent and collaborative,
• risk taking and learning are modeled and encouraged, and
• leaders excel in leading change and fostering ownership and commitment for exemplary results.

Inspiration, Infrastructure, Education, Evidence (I_2E_2): A formula for leading transformative change. The desired change begins with a clear values-driven vision. Then I_2E_2 becomes the blueprint for designing, leading and managing sustainable change (Felgen, 2007).

Interdependence: Bringing to a team ones fully developed gifts and working collaboratively to blend each others perspectives and talents. Interdependence brings to our patients or customers the highest level of excellence. Achieving successful, empowered relationships requires leaders to move beyond the point of performing ones role independently to this higher level of maturity and function.

Interdisciplinary: The process whereby two or more professional disciplines work interdependently to accomplish shared goals. Members of each discipline bring their unique body of knowledge and best thinking to the planning. Final plans or decisions are the culmination of respectful communication and collaboration to achieve the best results.

Leading Change: Inspiring, designing and modeling a desired future. Knowledge and skill in problem-solving methodologies are an inherent aspect of successful leadership for change. Leading change includes:

• creating a shared vision,
• inspiring others to own and commit to the vision,

• designing and managing the infrastructure to achieve the vision,
• providing education and coaching to support the growth and development essential to own the change, and
• defining and measuring evidence of success.

Learning Organization: The concept of the learning organization is defined by Peter Senge in his book *The Fifth Discipline* (1994). Senge describes a learning organization as human beings cooperating in dynamic systems that are in a state of continuous adaptation and improvement. A successful learning organization is one in which people are open to changing their mindsets and continuously adapt and learn in order to respond to changes in the environment and to grow (Senge, 1994).

Levels of Authority: (see Authority)

Mentor: A person who guides another (or protégé) in becoming the best that he or she can be personally and professionally. This relationship may take place in multiple settings and generally occurs over an extended period of time. A mentor is someone who influences the thinking/behaviors of others through a mutually beneficial relationship (Taylor, 2001).

Model: A structural representation designed to promote understanding of the relationship of parts in creating a whole; a way of conceptual abstraction that aids in communication and problem solving.

Outcomes Measurement: A basic premise of effective outcomes measurement is that data need not only be meaningful, but also motivating for leaders and practitioners to improve the way they work (Kinnaird & Dingman, 2004).

Ownership and Commitment: Individual ownership and commitment emerge when one feels fully responsible for making change happen. Committed individuals embrace the future vision and are willing to do whatever it takes to make the vision real. The groundwork includes self-awareness of one's potential to influence others toward the greater good, clarity about the desired direction and the necessary competence to get the job done. When this groundwork is in place, individuals have the self-confidence to take ownership and commit to the desired direction. Fully committed leaders accept accountability and are honest about their strengths and weaknesses. Leaders foster ownership and commitment in others through meaningful dialogue in forming a shared vision and through conscious involvement every step of the way. *(Leading and Empowered Organization, 2007)*

Patient-Centered Care: A concept defined by the Institute for Healthcare Improvement (IHI) as follows: *Care that is truly patient-centered considers patients' cultural traditions, their personal preferences and values, their family situations and their lifestyles. It makes the patient and their loved ones an integral part of the care team who collaborate with health care professionals in making clinical decisions. Patient-centered care puts responsibility for important aspects of self-care and monitoring in patients' hands—along with the tools and support they need to carry out that responsibility. Patient-centered care ensures that transitions between providers, departments and health care settings are respectful, coordinated and efficient. When care is patient centered, unneeded and unwanted services can be reduced.* (http://www.ihi.org/IHI/Topics/PatientCenteredCare/PatientCenteredCareGeneral/)

Point of Care: Describes the juncture at which patient care delivery occurs. In hospital settings it is often referred to as "at the bedside." Other point of care junctures include the patient's home, outpatient clinic settings, long-term care facilities, rehabilitation centers.

Preceptor: A person who guides the development of another person in a particular work setting for a specified period of time. The relationship is agreed upon by the two parties and is visible to others. The preceptor teaches and demonstrates specific work processes, policies and procedures for the work area. The preceptor provides support and encouragement for the other to acquire the competencies essential to function with confidence in the work area. The preceptor role models desired behaviors and assures that the person understands the work area norms and expectations.

Primary Nursing: A care delivery system and role defined by a responsibility relationship in which a registered nurse accepts responsibility, authority and accountability for establishing and maintaining a therapeutic relationship and an individualized plan of care with the patient and family. The Primary Nurse is responsible for coordinating the plan with other members of the health care team. The four elements of a care delivery system in Primary Nursing are defined as follows (Person, 2004):

1. **Clinical decision making:** The Primary Nurse makes decisions about nursing care for individual patients based on their therapeutic relationship, which is sustained for the length of stay.
2. **Work allocation:** Assignments are patient based to ensure continuity of relationships and care.
3. **Communication:** There is direct communication between the Primary Nurse and the attending physician as well as all health care team members.
4. **Management:** Managers promote the nurse-patient relationship and the professional nursing role. They influence care by creating a healthy work environment and empowering the staff to make decisions and solve processes of care.

Problem Processing: Various efforts toward fixing a problem that prove ineffective in truly solving the problem. Processing of problems may take the form of quick and superficial fixes or extensive committee meetings with minimal results. In the context of empowerment, problem processing can be related to lack of clear responsibility, authority and accountability (R+A+A) and/or not having the right team members involved who are closest to the situation and therefore most able to achieve workable results. (*Creative Health Care Management*, 2007).

Professional: One who possesses a well-defined body of knowledge and specialized skills derived from extensive academic and practical education. Professional knowledge and skills are important to the well-being of society. Professionals are self-regulating, possess autonomy in the workplace, are held to a code of ethical principles, base their practice on research and are expected to utilize independent judgment in carrying out their professional responsibilities. At all times a professional is cognizant that his or her first and foremost responsibility is to the well-being of those served.

Professional Practice: The exercise of a care provider's autonomous decision making within the parameters of his or her discipline. Professional practice occurs within the context of a responsibility relationship with the patient and is built upon ethical principles, clinical standards and a body of knowledge and skills.

Protégé: A person under the patronage, protection or care of someone interested in his or her career or welfare; an individual who willingly enters into a relationship with a mentor and accepts the help and support offered by the mentor (Taylor, 2001).

Punishment: The temptation to assign blame or guilt to others when they make decisions or have outcomes different from those expected. Punishment stifles initiative, new ideas, and risk taking and limits empowerment (*Leading an empowered organization*, 2007).

Relationship-Based Care: An overarching philosophy, model and system that focuses on three crucial relationships for the provision of humane and compassionate health care. These three relationships are with the patient/family, with colleagues and with the self. Relationship-Based Care serves as a framework for transformation of the organizational culture; presents a care delivery model for a responsibility relationship between professionals (nurses, other disciplines and care givers) and patients/families; provides principles that shape caring behaviors; supports collaboration among all members of the health care team; and is a way of being that is present in the moment in each relationship (Koloroutis, 2004).

Resource Driven Practice: Decision making based on patient requirements, time and human and fiscal resources. Requires practitioners and managers to make choices about what to do as well as what not to do, balancing the needs of individual patients with the patient population as a whole. Constitutes a mindset in which clinical staff move away from thinking about their work as being determined by tasks and routines to thinking about their work being determined by prioritized caring (Manthey & Koloroutis, 2004).

Responsibility: The clear and specific allocation of duties and obligations. Responsibilities must be both allocated and accepted to achieve desired outcomes

Results Council: A steering team which serves as the sponsors and champions for transforming the culture to embody Relationship-Based Care. This council owns the responsibility and accountability for the design, implementation and the ongoing support necessary to achieve the desired vision and approved principles for Relationship-Based Care. This council monitors progress, provides encouragement, evaluates and celebrates achievement of defined outcomes, and assures continuous improvement and development over time.

Risk Taking and Learning: Risk taking is trying things in new and different ways to achieve positive results through creativity, innovation and learning. Empowerment requires leaders to establish a culture in which staff members feel it's safe to make decisions and speak honestly even in the face of differences of opinion. Risk taking results in group and individual growth, learning and empowerment (*Creative Health Care Management*, 2007).

Role: An assigned or assumed set of responsibilities. In a decentralized system, each responsibility has an identified level of authority and accountability.

Role Model: A person who serves as an example to someone else with or without a relationship with that individual. A role model may not be aware of his/her influence on others. All leaders are role models.

Self-Directed Work Team: A group of people working together toward a common goal. Members are responsible for planning, executing, evaluating the work, utilizing and managing resources, and managing relationships in healthy ways. Members of a self-directed team must understand the implications of their work on others and initiate interdependent, collaborative processes as necessary.

Shared Governance: A decentralized organizational structure with clearly defined scope and responsibility, authority and accountability. It is designed to promote professional autonomy and collaboration. It empowers professional staff and managers to collaborate on decision making to optimize patient care, clinical practice, quality improvement and ethical behaviors.

System: A set or arrangement of things, practices, processes or behaviors that are related or connected in a way that these form a unity or organic whole, such as a solar system, a quality improvement pathway, financial reporting approaches and care delivery practices.

Team: A group of people with complementary skills who are committed to a common purpose, performance goals and behavioral standards for which they hold themselves mutually accountable.

Teamwork: Requires a group of diverse members to focus on a shared purpose and to work together to fulfill that purpose. In healthy and productive teams, each member contributes his or her unique knowledge and skills within a clearly defined scope of responsibility, authority and accountability (R+A+A) (Wright, 2004).

Theory: A general principle that is based on evidence and research, and has been verified by observation.

Therapeutic Relationship: One in which the patient's and family's healing is the purpose for the relationship. All interactions within the therapeutic relationship are for the purpose of providing safe and compassionate care to patients and their families. The three phases of the therapeutic relationships are receiving, engaging and transitioning (Koloroutis, 2004b).

1. **Receiving:** welcomes patients and their loved ones into a relationship that continues for the duration of the patient's stay in a particular unit or area, even when that stay lasts no more than a few moments or hours. Helps people cope with whatever they may be facing and conveys that they are seen and understood by somebody who has anticipated their arrival.

2. **Engaging:** core of the interaction, includes ongoing monitoring and assessment, planning, implementing and evaluating care.

3. **Transitioning:** anticipating what patients and their families need to know when they move to the next phase, whether that is discharge, moving to another area for care, or death.

Transformational Leadership: The ability to influence people to accomplish extraordinary things through conscious actions and embodying the desired change. This leadership happens at all levels of the organization (Koloroutis, 2004).

Unhealthy Behaviors: Nonproductive ways of relating to others that interfere with the ability of leaders to care for themselves and empower staff to increasing levels of performance. Unhealthy behaviors may range from excessive caretaking or failure to stand up for one's needs, to controlling or dominating behaviors (*Creative Health Care Management*, 2007).

Unit Practice Council: A unit or department-based group of staff members, chosen by their peers, who accept responsibility, authority, and accountability to plan, implement, evaluate and continuously improve the unit-specific Relationship-Based Care delivery model for their unit. The plans are based on approved principles and outcome measures as determined by hospital leadership. The council members are chosen by their peers and develop their plan through consensus decision making based on two-way communication with 100% of their peers. The plan includes measurement of their impact and methods for sustaining the change. The term Area Practice Council is used in lieu of Unit Practice Council for work areas outside of patient care units.

Vision: A picture, a dream, a description of something of value and importance and a desire to make it a reality. A vision takes form when it is put into words. It becomes real when choices are made and actions are taken that make it happen. A vision becomes substantive when it is lived every day—no matter what.

References

Dingman, S. et al. (1999). Implementing a caring model to improve patient satisfaction. Journal of Nursing Administration, 29(12), 30- 37.

Felgen, J. (2004). Caring and healing environment. In M. Koloroutis (Ed.), *Relationship-based care: A model for transforming practice* (pp. 23-52). Minneapolis, MN: Creative Health Care Management.

Felgen, J. (2007). I_2E_2: *Leading lasting change.* Minneapolis, MN: Creative Health Care Management.

Kinnaird, L., and Dingman, S. (2004). Outcome measurement. In M. Koloroutis (Ed.), *Relationship-based care: A model for transforming practice* (pp. 215-248). Minneapolis, MN: Creative Health Care Management.

Koloroutis, M. (2004). Leadership. In *Relationship-based care: A model for transforming practice* (pp. 53-90). Minneapolis, MN: Creative Health Care Management.

Koloroutis, M. (Ed.). (2004). *Relationship-based care: A model for transforming practice.* Minneapolis, MN: Creative Health Care Management.

Creative Health Care Management. (2007). *Leading an Empowered Organization:* Participant Manual. Minneapolis, MN.

Manthey, M., & Koloroutis, M. (2004). Resource driven practice. In M. Koloroutis (Ed.), *Relationship-based care: A model for transforming practice* (pp. 183-214). Minneapolis, MN: Creative Health Care Management.

Person, C. (2004). Patient Care Delivery. In M. Koloroutis (Ed.), *Relationship-based care: A model for transforming practice* (pp. 159-182). Minneapolis, MN: Creative Health Care Management.

Senge, P. (1994). *The fifth discipline.* New York: Currency.

Taylor, L. J. (2001). Mentorship. In A. J. Lowenstein & M. J. Bradshaw (Eds.), *Fuzard's innovative teaching strategies in nursing* (pp. 251-260). Gaithersburg, MD: Aspen.

Wright, D. (2004). Teamwork. In M. Koloroutis (Ed.), *Relationship-based care: A model for transforming practice* (pp. 91-116). Minneapolis, MN: Creative Health Care Management.

Wright, D. (2005). *The ultimate guide to competency assessment in health care, third edition.* Minneapolis, MN: Creative Health Care Management.

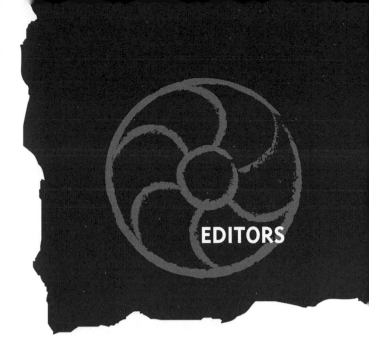

EDITORS

Mary Koloroutis, BSN, MS, RN

Mary is the editor and a co-author of *Relationship-Based Care: A Model for Transforming Practice*, the precursor to this Field Guide. Mary also champions the Relationship-Based Care (RBC) Practicums for Creative Health Care Management. These Practicums are intensive five day programs where hospitals from around the US gather to discuss success strategies and their experience with RBC.

Mary is passionate about helping individuals embody the knowledge and skills necessary to bring RBC to life in everyday practice. Mary has more than 20 years of health care experience helping organizations emphasize the "care" aspect that is so important to hospitals and helps strengthen all professional nursing models.

Jayne A. Felgen, MPA, RN

As President of Creative Health Care Management (CHCM), an international health care consultation company, Jayne works to improve patient and family care through the design and implementation of world-class patient care delivery systems. Grounded by the healing principles of Relationship-Based Care, CHCM provides executive, leadership, and team development consultation to become providers of choice in their communities.

Jayne is a specialist in organizational management and work redesign, focusing on patient outcomes. Passionate about patient and family care—those who touch them as care providers and the systems that value and support them—Jayne works to strengthen the therapeutic relationships at the core of care delivery. She provides direction for executives, physicians, trustees, nurses, allied health professionals and teams using her unique ability to inspire and galvanize organizations. She creates common goals and a clear structure that helps achieve measurable objectives. In her recent book I_2E_2: *Leading Lasting Change*, Jayne shares this in-depth, yet elegantly simple formula for managing the change process.

The American Organization of Nurse Executives' (AONE) prestigious Community Partnership Award was given to Jayne for her work as founder and president of the Nightingale Awards of Pennsylvania, a nonprofit organization that has recognized more than 1800 nurses and grants scholarships throughout the state. Jayne was recently awarded the honorary lifetime title of President Emeritus for all of her contributions to the organization. Jayne is a graduate of The Johns Hopkins Hospital School of Nursing, The Johns Hopkins University, and Penn State where she earned a Master of Public Administration, Health Care.

Colleen Person, MMA, RN

Using innovative strategies grounded in Relationship-Based Care, Colleen provides facilitation, consultation, and education services for the health care industry. From extensive clinical, administrative and consultative experiences in settings throughout the continuum of care, she provides practical orientation and positive practices that help with the many challenges and change processes in health care today.

Colleen Person is the Vice President of Creative Health Care Management, providing direction for the company in its mission to improve patient care through the design and implementation of world-class patient care delivery systems. Among these delivery systems are leadership programs, staff development, and transformational change processes that help create and maintain healthy work environments.

Susan Wessel, MS, MBA, RN, CNAA

Susan Wessel serves as a Consultant with Creative Health Care Management (CHCM), where she specializes in organizational assessment. In her assessments, she uses an Appreciative Inquiry methodology to build professional practice environments consistent with Magnet Recognition criteria and other organizational excellence programs. She currently champions *Leading an Empowered Organization (LEO)* for CHCM, a leadership program with more than 100,000 participants worldwide.

Susan holds a national certification for Nursing Administration, Advanced, and has completed a Fellowship in the J & J Program in Management for Nurses at the Wharton School of Business. Susan served as Chairman of the Board for Hospice Partners in Chicago and is currently on the American Nurses Credentialing Center Nursing Administration content expert panel. Her professional memberships include Sigma Theta Tau, American Organization of Nurse Executives, and the Illinois Coalition for Nursing Resources.

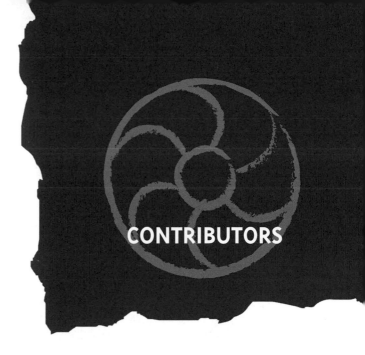

CONTRIBUTORS

Diane E. Allen, MN, RN, BC, is a leader of nurses in a state psychiatric hospital that provides Relationship-Based Care for patients with acute mental illness.

Ronald J. Bachman has served as President and CEO of Marion General Hospital in Marion, Ohio since February, 2000.

Vicki L. Bailey is a writer, Catholic chaplain and mental health counselor who lives on a small ranch in Sacramento, CA.

Diane K. Bradley, MS, MPA, RN, CNAA, BC, LNHA, is a consultant with Creative Health Care Management, specializing in The Caring Model, the *Caring Manager, Leadership at the Point of Care* and *Relationships at the Point of Care.*

Susan Bullock, MEd, RN,C, in an Education Specialist with Centra Health in Lynchburg, VA. Susan has been a geriatric nurse for 24 years, serving as a director of nursing, a practicing clinician, geriatric nurse specialist and educator, as well as public speaker, in both long term care and acute care settings.

Cheryl Burnette, RN, Med, CPLP, is the Nurse Retention Coordinator at Centra Health with over 12 years experience in nursing education and a certified professional in learning and performance.

Michelle Cabell, BSN, MEd, is a Certified Life Coach/Life Plan Facilitator.

Agnes Cappabianca RN, BSN, is a nurse manager at Lutheran Medical Center on a neuro-orthopedic unit. She is a champion for the facilitation of Relationship Centered Care.

Michael Henry Cohen is President of a leadership & employee relations consulting firm, has a Master of Arts degree from Northwestern University and has written three books, *On The Job Survival, The Power of Self Management,* and *What You Accept is What You Teach.*

Scott Louis Diering, MD is an emergency department physician at Walter Reed Army Medical Center in Washington, DC. He is the author of *Love Your Patients.*

Marlene Dufault, PhD, is a research consultant at Newport Hospital (Newport, RI) Nursing Department, Professor of Research, Theory, and Leadership: Graduate and Undergraduate Programs and Director of Onsite Master's in Nursing Administration Program at the University of Rhode Island College of Nursing (Kingston, RI). She is also a member of the Editorial Board for Advances in Nursing Science and Worldview on Evidence-Based Practice in Nursing.

Susan Edstrom, BSN, MS, RN, is a consultant with Creative Health Care Management where she facilitates both *Work Complexity Assessment* and *Reigniting the Spirit of Caring.*

Paula Ellis, MSN, RN, CARN, , a nurse with a variety of health and behavioral health care experiences, works at St. Francis Health Center in Topeka, Kansas directing Home Care, Medical Staff Office, Case Management, and Alcohol/Drug/Gambling Services.

Kathryn Ewers is an Educator and Project Leader for Evidence-Based Nursing at Jackson Health System, Miami, FL.

Kathleen Fedoronko, BSN, RN, OCN, serves as the Director of Patient Services at the Karmanos Cancer Center in Detroit Michigan. She received her BSN from Wayne State University in 1989.

Gayle Garland is the programme director for the Centre for the Development of Healthcare Policy and Practice at the Univerisity of Leeds in the United Kingdom.

Dorothy Anne Garman, MSN, RN, is the Coordinator of Nursing Professional Development and Patient Education and Magnet Coordinator for Newport Hospital (Newport, RI).

Frances Glosson, EdD, RN is the Director of Community Learning Strategies for Centegra Health System and is a specialist in leadership, learning, service and research with 40 years of progressive health care experience with a focus on organizational development.

John O. Hardiman, MD, a physician for 50 years, recently had an eight day stay in a hospital and received such superior nursing care he felt compelled to explain the basis for the difference between "nursing care" and "excellent nursing care".

Sandra Hoffman, MS RN, is a Clinical Nurse Specialist for the Birth Center of Abbott Northwestern Hospital in Minneapolis, Minnesota. Her Master's Degree is in Childbearing Childrearing Family Nursing for the University of Minnesota, she is certified in Health Risk Management, and has worked in perinatal nursing for over 25 years.

Teresa Kellerman, MSN, BSN, ARNP, CWON, OCN, is an advanced practice nurse and a *Reigniting the Spirit of Caring* facilitator at St. Francis Health Center in Topeka, KS.

Carolyn Kile, RD, is the Director of Customer Service and Operations Improvement and coaching facilitator for Marion General Hospital in Marion, OH.

Leah Kinnaird, EdD, RN, is a consultant with Creative Health Care Management. Leah specializes in fostering healthy interpersonal relationships, developing measurable outcomes, creating and implementing programs, and fostering leadership development.

Ellen Kissinger MSNc, RN,C is an Assistant Nurse Manager in Pediatrics at the University of California Davis Medical Center in Sacramento, California and chair of the Pediatric Primary Nursing Steering Committee and a member of the hospital wide Primary Nursing Steering committee.

Mary Jo Kreitzer, PhD, RN, FAAN is the Director of the Center for Spirituality and Healing and a Professor in the School of Nursing at the University of Minnesota.

Susan Lampe, RN, MS, is the author of *Focus Charting* and is currently retired from Minnesota State University Mankato School of Nursing.

Michael Leonard, MD, is the Physician Leader for Patient Safety, Kaiser Permanente; Faculty, Institute for Healthcare Improvement.

JoAnn Maklebust, APRN-BC, MSN, AOCN, FAAN, is a Nurse Practitioner in Oncological Surgery and the Administrative Liaison to the Oncology Nurse practice Committee at Karmanos Cancer Center, Detroit, MI.

Marie Manthey, MNA, FRCN, FAAN, PhD (hon.), is founder and president emeritus of Creative Health Care Management and author of *The Practice of Primary Nursing*.

Matt Marchbanks is the General Manager of Sodexho Services at Faxton–St. Lukes Healthcare in Utica, NY. He is an Executive Chef and currently certified as a Master Certified Food Executive (MCFE–International Food Service Executives Association).

Karen McGlynn is the director of Oncology Surgery at North Shore University Hospital in Manhasset, NY.

Sharon E. Melberg directed General Nursing and Social Services and the Center for Nursing Research at the University of California, Davis Medical Center until her retirement in 2006; currently she writes and edits The Way of St. Francis in Sacramento.

Kim Moore, MSN, RN, CNAA, BC, is the Chief Nursing Officer for Saint Elizabeth Regional Medical Center, Lincoln, NE.

John W. Nelson, MS, RN, is the President of Healthcare Environment and an adjunct faculty with Creative Health Care Management, specializing in evaluating the work environment of health care as perceived by the health care employee. He also works with organizations to manage other indicators, including employee, financial and patient outcomes.

Lynda Olender, MA, RN, ANP, is a consultant with Creative Health Care Management and Chief Nurse Executive at the Bronx VA Medical Center. She has served as Assistant Clinical Professor, Division of Nursing at NYU for many years and is currently in pursuit of her Doctorate in Nursing at Columbia University.

Peter E. Person, MD, is a physician and the Chief Executive Officer at SMDC Health System in Duluth, MN.

Margaret (Peg) Pierson MSN, RN, CNA, BC, is the Professional Practice/Magnet Coordinator at Saint Elizabeth Regional Medical Center in Lincoln, NE.

Linda Pullins, MS, RN, is Vice President of Patient Care at Marion General Hospital in Marion, OH.

Patricia A. Roach MS, RN, OCN, CNAA, is the Senior Vice President & Chief Nursing Officer at Faxton-St. Lukes Health care in Utica, NY. She has over 19 years of healthcare experience, having held positions as Staff Nurse, Charge Nurse, Nurse Recruiter, Nurse Manager and Cancer Program Director.

Gary L. Saltus DO, FACOS, is the Founder and President of Longevity Guide LLC and is a Physician/Health Care Consultant and Adjunct Faculty with Creative Health Care Management.

Laurence A. Savett, MD, author of *The Human Side of Medicine: Learning What It's Like to be a Patient and What It's Like to be a Physician,* practiced primary care internal medicine for 30 years, first in Gloucester, MA, and then in St. Paul, MN and currently helps advise pre-medical and other pre-health professions students at Macalester College and University of St. Thomas in St. Paul, MN.

Philip Schwartzkopf, is currently the director of marketing for Creative Health Care Management. Phillip has helped develop mind maps for company programs such as Work Complexity. These mind maps give clients a better understanding of their many complex processes and ultimately provide direction for system-wide improvements.

Sandra Seagal, PhD, has been a leader in the field of Human Dynamics since 1979 and is the founder of Human Dynamics International.

Katherine Smith, RN,C, BSN is Project Manager for the University of California Davis Medical Center.

Rebecca Smith is the author of *SHOULD: How Habits of Language Shape Our Lives*; she is a writer, ghost-writer and editor in Minneapolis, MN.

Kristen Swanson, PhD, RN, FAAN, is Chair of Family and Child Nursing at the University of Washington Medical Center in Seattle, WA.

Beth Ware, RN, BSN, Director of Patient Care Services at Eliza Coffee Medical Center, in Florence, AL.

Alice Weydt, RN, MS is a consultant with Creative Health Care Management. Alice facilitates both *Work Complexity Assessment* and *Leading an Empowered Organization*.

Donna Wright, RN, MS, a consultant with Creative Health Care Management, helps health care organizations create valuable competency and staff development programs for all departments. She is the author of *The Ultimate Guide to Competency Assessment in Health Care.*

RESOURCES

Books and Articles

Alfaro-LeFevre, R. (2005). *Critical thinking in nursing: A practical approach.* (3rd ed.). Philadelphia: W. B. Saunders.

American Nurses Association. (1994). *Registered professional nurses and unlicensed assistive personnel.* Washington, DC: American Nurses Publishing.

American Nurses Association. (2001). *Code of ethics for nurses with interpretive statements.* Silver Springs, MD: ANA Publishing.

American Nurses Association. (2003). *Nursing's social policy statement.* (2nd ed.). Silver Springs, MD: ANA Publishing.

American Nurses Association. (2004). *ANA nursing standards.* Silver Springs, MD: ANA Publishing.

Baldwin, C. (1998). *Calling the circle: The first and future culture.* New York: Bantam.

Baldwin, C., & Linnea, A. (1999). *PeerSpirit council management: Calling the circle.* Langley, WA: PeerSpirit. www.peerspirit.com

Benner, P., Tanner, C., & Chesla, C. (1996). *Expertise in nursing practice: Caring, clinical judgment and ethics.* New York: Springer.

Block, P. (2002). *The answer to how is yes: Acting on what matters.* San Francisco: Berrett-Koehler.

Brown, J., & Isaacs, D. (2005). *The world café: Shaping our futures through conversations that matter.* San Francisco: Berrett-Koehler.

Buresh, B., & Gordon, S. (2000). *From silence to voice: What nurses know and must communicate to the public.* Ithaca, NY: Cornell University Press.

Editors' note: *The following references are books, articles and videos we have found helpful when helping organizations implement Relationship-Based Care.*

Cashman, K. (1999). *Leadership from the inside out: Becoming a leader for life.* Minneapolis, MN: Leadersource.

Cashman, K. (2003). *Awakening the leader within: A story of transformation.* New York: John Wiley & Sons.

Collins, J. (2001). *Good to great.* New York: HarperCollins.

Cooperrider, D., & Whitney, D. (1999). *Appreciative inquiry: Collaborating for change.* San Francisco: Berrett-Koehler.

Creative Health Care Management. (2002). *Staffing: Changing the way we think.* Minneapolis, MN: Author

Dandrinos-Smith, S., Garman, D., Baranowski, S., Davol, L., & Person, C. et al. (2000). The making of the supermodel. *Nursing Management.*

De Pree, M. (2003, October). *Leading without power: Finding hope in serving community.* San Francisco: Jossey-Bass.

Dingman, S., Williams, M., Fosbinder, D., & Warnick, M. (1999). Implementing a caring model to improve patient satisfaction. *Journal of Nursing Administration,* 29(12), 30-37.

Ellison, S. (2007). *Taking the war out of words: The art of powerful non-defensive communication.* Berkeley, CA: Bay Tree. www.pndc.com

Felgen, J. (2000). Patient as CEO: Passion in practice. *Journal of Nursing Administration,* 30(10), 208-214.

Felgen, J. (2007). *I_2E_2: Leading lasting change.* Minneapolis, MN: Creative Health Care Management.

Goleman, D. (1997). *Emotional intelligence.* New York: Bantam.

Greenleaf, R. (1998). *The power of servant leadership: Collection of essays by Robert Greenleaf.* San Francisco: Berrett-Koehler.

Guanci, G. (2005). Destination magnet: Charting a course to excellence. *Journal for Nurses in Staff Development,* 21(5), 227-235.

Haase-Herrick, K. (2004). Letter from the leadership. *Voice of Nursing Leadership,* 2(5), 1, 10.

Hansten, R. I., & Jackson, M. (2004). *Clinical delegation skills.* (3rd ed.). Sudbury, MA: Jones and Bartlett.

Johnson, M., Maas, M., & Moorhead, S. (Eds.). (2000). *Nursing outcomes classification.* St. Louis, MO: C. V. Mosby.

Keeling, B., Adair, J., Seider, D., & Kirksey, G. (2000). Appropriate delegation. *American Journal of Nursing,* 100(12):24A,24C-24D

Koloroutis, M. (Ed.). (2004). *Relationship-based care: A model for transforming practice.* Minneapolis, MN: Creative Health Care Management.

Kouzes, J., & Posner, B. (2003). *Encouraging the heart: A leader's guide to rewarding and recognizing others.* San Francisco: Jossey-Bass.

Lee, F. (2004). *If Disney ran your hospital: 9 1/2 things you would do differently.* Bozeman, MT: Second River Healthcare.

Leider, R. (1997). *The power of purpose.* San Francisco: Berrett-Koehler.

Manthey, M. (2001). Two miracles in one career. *Nursing Administration Quarterly,* 25(2), 55-60.

Manthey, M. (2002). *The practice of primary nursing: Relationship-based, resource-driven care delivery.* Minneapolis, MN: Creative Health Care Management.

Manthey, M. (2004). *Changing the staffing mindset.* Minneapolis, MN: Creative Health Care Management.

Manthey, M. (1994). Issues in patient care delivery. *Journal of Nursing Administration,* 24(12):14-6.

McCloskey, J., & Bulechek, G. (Eds.). (2004). *Nursing interventions classification.* (4th ed.). St. Louis: C. V. Mosby.

Meier, D. (2000). *The accelerated learning handbook.* New York: McGraw-Hill.

National Quality Forum. (2004). *National voluntary consensus standards for nursing-sensitive care: An initial performance measure set.* Retrieved November 20, 2005, from http://www.quality-forum.org/txNCFINALpublic.pdf

Nelson, J. W., & Venhaus, E. (2005). Improving retention through nurse/physician communication. *Nurse Leader,* 3(1), 54-56.

Patterson, K., Grenny, J., McMillan, R., & Switzler, A. (2002). *Crucial conversations: Tools for talking when stakes are high.* New York: McGraw-Hill.

Patterson, K., Grenny, J., McMillan, R., & Switzler, A. (2004). *Crucial confrontations: Tools for resolving broken promises, violated expectations and bad behavior.* New York: McGraw-Hill.

Quinn, R. (1996). *Deep change: Discovering the leader within.* New York: John Wiley & Sons.

Rosenstein, A. H. (2002). Nurse-physician relationships: Impact on nurse satisfaction and retention. *American Journal of Nursing,* 102(6): 54-64

Ruiz, D. M. (1997). *The four agreements: A practical guide to personal freedom.* San Rafael, CA: Amber-Allen.

Savett, L. (2002). *The human side of medicine: Learning what it's like to be a patient and what it's like to be a physician.* Westport, CT: Greenwood.

Schwerin, J. I. (2004). The timeless caring connection. *Nursing Administration Quarterly,* 28, 265-270.

Seagal, S., & Horne, D. (1996). *Human dynamics: A new framework for understanding individuals and realizing potential in our organizations.* Waltham, MA: Pegasus Communications. www.humandynamics.com

Senge, P., Kleiner, A., Roberts, C., Ross, R. & Smith, B. (1994). *The fifth discipline fieldbook.* New York: Currency.

Stone, D., Patton, B., & Heen, S. (2000). *Difficult conversations: How to discuss what matters most.* New York: Penguin.

Stone, R. (1996). *The healing art of storytelling: A sacred journey of personal discovery.* Lincoln, NE: iUniverse.

Swanson, K. (1993). Nursing as informed caring for the well-being of others. *IMAGE: Journal of Nursing Scholarship,* 25, 352-357.

Watkins, J., & Mohr, B. (2001). *Appreciative inquiry: Change at the speed of imagination.* New York: John Wiley & Sons.

Watson, J. (2002). *Assessing and measuring caring in nursing and health science.* New York: Springer.

Wheatley, M. (2002). *Turning to one another: Simple conversations to restore hope to the future.* San Francisco: Berrett-Koehler.

Wheatley, M. (2005). *Finding our way: Leadership for uncertain times.* San Francisco: Berrett-Koehler.

Wheatley, M. (2005). *Leadership and the new science: Discovering order in a chaotic world.* San Francisco: Berrett-Koehler.

Wright, D. (2005). *The ultimate guide to competency assessment in health care.* (3rd ed.). Minneapolis, MN: Creative Health Care Management.

Wright, S. G., & Sayre-Adams, J. (2000). *Sacred space.* Edinburgh, Scotland: Churchill Livingstone.

Videos and Audios

Leadership for Relationship-Based Practice: Magnet Keynote Address, 2004, Marie Manthey

Healing Environments: Passion in Practice, Jayne Felgen

Moments of Excellence Video Series, 4 programs, Donna Wright

Primary Nursing: Making a Difference, Center for Nursing Education, UC Davis Health System

Patients Love their Nurses

Available from the Resources Division of Creative Health Care Management: (800) 264-3246 or online at www.chcm.com

Relationship-Based Care Services

Relationship-Based Care (RBC) is the most direct route to world-class care and service to patients and families.

Creative Health Care Management can help you implement Relationship-Based Care in many ways:

- *Education Session. How does RBC work on individual units and system wide? What outcomes can be expected? (Half day or one day)*

- *Design Day. A customized design for your organization and the infrastructure needed to support the implementation of the RBC model. (One day)*

- *Appreciative Inquiry Organizational Assessment. Identifies organizational strengths and desired outcomes. (One to two days)*

The Relationship-Based Care Leader Practicum

Sharing the RBC concept with peers and employees, helping managers understand its benefits, and making it a success in your organization is a true challenge. Whether you're a new or experienced RBC Leader, this program will help give you the direction you need to make RBC succeed at your organization.

The Relationship-Based Care Practicum was developed specifically to help with the challenges you face in implementing Relationship-Based Care. This practical five day course will provide RBC Leaders with the clarity and competence essential for assembling a collaborative team of change leaders. The program blends a variety of experiential methodologies to develop competencies, integrate learning relative to RBC, and design customized strategies and outcomes in your individual organizations.

For more information visit: www.chcm.com

Relationship-Based Care:
A Model for Transforming Practice

—Mary Koloroutis, editor

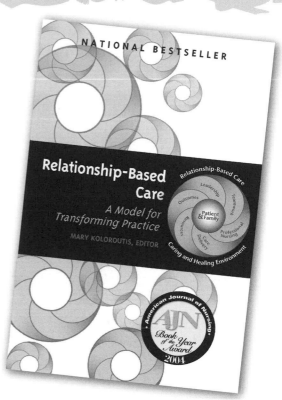

Designed to help health care leaders create lasting change in their organizations, *Relationship-Based Care: A Model for Transforming Practice*, edited by Mary Koloroutis has evolved from over 25 years of work in the health care field working in a variety of hospitals and settings across the United States and around the world.

While reflecting the integrated work of Creative Health Care Management over the past twenty-five years, this book honors the deep knowledge and experience of the individuals within the company. In each chapter, readers will benefit from the interest, expertise and, most importantly, the passion of the authors. Authors and chapters include:

- *A Caring and Healing Environment — Jayne Felgen*

- *Leadership — Mary Koloroutis*

- *Teamwork — Donna Wright*

- *Professional Nursing Practice — Mary Koloroutis*

- *Nursing Care Delivery System — Colleen Person*

- *Resource Driven Practice — Marie Manthey and Mary Koloroutis*

- *Outcome Measurement — Leah Kinnaird and Sharon Dingman*

Item # B510 • Softcover, 288 pages. (2004)

ISBN 13: 978-1-886624-19-1.
ISBN 10: 1-886624-19-4.

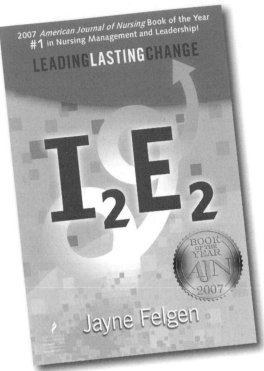

I$_2$E$_2$: Leading Lasting Change

—Jayne Felgen

In *I$_2$E$_2$: Leading Lasting Change*, author Jayne Felgen shares her in-depth and elegantly simple formula for inspiring and leading real change at all levels of any organization.

I$_2$E$_2$ is not a step-by-step guide to re-creating the newest business model; rather it is a new way of thinking about change. Leaders learn to visualize the whole process, from shared vision to detailed changes in infrastructure. I$_2$E$_2$ is a simple and elegant formula for initiating and sustaining lasting change over time.

Jayne Felgen, MPA, RN, has the gift of creating clarity out of chaos and discovering practical solutions that benefit patients as well as families. Her approach is data driven, grounded in appreciative inquiry, organizational principles, along with strong process skills. She is passionate about patients and families, those who touch them as care providers, and the systems that value and support the therapeutic relationships at the core of care delivery.

Item # B560 • Softcover, 136 pages. (2007)

ISBN 13: 978-1-886624-12-2
ISBN 10: 1-886624-12-7

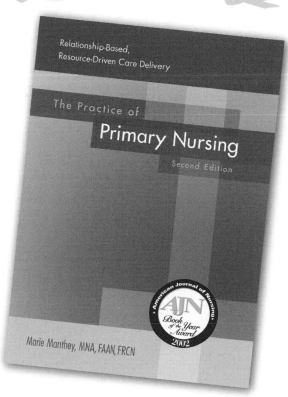

The Practice of Primary Nursing: Relationship-Based, Resource-Driven Care Delivery

—Marie Manthey

The Practice of Primary Nursing: Relationship-Based, Resource-Driven Care Delivery is an update to Marie Manthey's classic work. Primary Nursing was the first delivery system in hospital nursing that created a professional role for the Registered Nurse at the bedside. Under Primary Nursing, patients in hospitals receive coordinated care, delivered with continuity over time and place, managed by an RN known to the patients and families. Today's hospital needs the type of Relationship-Based Care delivery that Primary Nursing provides.

This new edition thoroughly explains the four important operating elements of Primary Nursing and outlines the actual steps taken at the unit level for successful implementation. The insights of other Primary Nursing pioneers as well as Marie's most current thinking about Primary Nursing help readers see how Primary Nursing fits in today's health care climate. Originally started at the University of Minnesota Hospitals in 1968, Primary Nursing has been used by many hospitals in the U.S. and throughout the World and remains applicable even today.

Item # B240 • Softcover, 136 pages.
ISBN 13: 978-1-886624-17-7
ISBN 10: 1-886624-17-8

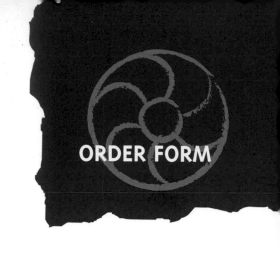

1. Call toll-free 800.264.3246 and use your Visa, Master-card or American Express or a company purchase order.

2. Fax your order to: 952.854.1866.

3. Mail your order with pre-payment or company purchase order to:

CREATIVE
HEALTH CARE
MANAGEMENT

Creative Health Care Management
1701 American Blvd East, Suite 1
Minneapolis, MN 55425
Attn: Resources Department

4. Order Online at: www.chcm.com, click Online Store.

Product	Price	Quantity	Subtotal	TOTAL
B510—*Relationship-Based Care: A Model for Transforming Practice*	$34.95			
B600—*Relationship-Based Care Field Guide*	$99.00			
B560—*I_2E_2: Leading Lasting Change*	$24.95			
B240—*The Practice of Primary Nursing, 2nd Edition*	$19.95			
M501—*Commitment to My Co-worker* for Health Care Cards (Pack of 25)	$15.00			
Shipping Costs: 1 item - $6.50, $1.00 for each additional item • Call for express rates				
Order TOTAL				

Need more than one copy? We have quantity discounts available.

Quantity Discounts (Books Only)		
10–49 = 10% off	50–99 = 20% off	100 or more = 30% off

Payment Methods: ☐ Credit Card ☐ Check ☐ Purchase Order PO# _____

Credit Card	Number	Expiration	AVS (3 digits)
Visa / Mastercard / American Express	– – –	/	
Cardholder address (if different from below):	Signature:		

Customer Information	
Name:	
Title:	
Company:	
Address:	
City, State, Zip:	
Daytime Phone:	
Email:	

Satisfaction guarantee: If you are not satisfied with your purchase, simply return the products within 30 days for a full refund.

For a free catalog of all our products, visit www.chcm.com or call 800.201.0210.